Fit to Serve Him Longer... and Better

Dick Couey

Tommy Yessick

LifeWay Press
Nashville, Tennessee

ISBN 0-7673-9123-3

Dewey Decimal Classification: 613.7
Subject Heading: PHYSICAL FITNESS

Printed in the United States of America.

Pastor-Staff Leadership Department
LifeWay Christian Resources
of The Southern Baptist Convention
127 Ninth Avenue, North
Nashville, Tennessee 37234

Cover Images:
Tony Stone Images—male swimmer, assorted fruits and vegetables, tennis couple
FPG—woman hiker with puppy in backpack
Comstock Inc.—senior adult couple walking and male runner

Contents

Preface

God created for every individual a uniquely different and highly complicated body in which to live during his or her limited existence. He expects us to care for His temple (our bodies) from our first to our last breath. He expects us to protect and feed our bodies properly and exercise regularly. Christians must grow not only spiritually, mentally, socially, and emotionally but also physically.

This book is intended to improve the physical well-being of both Christians and non-Christians. The most current medical information concerning physical fitness is presented, along with personal research and experiences, which should help readers develop an intelligent understanding of their physical well-being.

My loving and appreciative thanks to Elray, my wife, who sacrificially kept the family together; and to my children, Suzanne and Paul; and to my grandchildren Will and Mallory, for their patience and understanding during the long months of study and writing.

—Richard B. Couey

Dedication

To
Elray, Suzanne, Paul, Brad, Will, and Mallory
Whom I truly love

——Dick

[CHAPTER 1]

Becoming a Whole Person

One of my favorite hymns is "Jesus Is Tenderly Calling." I picture Jesus tenderly calling us to live our lives according to His will. God created us. The Bible tells us that He knows our innermost being, and He knows what makes us happy. I picture Jesus encouraging us to put away all our worldly sins and to follow His teachings. Yet many Christians neglect this plea and allow their lives to be dominated by sins that destroy their bodies, their mental health, their spiritual worship, their love for one another, and consequently their happiness. It must be sad for Jesus to see His immaculate creation being destroyed and suffering from poor health, mainly because of physical neglect. God wants us to be happy, to have abundant life. He tells us in the Bible that for us to be happy we have to learn to love God with all our heart, soul, mind, and strength, and to love our neighbor as ourselves. My prayer is that from reading this book you will hear the call of Jesus tenderly pleading for you to develop your life according to His will so that you might serve Him better and longer.

What Is Wholeness?

The definition of *wholeness* does not imply physical, emotional, or spiritual perfection; a state of complete serenity or euphoria; or a state of perpetual bliss or contentment. Being whole implies being healthy in mind, body, and spirit and having healthy relationships and attitudes. We can, therefore, define a *whole person* as one who lives in conformity with God's will and standards and is happy to do so.

You may ask, "How does one develop wholeness?" Only one person ever developed perfect wholeness. As we so often do, let us focus our attention on Jesus, examine His lifestyle, and draw from it perfect examples of how we should live our lives.

Several Scriptures emphasize the "whole person." In 1 Thessalonians 5:23, Paul wrote, "Now may the God of peace Himself sanctify you entirely; and may your spirit and soul and body be preserved complete, without blame at the coming of our Lord Jesus Christ."

Luke 2:52 summarizes the life of Jesus. From close examination of that Scripture, we can find some revealing hints that can be useful for us in developing into the whole person. This Scripture discloses that Jesus developed in four areas of His life: "And Jesus kept increasing in wisdom (mentally) and stature (physically), and in favor with God (spiritually) and men (socially)." Jesus' development was not only spiritual but also physical, mental, and social.

A human being is not just a soul with spiritual needs but a creature of many dimensions. We all have physical, mental, emotional, vocational, and social dimensions and must grow and develop continuously in each area. If we neglect one of these areas, that area will experience decay. This decay will affect other dimensions of our person. For example, many Christians may be healthy spiritually and socially but unhealthy mentally and physically. The confusions and frustrations caused from being unhealthy in these areas will affect the spiritual and social dimensions. For instance, many Christians may have developed a close relationship with God or acquired many friends; but because they have become overweight, which often leads to poor health and low self-esteem, they lose their enthusiastic desire to continue their spiritual and social development. We must learn to develop our health and total well-being in all four areas so that we can develop into the whole person, just as our Savior did

Many Christians fail to cultivate their mental potential and have allowed their minds to become stagnant.

while He lived on this earth some two thousand years ago.

Let us review some ways in which we can develop into the whole person, for we have tremendous growth potential in all four areas.

Mental

"And Jesus kept increasing in wisdom." During His life, Jesus demonstrated scholarly growth and development many times. According to Luke 2:42–47, Jesus, at age 12, amazed even the scholarly priests with His knowledge of Old Testament Scripture. This would have been impossible if He had not spent considerable time in concentrated study of the Scriptures. We should follow the example of Jesus and improve our mental faculties to their fullest potential.

The potential for our mental development is almost unlimited. For example, our brain contains approximately 30 billion neurons which are interconnected. This means the possible interconnections are approximately 30 billion to the 30 billionth power. Scientists theorize that if our brains could be stimulated properly we could recall everything we have ever seen and heard. Yet everything we have experienced during our lifetime would comprise only about 10–15 percent of the brain's potential.

Many Christians fail to cultivate their mental potential. Watching soap operas on television, reading romance magazines, or attending movies that portray violence and sex does not contribute to mental growth. Many Christians have allowed their minds to become stagnant. They go to work, work at the same job every day, return home, and watch the same television programs. They get into a routine which becomes boring. God has created in the brain tremendous potential for mental development. It is up to you to develop your mental abilities.

"For as he thinks within himself, so is he" (Prov. 23:7). To learn effectively, a mental overload must be placed consistently on your mental capabilities. This overload should contribute positively, not negatively, to mental development. "Wise men store up knowledge" (Prov. 10:14). Read educational books, watch television programs that contribute to your knowledge, and attend lectures or seminars that can broaden your education. Do not allow this immeasurable potential to go stagnant. Do not be afraid or too lazy to learn about new areas of life. Develop your God-given potential by consistently stretching your mind with positive educational thoughts. Only when you develop your mental abilities will you become a whole person.

Social

"And Jesus kept increasing . . . in favor with men." God created human beings with social needs, and we cannot hide from or neglect these needs. The Bible tells us that Jesus developed His social needs by attending weddings, religious functions, and, on many occasions, dining with friends. Our social needs can be satisfied with positive interpersonal relationships.

To establish positive interpersonal relationships, you first must learn to love yourself. This doesn't mean loving yourself in a selfish manner. It means you must like the way you are, the way you feel, the way you think, and the way you behave. If you don't like yourself in these areas, you will not be able to love others because they will conflict with you in these areas. For example, I've known many Christians who became overweight, which caused them to dislike their appearance, which in turn caused emotional conflicts within their personality. They might resent others who are physically fit. This resentment could cause them to lose their witness for Him. Jesus understood this when He gave the directive, "You shall love your neighbor as yourself" (Matt. 22:39).

The second thing you must do to improve your interpersonal relationships is to learn to love everyone. This includes learning to love the unlovely. Jesus loved every type of person during His time on Earth. He loved the rich, the poor, the intelligent, the mentally challenged, His friends, and His enemies. We should adhere to His teachings and "through love serve one another" (Gal. 5:13).

Your family is an important part of your social well-being. Among all the people who need your attention, family members should rank high on the list. In the long run, time invested in family pays some of the biggest return to your total well-being. No matter where you are, how many times you change jobs, or how many times you move, your family is the constant which helps you through all circumstances. They are the ones for sharing celebrations and troubles.

Always welcome new friends. Seek out people with varied interests, backgrounds, and cultures. Learn and share ideas with them. This giving and receiving from new relationships will enhance your social well-being. Only when you make a concentrated effort to make friends will you ever develop into a whole person.

Spiritual

"And Jesus kept increasing in . . . favor with God." The most important decision a person can make in life is to trust Jesus Christ as Lord and Savior. Every other decision in life pales into insignificance compared with this important decision. Acceptance and confession that Jesus is God's Son will provide eternal life with God for the believer (see Rom. 10:9-10). After accepting Jesus as Savior, the next primary goal of all Christians should be to serve God as long and as well as they can. This includes developing a close personal relationship with Him. Jesus learned early in life about the tremendous potential that was given to Him for developing a close relationship with God, and He spent many hours of His life developing this close relationship with His Father. His growth toward attaining a close relationship with God is one we should try to emulate.

Many Christians are unaware of the resources God has provided for leading a rich and exciting life. The untapped potential lies within our grasp; yet we lead a mediocre, roller-coaster existence of occasional mountaintop experiences followed by slides back into the same rut. A few, having never experienced anything else, conclude this must be the normal Christian life. But Jesus came so that believers might have "abundant" life (see John 10:10). Abundant living is not all "peaches and cream" experiences. If we are willing to pay the price, God will lead us into fulfillment and adventure with Him. The following principles and guidelines can help us develop our spiritual growth.

Growth involves reliance on both God's resources and our own personal effort.—The purpose of growing in Christ is to reflect His character to others and to minister to them that they may come to know Him. According to the Bible Christians do not grow just by their own strength but by the actions of God's Spirit within. It is, however, the believer's responsibility to spend time and energy fulfilling God's requirements for growth (see Phil. 4:6).

Frantic efforts to develop spiritual wholeness or a lackadaisical "leave all the rest to God" attitude does not produce growth. We, as Christians, are called both to rely on God's resources and to respond in obedience to Him.

Growth means living in the fullness of the Holy Spirit.—Upon acceptance of Jesus as Savior, God's Holy Spirit enters into our bodies. However, many Christians still do not yield to Him or rely on the resources He brings into their lives. Through ignorance or rebellion, they miss the abundant life Christ promised and enter a cycle of frustration and depression.

If we are to live in the fullness of the Holy Spirit, we must confess all known sin and accept God's cleansing by faith. Confession of sin brings cleansing from all unrighteousness (see 1 John 1:9). This will bring a feeling of peace and freedom to your life.

Another way to live in the fullness of the Holy Spirit is to yield all areas of life to Jesus (see Rom. 12:1-2). Many Christians are afraid to yield their lives totally to Christ. They have pet sins they desire to retain. Or they fear God will cheat them out of a really full life if they submit to Him. God intends what is best for us (see Jer. 29:11). God desires that we spend our lives on things of everlasting value, not on impressive and attractive things the world offers us. If you really want to live life to its fullest, yield your life in its entirety to His control, asking Him to fill you and take charge. With the help of His power, commit yourself to break with those things displeasing to Him and to develop in your life those patterns that honor Him.

Abundant living is not all "peaches and cream" experiences. If we are willing to pay the price, God will lead us into fulfillment and adventure with Him.

Growth means increasing personal knowledge of God.—To get to know God you must spend time with Him and learn more about Him. Develop a daily time with God. Personal relationships demand personal time together. Even Jesus found it necessary to set aside a special time for communication with the Father (see Mark 1:35). Our time with God before the day starts will set the tone for all we do that day. Yield to God in prayer for control and filling of your life. Express thanks and praise to Him. Pray over matters that will affect you that day.

Growth means gaining a practical grasp of God's Word.—An understanding of the Bible will help you develop a closer relationship with God. One of the major reasons many Christians do not live a fuller life is that they are ignorant of the Bible's teachings. Listening, reading, studying, memorizing, and meditating are excellent methods to achieve a knowledge of God and obedience of His way.

Growth means ministering to others.—Read God's Word. A key part of God's plan for our growth is service. What we receive

We can see Jesus' strength and condition on the day He was beaten and crucified.

from Him, He desires that we pass on to others. We can minister to others about God's grace by becoming a part of a fellowship of Christians. When you join a local church, you will have the opportunity to help others and be helped by them, as they teach and encourage you. Learn to share Christ with others around you. If you ask Him to guide you into ministry opportunities and you yield yourself to Him, God will use you to share the good news about Christ.

Use God's resources (His promises, His Spirit, His Word, and His church) for spiritual growth. These resources will help you develop into the whole person.

Physical

"And Jesus kept increasing in . . . stature." I picture Jesus as a highly conditioned person. I base my judgment on a study of His lifestyle. Jesus possessed a high oxygen intake which was evident from the long distances He and His disciples walked. Just read the Gospels (Mark 5—6, for example). A number of towns are named where Jesus visited, taught, and healed people. To go to these places, Jesus walked. Often these towns were 10–20 or more miles apart. Some areas he visited were as much as 50 miles apart. He could not have walked such distances had He not been in excellent cardiovascular condition.

In His early life Jesus was a carpenter. His work required Him to possess a great amount of strength. He didn't have power tools to aid Him, and His tools were not sharpened by power-driven machines. He needed strength and muscular endurance just to saw a board. We can see Jesus' strength and condition on the day He was beaten and crucified. Only a well-conditioned man could have survived the beating and torture that preceded the crucifixion.

God has created tremendous physical potential in the human body. This physical potential that each person possesses can be reached only through what one exercise physiologist describes as the "overload principle." To gain strength or skill, an overload, whether a heavy weight or a long practice, must be placed on our present physical ability. The degree of overload will determine the increase in our physical ability. The smaller the overload, the smaller the increase. Conversely, the larger the overload, the larger the increase in physical ability.

For us to develop wholeness, we must consistently place an overload on the four areas of growth in a balanced manner. We should not neglect one area of growth or place too much emphasis on another. Any imbalance will cause deterioration in the other three. To serve Him longer, we must become fit in all four areas.

Vocational

What you do, your vocation, is part of your wholeness. Well-being in this area involves working in an area where God has given you gifts, talents, and training. Your vocation should be in line with what God has equipped you to do. Minister, teacher, lawyer, accountant, construction worker, stay-at-home mom, songwriter, researcher, social worker, medical professional, or administrator, or any other job should be according to His will for your life.

Jesus was about His Father's work as He continually sought to do the right thing at the right time. You, too, can follow God's lead in your vocation.

Emotional

The way you deal with your emotions indicates a level of emotional well-being and in turn a degree of total well-being. The way you express the primary emotions of glad, sad, mad, and scared contributes to your overall condition.

Resilience contributes to and nurtures your well-being. Resilience is your ability to navigate the storms of everyday life and remain unscathed for the long run. It includes knowing and understanding your strengths, which are a resource in any situation.

Emotional well-being also includes stress management. Stress is a part of everyone's life, from the youngest to the oldest. Those in the two extremes, youngest and oldest, may deal with stress the best. Those in the ages in between have the hardest time managing stress. Chapter 9 will talk more about stress management.

References

Brand, P., and P. Yancey. *Fearfully and Wonderfully Made.* Grand Rapids, Michigan: Zondervan Publishing House, 1980.

Couey, Richard. *Lifelong Fitness and Fulfillment.* Nashville, Tennessee: Broadman, 1980.

Couey, Richard. *Building God's Temple.* 2nd edition. Edina, Minnesota: Bellwether Press, 1987.

Couey, Richard. *Happiness Is Being a Physically Fit Christian.* Nashville, Tennessee: Broadman Publishers, 1985.

Yessick, Tommy. *Building Blocks for Longer Life and Ministry.* Nashville, Tennessee: Convention Press, 1997.

[CHAPTER 2]

Developing a Positive Philosophy Toward Fitness

Several times throughout my travels concerned people have asked me to elaborate on the question, Why should Christians develop fitness? Most of their concerns stem from the philosophy that Christians should develop only their spiritual dimensions. My belief is that we can't develop our spiritual dimensions to their fullest until we develop all our other dimensions (mental, physical, and social) equally. Let's turn to the Bible and search for reasons Christians should develop fitness.

Our Body Is God's Greatest Creation

It is hard to believe, as some scientists theorize, that by chance two small cells floating in the ocean, each with the exact necessary chemicals, could have fused together and, through millions of years, mutated into the wonderfully made human form. Only God could have created this complex, beautifully synchronized body He called His temple.

God made man in "His own image" (Gen. 1:27), and "man became a living being" (Gen. 2:7). Every system in his body, including every cell, was in perfect working condition. This was the ultimate in wholeness. There was no air pollution, noise pollution, junk food, stressful situations, or automated labor-saving devices to deteriorate this perfection. One can almost sense the pride that God felt as He viewed His wonderful creation and remarked, "It was very good" (Gen. 1:31).

One of my favorite Scriptures is found in Psalm 139:13-14. The psalmist was trying to praise God's greatest creation: "You created my inmost being; you knit me together in my mother's womb. I praise you because I am fearfully and wonderfully made" (NIV).

As a professor of exercise physiology and nutrition, I am amazed at how complicated the body is, how intricate each part, how diversified each system; yet each system lives in harmony, efficiently performing specific tasks. To me, the human body is perhaps the supreme wonder of the universe.

For example, let us look at some of the marvels of the body as God created it. Let's begin by examining the human cell, often called the basic element of life.

The human body begins with the fertilization of a single female egg, which is the ultimate wonder among cells. After ovulation, the egg takes three to five days to travel down the fallopian tubes, a distance of four inches. In contrast to the egg's

The human body begins with the fertilization of a single female egg, which is the ultimate wonder among cells.

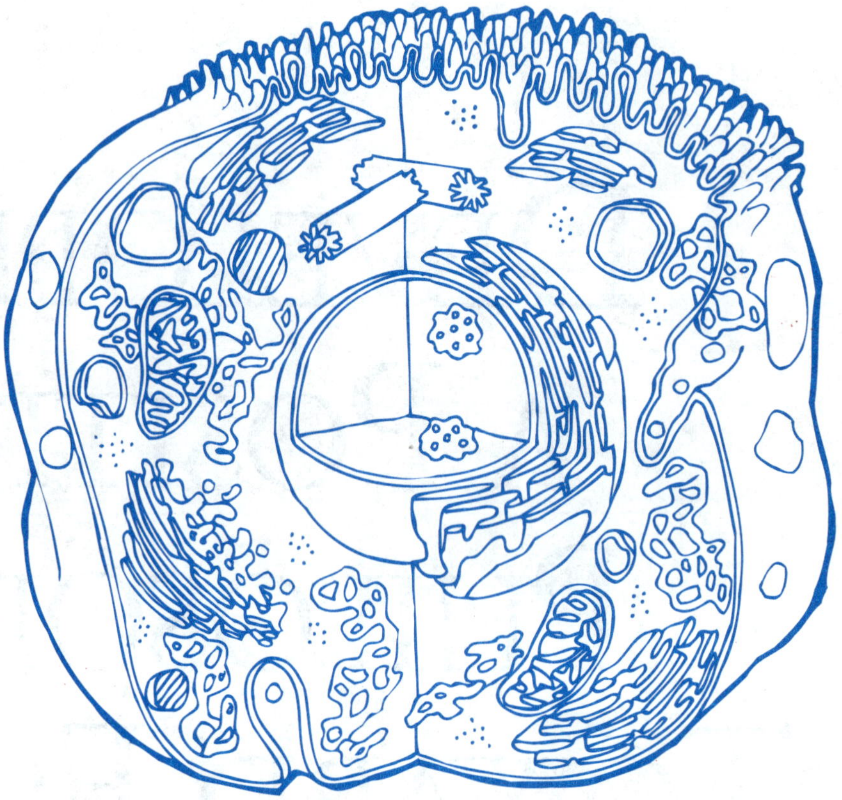

quiet, easy movement, the male's tiny sperm cells (1/500th of an inch long) are continuously active, like tadpoles with large heads and skinny tails. Sperm scramble for position around the egg as if competitively aware that only one of almost three hundred million will fertilize the egg. During the next nine months, the egg cell will divide into various types of cells: blood cells, brain cells, nerve cells—almost three trillion cells comprise that clay-colored, wrinkled package of screaming cells we call a baby. A baby is composed of many cells but is only one organism, and all the baby's three trillion cells know that.

Inside the cell are numerous anatomical structures that regulate the cell's various functions. Each cell has a nucleus that contains chromosomes, which are made up of genes, which are composed of DNA and amino acids. DNA is the substance that binds cells together. DNA determines how cellular components behave, what each manufactures, seeks, and avoids. It coordinates the activities of an adult's one hundred trillion cells as we move, see, think, and feel. DNA is so narrow and compact that all the genes in a person's cells would fit into an ice cube; yet when unwound and joined together end to end, the DNA strand would extend from the earth to the sun and back (186 million miles) more than four hundred times.

Cells constantly divide and reproduce themselves throughout life. Every second, millions of cells die, and millions are formed as old cells divide to create two identical new cells.

Cells manufacture almost three thousand enzymes, which are remarkable substances. In harmony with DNA , these enzymes, sometimes called master chemists, instantly and effortlessly synthesize proteins. A cell can produce more than one hundred thousand different chemical compounds. A cell can extract protein from digested fish, break it down into its components, and rearrange the amino acids to produce human protein needed for a toenail or an eyelash. The cellular enzymes also build complex hormones and disease-fighting antibodies and perform many tasks beyond the capabilities of the world's most gifted chemists.

Each day millions of skin cells are formed in the innermost epidermis and push outward, changing from jelly-like cellular material to firm tissue called keratin. This layer, approximately 30 cell layers thick, consists of flattened, inert, shingle-like cells that are all dead. This tissue is waterproof and resistant to friction and abrasions. Fragile living cells could not survive exposure to the hostile external environment. Each day millions of cells are washed away by a shower, or rubbed away by clothing. Almost 90 percent of all household dust contains dead skin. Because of this continuous process, a new outer skin is developed every 27 days.

If we were to cut a one-inch cube of flesh from the palm of our hand and examine it under an electron microscope, we would observe amazing proof of God's wonderfully made temple. Upon examination, we would find approximately 19,500,000 cells. If we linked the blood vessels together in that

For Christians, care of the body is a matter of stewardship.

one-inch cube, they would extend 56 yards. If fact, if we linked all our body's blood vessels together, depending on one's size, they would extend 100,000 miles, or reach four times around the equator of the earth.

Perhaps the story of cells can best be summed up by stating that the cell is responsible for everything from the beginning to the end. That one hundred trillion cells can live in such harmony, efficiently performing specific tasks, is wonderful to contemplate. The psalmist expressed himself beautifully when he wrote that we are fearfully and wonderfully made.

The Scriptures Teach Fitness

Another reason Christians should develop fitness is because the Bible teaches it. Let us examine what the Scriptures tell us about wholeness.

God knows every minute detail about the human body, His temple. He instructed Paul to record His doctrine concerning our behavior toward His creation. Paul recorded this doctrine in 1 Corinthians 6:19-20. Every Christian, regardless of doctrinal or denominational beliefs, should adhere to the principles described in these outstanding verses: "What? know ye not that your body is the temple of the Holy Ghost which is in you, which ye have of God, and ye are not your own? For ye are bought with a price: therefore glorify God in your body, and in your spirit, which are God's" (KJV).

Three distinct principles can be delineated from this Scripture: ownership, occupancy, and obedience. Let us analyze these verses that were divinely written nearly 2,000 years ago by an ex-tentmaker.

Ownership

This Scripture clearly reveals that your body does not belong to you. Examine this Scripture again. "Know ye not that your body is the temple of the Holy Ghost . . . which ye have of God, and ye are not your own? For ye are bought with a price." God created your body in His likeness. He breathed the breath of life into you, and He paid a great price in proving His love for you and redeeming you from sin. If you are a professing Christian, you have greater reason than others to take care of your body until you take your last breath.

For Christians, care of the body is a matter of stewardship. *Steward* refers to a supervisor who manages an estate or property for someone else. God has given us a body, and He expects us to feed it properly, to rest it properly, to grow in mind and spirit, and to exercise it properly. He wants us to use our body to give glory to Him, because He owns it. If we do not keep our bodies in the best possible physical condition, they are incapable of honoring God as they should.

Therefore, as professing Christians and good stewards, we have the responsibility to maintain internally and externally the temples God created. We should continually and consistently develop our bodies mentally, emotionally, spiritually, and physically for the best possible performance and production capability.

Occupancy

God expressed His love by giving His Son to die for our sins so that those who accept His redeeming love might have eternal life. When we accept Christ, the Holy Spirit comes to live in us. This means, as Christians, our flesh and blood is the earthly dwelling place for the Spirit of God. "Do you not know that you are a temple of God and that the Spirit of God dwells in you? If any man destroys the temple of God, God will destroy him, for the temple of God is holy, and that is what you are" (1 Cor. 3:16-17).

This expression of God's love honors us. God honors each of us by allowing His Spirit to live within our bodies. What an overwhelming privilege and responsibility we Christians have to house the Spirit of our God! When I think of God dwelling in my body, pride, a sense of responsibility, and feelings of humility fill my mind. I am proud that God chose to live in my body. Knowing that God lives in my body gives me confidence in myself. I am not afraid of taking on life's challenges, for I know God is with and within me. With this feeling of pride and confidence also comes a sense of responsibility. I realize that my body will function more effectively and efficiently if I care for its development and maintenance. I am committed to the principle of continually and consistently keeping my body at its optimum operating efficiency. This means I must eat properly, rest properly, continue educational development, and exercise properly. It is difficult to understand why some Christians drink alcohol, smoke tobacco, consume harmful drugs, fill their minds with junk, and overeat when the Holy Spirit of God is present within their bodies. Our Christian responsibility is to maintain optimum physical wholeness for His temple.

When I remember how wonderfully God made His temple

It is difficult to understand why some Christians drink alcohol, smoke tobacco, consume harmful drugs, fill their minds with junk, and overeat when the Holy Spirit of God is present within their bodies.

and how God expressed His love through His Son, reverence and humility overwhelm my thoughts. How can God, who created the heavens and earth and breathed life into all life forms, love and honor me by living within my body? All of life's obstacles seem insignificant when compared to the omnipotent presence of God's Spirit within us. The fact that God indwells the body is reason enough to develop fitness in our bodies to their fullest potential.

Obedience

The last principle is found in 1 Corinthians 6:20: "Therefore glorify God in your body and in your spirit, which are God's" (KJV). Our option to choose whether we will care for our bodies and spirits is shown in this verse. God has given us free will to choose for ourselves. But He has also given us rules by which to live. God knows that for us to be truly happy we must obey and live our lives according to God's directions. Many Christians who stray from His directions experience unhappiness for choosing the wrong lifestyle. We all stray, and many of us are still learning to put God first in our lives.

In this verse God provided the rule that will make us truly happy. He is directing us to glorify God in our bodies to the best of our abilities and to condition our bodies to their optimum physical capability. If we obey this directive, we will remain healthy throughout our lives. Good health will enhance our service for Him, and we can serve more effectively without stress and fatigue.

Many Christians choose to neglect this directive. They let false pleasures dominate their bodies. Many overeat, eat foods without nutritional value, drink alcohol, smoke tobacco, worry unnecessarily, and avoid every opportunity to exercise. This lifestyle is prevalent among Christians of all denominations. Some studies suggest a relationship between the practice of religion and being overweight. Since extra pounds are a major health risk factor, this is a sad note. Many Christians are shortening or limiting their ministry because of the increased risk of diabetes, hypertension (high blood pressure), cardiovascular disease, and some cancers. Obesity relates strongly to these diseases.

This is an attitude of negligence of God's directive. Many Christians obey God's spiritual laws, attend church regularly, tithe, serve others with compassion and concern, but do not glorify God in their bodies. This lack of obedience to God's command is sin. I feel it is sin to neglect the physical needs of God's temple. The Holy Spirit inspired Paul to write: "I urge you therefore, brethren, by the mercies of God, to present your bodies a living and holy sacrifice, acceptable to God, which is your spiritual service of worship. And do not be conformed to this world, but be transformed by the renewing of your mind, that you may prove what the will of God is, that which is good and acceptable and perfect" (Rom. 12:1-2).

Just like any other, sin against the body ruins God's temple. Christians need to start practicing self-discipline and learn to overcome lazy attitudes toward physical exercise and mental and spiritual development. When we obey God's directive, we will feel better and experience a happier life and better health. We have the option to neglect our body's physical needs, which leads to poor health, or to glorify God in our bodies, which leads to good health.

Don't use the excuse of "I can't." I can't because I'm too old, too tired, or don't have time. Every time you find yourself making excuses, remember this Scripture: "For God has not given us a spirit of timidity, but of power and love and discipline" (2 Tim. 1:7).

God did not give you a weak (timid) spirit but a spirit of power and self-discipline. God will help you overcome your weak spirit. Don't say, "I can't." Say, "I can!"

References

Brand, P., and P. Yancey. *Fearfully and Wonderfully Made.* Grand Rapids, Michigan: Zondervan Publishing House, 1980.

Couey, Richard. *Building God's Temple.* 2nd edition. Edina, Minnesota: Bellwether Press, 1987.

Couey, Richard. *Happiness Is Being a Physically Fit Christian.* Nashville, Tennessee: Broadman Publishers, 1985.

Greer, E. *Toward Physical Excellence for the Glory of God.* Fort Worth, Texas: Harvest Press Inc., 1976.

Guyton, A. *Textbook of Medical Physiology.* Philadelphia: W. B. Saunders Co., 1991.

[CHAPTER 3]

Understanding the Benefits of Becoming a Fit Person

More than two thousand years ago, Hippocrates said, "Exercise strengthens while inactivity wastes." Today it is a basic physiologic law that an organ or system improves with use and deteriorates with disuse. From reading this chapter you will better understand the benefits received from developing fitness. Understanding these benefits will better motivate you to achieve a higher degree of fitness in each wholeness area. Let us examine each area.

Physical

Let us begin by gaining an understanding of the benefits received when people develop their bodies through physical exertion.

Cardiovascular-Respiratory System

The function of the cardiovascular-respiratory system is to provide the necessary flow of blood and oxygen to the various tissues of the body in response to their activity needs. The cardiovascular-respiratory (CVR) consists of the heart, blood, arteries, capillaries, veins, and lungs. The benefits received from exercising the cardiovascular-respiratory system are too numerous to mention in this book. Let us review some of the most beneficial ones.

Effects on the heart.—One of the most beneficial long-term effects is an increase in the size and strength of the heart muscle (myocardium) and a high stroke volume (amount of blood pumped per beat) at all levels of activity. With increased stroke volume, the heart does not have to pump as fast in order to supply the body with a given amount of blood for a particular level of activity. The slower heart rate at all levels of activity, resting and during exercise of heavy work, allows the heart more rest between contractions. This slow heart rate is evident in well-trained individuals. Studies done on American Olympic track athletes revealed a resting heart rate in the lower 30s per minute, much slower than that of the average American (72 beats per minute for males; 80 beats per minute for females).

In a well-conditioned individual, the heart rate also responds more quickly to various workloads and recovers faster to its normal resting rate. Because of its ability to supply an adequate amount of blood at a lower heart rate, the heart is able to tolerate greater workloads before reaching its maximum rate. For the average person, this can provide a reserve capacity to cope with sudden physical or emotional stresses that accelerate the heart rate.

Effects on the vascular system.—The size and elasticity of the arteries increase throughout the body as do the size and number of capillaries in the various tissues. Collateral circulation between all major arteries increases, and there is better diffusion between the capillaries and the working tissues. Improved blood flow takes an additional load off the heart. The enlargement and increase in the number of blood vessels decrease resistance to blood flow and lower an abnormally high blood pressure. The effect also helps blood pressure to return to normal faster following an increase from any cause. By increasing the size and helping to maintain elasticity of the large arteries, hardening of the arteries can be prevented or delayed.

Effects on the blood.—Red blood cells are significantly increased through regular exercise. Studies comparing well-trained with untrained individuals have shown that well-trained

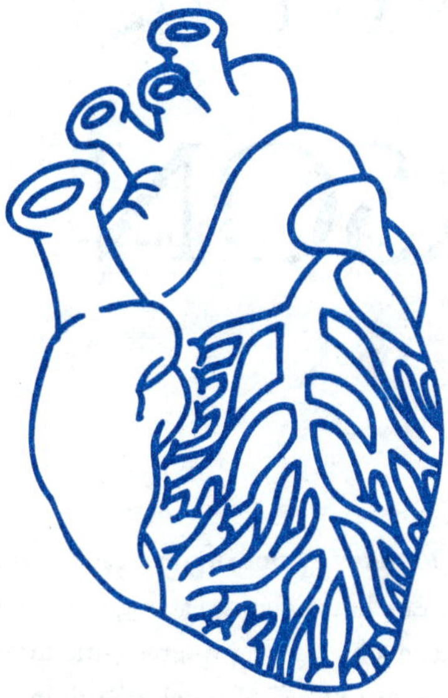

individuals have between seven and eight million red blood cells per cubic millimeter of blood, whereas untrained individuals have between five and six million. Because red blood cells combine with oxygen, the well-trained individual is better able to transport more oxygen to the starved cells.

Two other beneficial effects relate to the formation of blood clots and the level of fatty acids in the blood. Exercise affects the clotting time of blood in two ways: The blood coagulates more quickly when it leaves the vascular system, such as from a cut; and the blood plasma activity increases, which breaks up blood clots forming within the blood vessel. This lessens the chance of a blood clot forming in the heart, brain, or other vital organs.

Numerous studies have shown that residual levels of cholesterol and other fatty lipids in the blood can be significantly reduced with vigorous exercise. Reducing cholesterol and triglycerides significantly reduces your chance of atherosclerosis. Vigorous exercise also increases high-density lipoproteins (HDL), which can reduce atheroscleric plaque buildup in the arteries.

A study done by Dr. Ken Cooper, an authority on aerobic research, found that the ratio between total cholesterol level and HDL level should be under a 4.5 to 1 ratio to afford better protection against heart disease. Dividing the HDL level into the total cholesterol level will determine this ratio. For example, the HDL level was determined to be 60, whereas the total cholesterol was determined to be 180. The ratio would be 3:1. Lowering this ratio to 3.1 would better protect against heart disease. A simple blood test conducted by a physician can determine your HDL and total cholesterol level.

The question arises, How do you improve HDL level while reducing the total cholesterol level? To improve the ratio of cholesterol to HDL, diet remains important. By eating less cholesterol and saturated fat (contained in such foods as red meats, dairy products, palm oil, and coconut oil), you may change the ratio in your favor. It is also important to stop smoking and drinking alcohol and to get regular aerobic exercise. Exercise is the most beneficial way to increase HDL.

Effects on the lungs.—The immediate effect of exercise, of course, is an increase in the rate and depth of breathing in response to the body's need for more oxygen and the removal of increased levels of carbon dioxide. Increased breathing depth forces the use of more alveoli, the tiny air sacs in the lungs that connect to the capillaries where the actual exchange of gases takes place.

Because of the increased blood supply, the muscles of respiration increase in size, strength, and endurance. Their increased strength and tone increase the size of the thoracic cage (chest cavity) at all levels of activity, allowing more air to enter the lungs with each breath. And they become more efficient, requiring less oxygen to perform a given amount of work. The size and number of capillaries in the lungs also increase, allowing more oxygen to be absorbed and more carbon dioxide to be removed. In addition, the greater number of alveoli that are used bring about an even greater exchange. The combined effect of deeper and more efficient breathing results in a slower rate of breathing in the resting state and during submaximal levels of activity. The respiration rate returns to normal more quickly following exercise. The overall effect, in terms of physical performance, is the ability to do more work and to work for longer periods of time without fatigue.

The beneficial effects of regular exercise demonstrate why the incidence of cardiovascular disease has consistently been lower in physically active people than in those who lead more sedentary lives. The effects also explain why an increasing number of doctors prescribe exercise for patients showing signs of degenerative cardiovascular disease and even patients who are recovering from certain types of heart attacks.

Muscular System

When muscles are exercised, the blood flow through the capillaries into the muscle tissue is increased. Depending on the type and severity of the exercise, this causes a temporary expansion of the muscle size. Increased metabolic activity in the muscle tissue produces more heat, which is reflected in a rise of body temperature. This higher temperature causes the muscle to become more pliable, so it is able to contract and relax faster and more easily. Vigorous exercise also has been shown to reduce levels of neuromuscular tension as measured by the amount of electrical activity in the muscles before and immediately after exercise. Exercising the muscles is an excellent way to reduce stress that has built up during the day.

Depending on the type and amount, regular exercise increases the size, strength, and endurance of the muscles. In activities such as walking, running, and cycling, the major effect is on the blood flow through the tissues. More efficient delivery of oxygen and removal of waste products allow the muscles to work longer without fatigue. The improved nourishment helps to keep the muscles in good tone. In power-type activities, such as weight training and heavy calisthenics, thickening and increased size of both the muscle and connective tissue (called hypertrophy) are more prominent. With this comes increased strength. Contributing to strength is the activation and development of additional motor units in the muscle. The increased strength and number of motor units improve the efficiency and endurance of the muscles in another way; motor units work in relays. As strength increases, fewer units are needed to perform submaximal efforts. This allows the other units to rest. When the working units become fatigued, additional units are brought into operation, allowing the tired units to rest. The result is a significant increase in muscle endurance.

Effects on the skeleton system.—A normal adult has about 206 bones of various shapes and sizes. Besides supporting and giving general shape to the body mass, the bones serve as a protection for the softer and more vulnerable organs and systems such as the brain, lungs, and spinal cord. Vigorous exercise, by improving the supply of blood, helps bones to grow in size, thickness, and strength and to maintain their vital inner activity. Light resistive exercise has been shown to prevent or delay the onslaught of osteoporosis (softening of the bone tissue).

Effects on the digestive system.—Vigorous exercise approximately one hour before or after the intake of food interferes with the digestive process. Blood supply is diverted from the digestive system to the active muscles. Secretion of digestive juices is inhibited. In addition, the wavelike contractions of the smooth muscles along the alimentary canal are inhibited. The most notable effects are cramps and a delay in the stomach's emptying time. Therefore, it is best to wait at least three hours after a heavy meal before vigorously exercising. Regular exercise, by strengthening the smooth muscles along the digestive pathway, can regulate bowel movement and prevent or relieve constipation.

The beneficial effects of regular exercise demonstrate why the incidence of cardiovascular disease has consistently been lower in physically active people than in those who lead more sedentary lives.

Effects on the endocrine system.—Vigorous exercise stimulates production of certain hormones that have significant effects on the body. Stimulation of the adrenal glands produces two substances called adrenaline and noradrenaline. These adrenalins are partly responsible for increased heart rate, blood pressure, and blood sugar needed for a response often called "fight or flight." Increased production of adrenaline can be triggered by mental or emotional stress such as fear, anger, and anxiety. Unreleased energy is built up and muscles tighten. This causes an unnecessary waste of energy and taxing of the heart and certain organs of the body.

Exercise is valuable in lessening the detrimental effects of adrenaline produced by emotional stress in several ways. According to Hans Seyle, a Canadian endocrinologist, when stress is disproportionately greater on one organ or system, exercise may help by distributing the stress over a wider area.

Vigorous exercise also reduces the physiologic effects of emotional stress. Another important value of exercise in combating the effects of emotionally produced adrenaline is strengthening of the body, particularly the heart, to handle the increased workload. Because it is stronger, the heart may be able to resist attacks of emotional stress that might otherwise bring about heart failure and death.

Vigorous exercise also stimulates the thyroid gland, which produces a substance called thyroxin. Thyroxin releases caloric energy and activates cells in all parts of the body. The increased metabolic rate lasts for hours (sometimes as long as 24 hours), even after exercise is stopped. The caloric expenditure resulting from this general rise, combined with the expenditure produced by the adrenalins, is an important factor in weight loss.

Over a period of time, by its effect on thyroid gland activity, exercise can help normalize an individual's basal metabolic rate (the minimum amount of energy used by the body in its resting state). A low rate may be raised and a high one lowered. Persons with a low basal metabolism tend to be lethargic and overweight. By raising the metabolic rate, lethargy and obesity can be reduced. Tense people tend to have a high metabolic rate. Lowering it may reduce tension.

> **Do not grow old before your time; delay your aging processes with a program of regular exercise.**

Exercise also stimulates the secretion of cortisone from the adrenal cortex gland. Cortisone acts directly on the tissues of the brain and, therefore, can help stimulate better mental activity.

The beneficial stimulating effect of exercise on the endocrine glands is summarized by this quotation from the *Journal of the American Medical Association*: "The greatest value of exercise lies in its stimulating effect on endocrine activity, perhaps the thyroid, in particular, and in overcoming the tendency to sleep and snooze too much, a counterpart of obesity." Fatigue in old age is often the result of a drop in endocrine activity. Do not grow old before your time; delay your aging processes with a program of regular exercise.

Effects on aging.—After age 30, certain measures of physical performance gradually decline. The rate of decline varies both with different individuals and with different functions. Obviously some decline in physical performance can be expected with advanced age, but this decline can be slowed by a sensible program of diet and exercise. Furthermore, the decline is not enough to restrict reasonable physical activity as one grows older. In fact, research shows that persons in good health, particularly those who exercise regularly, require few restrictions.

A continuous program of physical activity throughout one's lifetime can delay the aging process. The major benefit of such a program is the slower rate of decline in the circulatory, respiratory, muscular, and other systems of the body. Inactivity causes a decrease in stroke volume; an increase in heart rate; lower cardiac output; lower oxygen consumption; and a loss of muscular size, strength, and tone. A sedentary life pattern brings about a faster decline than a life that includes regular, vigorous activity. Such an activity program will prevent or delay the onset of degenerative diseases usually associated with old age. Older persons who have continued a regular activity program show more energy, vitality, and higher levels of physical performance than many who are much younger. To illustrate this point, a humbling experience took place in my life when a 67-year-old man passed me at the 24-mile mark in a marathon race, patted me on the back, and said, "Hang in there, Sonny." I wished him well as he disappeared over the next hill!

Mental

Anyone who exercises regularly usually notices improved attitudes and feelings. Not everyone reports the same effects; but, as a group, exercisers assert that they have a more positive outlook on life and can concentrate better and cope with problems more effectively. They say they feel more assertive, think more creatively, and are more self-confident.

Dramatic mental benefits also have been observed, as exercise seems to help the psychologically disturbed. Several psychiatrists report remarkable results in the psychologically therapeutic value of exercise. Those with depression had fewer symptoms. Some schizophrenics could be taken off medication, and even some patients with anorexia nervosa (a condition in which people refuse food and can literally starve themselves to death) resumed eating.

Scientists do not know why exercise seems to have a beneficial effect on depression. It may be related to the fact that someone who is depressed generally feels better after successfully performing even one simple task, such as exercising for 10 weeks.

There may also be a chemical connection between exercise and the alleviation of depression. Researchers have found evidence that exercise promotes production in the brain of the hormone norepinephrine, which seems related to emotional stability. By analyzing blood samples taken during exercise, researchers discovered that the level of norepinephrine in the blood increased on the average by more than three times. Other studies indicate that people with balanced emotions seem to enjoy high levels of this hormone and of a similar one called epinephrine. Depressed individuals have low levels. Other theories contend that exercise affects mood by increasing blood flow to the brain, perhaps because the brain thrives on the extra oxygen and nutrients it receives.

Recent studies reveal that the brain produces substances called beta endorphins. These substances relieve pain, calm nerves, suppress appetites, produce sensations of pleasure, and are extremely addictive. Vigorous sustained exercise causes the body to produce more endorphins, which may explain how

Exercising with someone can provide an excellent opportunity to develop lifelong friendships.

long-distance runners can tolerate pain for hours. It may also explain why some runners become addicted to the pleasurable feeling derived from running.

Placing an overload on our mental ability will also develop our brain's functional capacity. Research has shown that people who constantly exercise their brain through reading, studying, and concentrated effort are capable of performing more difficult mental tasks much later in life than those who do not challenge their mind. These people are also capable of retaining and recalling more of what they have learned. The bottom line might be expressed in this statement: "Use it, or lose it." If you don't try to improve your mental ability, then you may lose it faster than you anticipated. Always try to learn new and challenging things.

Social

"A friend loves at all times" (Prov. 17:17). One of the most prized possessions in the world is a good friend—someone you trust; someone who can share your inmost feelings; someone who will give you good advice; someone who will laugh, cry, and play with you. Exercising with someone can provide an excellent opportunity to develop lifelong friendships. For example, I will find someone who wants to run a marathon (a distance of 26 miles, 385 yards), and ask him to train with me. During the next three to four months of training, sometimes running two or more hours a day in all weather conditions, a long-lasting friendship develops. We share our problems, joys, beliefs, and philosophy of life. I cherish the many friendships I have developed through running.

Sometimes adults, especially senior adults and housewives, meet together for exercise sessions and afterwards have fellowship together. I have seen some beautiful smiles in those post-exercise gatherings.

Not only can exercising together develop good friendships, but it can also develop good family relationships. Exercising together as a family can bring about positive interpersonal relationships. I once saw a bumper sticker that read, "A family that prays and plays together, stays together." A family should not only worship God together but also develop ways to play and exercise together. One of the most significant and meaningful times in my life is when I exercise with my daughter. We enjoy running together, and through that association my daughter has shared parts of her life that most dads don't have the opportunity to share with their daughters. I would not trade those precious moments together for anything. Parents, teach your children through education and example how to take care of God's temple.

Accomplishing exercise goals can also bring about a healthy self-esteem. Losing weight, running your fastest mile, or breaking your record in the bench press can do wonders for a low self-esteem. A positive self-esteem will give you confidence in yourself, which will make you more outgoing, which will help you develop more friendships, which can help you become a better servant for God.

Spiritual

Exercise and a proper diet can change the physiology of the body in a positive manner. Both have a positive effect on every system in the body. Every cell in every system of the body works more proficiently, creates more energy, carries out its proper metabolic functions more effectively, and rids itself of waste more efficiently. When the body's physiology is working correctly, our mind is more alert, our emotions are more sensitive yet more controllable, and our spirit is more receptive to God's will for our lives. This all adds up to being able to serve God longer and better, which should be a basic goal of all Christians.

When we live our lives according to God's will, God promises us that we will have "abundant life." If we fail to live according to His will, we may experience unhappiness. Improper care of our body (God's temple) is a sin against God's will. Just like any other sin against God, it causes guilt, frustration, and unhappiness. You can't be the best Christian possible if you are not physically fit. Inactivity can cause you to become tired, lethargic, sick, and maybe even depressed. This will affect your service for Him. Happiness comes from being physically active, eating proper foods, and living your life according to God's will.

In summary, the following are some general health benefits that can be received through exercise and a proper diet:

1. Increased general feeling of health and well-being.
2. Higher fatigue levels and greater physical work capacity.
3. Prevention, delay, or a greater ability to withstand and recover from cardiovascular accidents and other degenerative diseases.
4. Controlled body weight.
5. Improved posture and appearance.
6. Relief of tension and stress.

7. Prevention of lower back pain.
8. Delayed aging process.
9. Delayed aging of brain cells.
10. Improved neuromuscular skill and physical performance.
11. Stimulation of mental activity.
12. Better digestion and bowel movement.
13. Improved functioning of the internal organs.
14. Better mental attitude.
15. Improved sense of accomplishment.
16. Better self-concept.

If we fail to eat properly and exercise regularly, we are highly vulnerable to a fatal heart attack. If we smoke cigarettes, natural law decrees that our lungs will be harmed. If we drink, our brain, liver, heart, and kidneys will suffer. If we eat sugar-filled food in excess of our energy expenditure, we will become obese. If our muscles become flabby and weak, we should not complain about lower back or musculoskeletal problems. We are responsible for giving up these self-destructive habits. We know the rules and the penalties for breaking them. Cause and effect, the underlying principle of natural law, is the first fundamental belief taught in the scientific method. To ignore it leads to our destruction.

We need to practice our own preventive medicine. To believe that "it can't happen to me" is foolish, dangerous, and unrealistic. Yes, it can happen to any of us who ignorantly or willfully defy God's natural laws. For God tells us in Matthew 5:45 that He does not make exceptions: "He . . . sends rain on the righteous and on the unrighteous."

Emotional

Exercise and fitness level can help you with your emotional well-being. Emotional well-being includes dealing with emotions, reilience, and stress. Expressing the emotions *glad, sad, mad,* and *scared* can better be moderated. Imagine you have become upset, angry at another person. What better way to gain perspective than to take a walk, pound a racquetball, or sweat out your frustrations? If you are scared about something, take a walk and talk with God.

The discipline of an exercise routine helps build the relilience to deal with a lifestyle that pulls you in all directions. Such a discipline can be transferred to other areas of your life competences which help you navigate the areas of challenge.

Stress creates good and bad by-products. The negative buildup of a day's worth of stress can be moderated through good fitness and an exercise routine. An individual accumulation of muscle tension, anxiety, and stress by-products can be relieved with moderate physical activity. The movement of large muscle groups actually relieves muscle tension. After exercise, which is repeatedly causing muscles to contract and extend, these muscles are much more supple, less tense, and relaxed. It also helps use up some of the physiological substances stress produces within your body. A great way to relieve the effects of stress is to take a walk, go for a run, or ride a bike—just move on a regular basis.

Vocational

Your level of physical fitness can impact your work. Exercise helps to clear your mind, enabling you to think better about the tasks you do related to work. Have you ever felt so overwhelmed by your workload that you could not think straight? A little movement helps. This may sound like intellectual or mental well-being. It is, but it impacts your ability to do your job. One philosopher said, "Never trust an idea you come upon standing still."

Many times, while exercising, I have come up with a new idea related to work. It may be a solution to a problem or a new approach to an old program.

Another connection between fitness and vocation is weight and advancement. Right or wrong, a deconditioned, overweight person does not get the same chances for new positions or advancement. Such persons may be equally qualified, but they must overcome the impression being overweight communicates.

A great way to give glory to God is to be prepared to serve Him longer and better. Taking care of yourself, including proper exercise and good nutrition, will help you do that. It will also help ensure that you will continue to live and enjoy good health so that you might enjoy more years with your family.

References

Astrand, I. *Aerobic Work Capacity in Men and Women with Special Reference to Age.* Acta physiol Scand 49:1-92, 1960.

Bortz, W. "The Disuse Syndrome." *Western Journal of Medicine,* 141:691-4, 1984.

Cooper, Ken. *The New Aerobics.* New York: Bantam Books, 1970.

Couey, Richard. *Building God's Temple.* Minneapolis: Burgress Publishing Co., 1987.

Couey, Richard. *Happiness Is Being a Physically Fit Christian.* Nashville: Broadman Publishers, 1985.

Cratty, B. *Psychology and Physical Activity.* Englewood Cliffs, N.J.: Prentice-Hall, 1968.

DeVries, H. *Physiology of Exercise for Physical Education and Athletics.* Dubuque, Iowa: W. C. Brown Co.,1985.

Falls, H. *Essentials of Fitness.* Philadelphia: Saunders College, 1980.

Selye, H. *Stress Without Distress.* Philadelphia: J.B. Lippincott Co., 1974.

[CHAPTER 4]

Understanding the Components of Fitness

Many Americans are confused about what physical fitness is. This confusion is brought about by what all the literature says about running, calisthenics, aerobic dancing, stretching, dieting, and lifting weights. People can easily become confused; for the media are flooded with information concerning what you should eat, not eat, how to jog, how to lift weights, and so forth. Regrettably, much of this information is contradictory; and some of it is not based on scientific information. This chapter can help you make a decision concerning your physical fitness needs.

Basically, fitness means being in good physical condition and able to function at one's best. It is the capability of the heart, blood vessels, lungs, and muscles to function at optimal efficiency. *Optimal efficiency* means the health needed for the most enthusiastic and pleasurable participation in daily life.

Many fallacies exist about the concept of physical fitness. Some think a physically fit person is the muscular bodybuilder who is capable of knocking down doors or kicking sand in anyone's face if he so desires. Others believe that persons who are slender and can run miles at a fast pace are physically fit; while others believe that a woman who wears a size 6 dress or a man who has a 30-inch waist is physically fit. Actually none of these may be classified as physically fit. For example, the muscular person may lack the ability to run a great distance, or the fast person may possess little strength, while the slender person may lack both. Being physically fit encompasses many components. Most exercise physiologists agree that there are 10 components of physical fitness. They have divided these components into two categories—health related and skill related.

The health-related components are those that best improve the physiological systems of the body, whereas the skill-related components are those essential for performance in games and sports, as well as for working efficiency. The skill-related components will not be discussed here; but they include agility, balance, coordination, power, reaction time, and speed. Having these skills is desirable but not essential for maintaining a good level of physical health. Your ability to dodge, to control your balance, to react and move quickly, and the ability of your muscles to function harmoniously and efficiently are all reflections of your general athletic skill. There is good news for those who have limited athletic prowess. You don't have to worry about being chosen last to become fit in the health-related components, for the health-related components do not require athletic skills (coordination, agility, etc.) in order to obtain fitness. Let's examine the health-related components.

Health-Related Components

The basic components with health-related fitness are cardiovascular-respiratory (CVR) endurance, body composition, muscular endurance, and flexibility. Each component and its health-related effects on God's temple are discussed below.

Overwhelming evidence supports the conclusion that exercise reduces the probability of contracting cardiovascular disease.

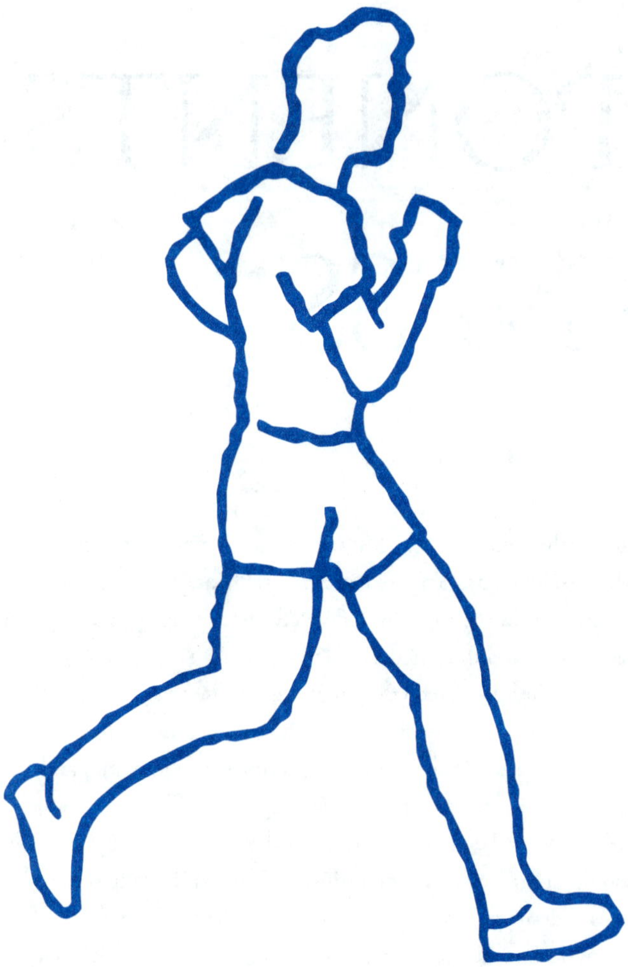

CVR Endurance

CVR endurance is the most important health-related component in the fitness area. As its name implies, CVR endurance means becoming fit in the heart, blood, blood vessels, and lungs. Obtaining fitness in these areas reduces the probability of having a cardiovascular disease such as heart attack or stroke. These circulatory diseases are the leading causes of death among the adult population of most industrialized countries throughout the world. The United States has the unenviable distinction of leading all 168 countries in the world in deaths from these circulatory diseases. Not only do American men lead the men of the world in cardiovascular diseases, but recent statistics show that American women also lead the women of the world in deaths from this disease. In 1995, nearly two million Americans suffered from a cardiovascular disorder, and nearly one million died from one. This means three hundred people die each day from circulatory diseases, and most people in our society don't seem too alarmed.

Americans should be concerned, embarrassed, and ashamed of these statistics because cardiovascular disease can be prevented in most cases. Most exercise physiologists, cardiologists, and other health professionals are convinced that exercise at high enough intensity will improve CVR fitness by either preventing the circulatory disease altogether or by reducing its effects if it does occur. Overwhelming evidence supports the conclusion that exercise reduces the probability of contracting cardiovascular disease. Research has clearly shown that sedentary individuals have a higher incidence of myocardial infarction (heart attack) and that the fatality rate among those who suffer such attacks is higher than in those who are physically active. High levels of CVR fitness lower the serum cholesterol, serum triglycerides, serum glucose, serum uric acid, blood pressure, and body fat percentage. Each of these areas is a risk factor in cardiovascular disease.

Some general and specific recommendations for setting up and carrying out an exercise program to improve CVR fitness are given in chapter 5.

Body Composition

Body composition refers to the relative percentages with fat and fat-free body mass. It is the relative makeup of body fat compared with lean body mass in muscle, fat, bone, and other vital parts. A fit person has a relatively low percentage of body fat.

Obesity in the United States is widespread. Public health records estimate that 40 percent (35 million) of Americans are overweight. Thirty-three percent of our schoolchildren are considered overweight. Retention of body fat is a serious health problem, especially among children and adolescents, because research has shown that the fatty tissue developed at an early age remains throughout a lifetime. This means that fat children often grow up to be fat adults. Life insurance companies claim that overweight individuals are poorer risks than persons with normal weight, as life expectancy is shorter with excessive body fat. The death rate is increased 30 percent for individuals who are 15–24 percent overweight and as much as 80 percent for those who are 35 percent or more overweight.

Diseases of the heart and circulatory system are often associated with obesity. High blood pressure is twice as frequent, and arteriosclerosis is three times more frequent in obese individuals. In addition to an increased incidence of coronary heart disease among obese persons, other health problems are manifest. These include diabetes mellitus, gallbladder disease, degenerative arthritis, some cancers, kidney disease, adverse postural deviations, delayed puberty in children, and decreased endurance and work capacity. Jean Mayer, distinguished professor of nutrition at Harvard, estimates that if all deaths from cancer were eliminated, two years would be added to the human life span; if all deaths related to obesity were removed, the life span would increase seven years. Being overweight is a threat to the quality and length of one's life. The effects of and remedy for obesity are discussed later in this book.

Muscular Strength and Endurance

Strength is defined as the capacity of a muscle to exert a maximal force against a resistance. Muscular endurance is the capacity of a muscle to exert a force repeatedly over a period of time. In other words, it is the ability to apply strength and sustain it. Even though there is a slight difference between the two, muscular endurance and strength will be used synonymously.

More and more Americans are beginning to see the need for a good exercise and recreational program. Many are joining recreational programs such as softball, tennis, racquetball, and golf. To be successful in competition, muscular endurance training is necessary. Stronger muscles better protect the bones and joints that they cross. As a result, people who are physically fit experience less susceptibility to strains, sprains, fractures, dislocations, and pulls that sometimes occur when playing in sports. This same protection carries over to your daily lifestyle activities.

The most important reason for developing muscular endurance is to prevent some of the more common postural deviations that plague the American population such as lower back pain, lordosis, scoliosis, round shoulders, and fallen arches in the feet. Developing muscular balance in all of the major muscle groups will help prevent or rehabilitate most of the postural deviations.

Also many psychological needs are met through toning up flabby muscles. Nearly everyone wants to have the strong lean appearance that can be provided by a good muscular endurance program and a proper diet. A strong healthy body improves one's self-esteem.

Developing muscular balance in all of the major muscle groups will help prevent or rehabilitate most postural deviations.

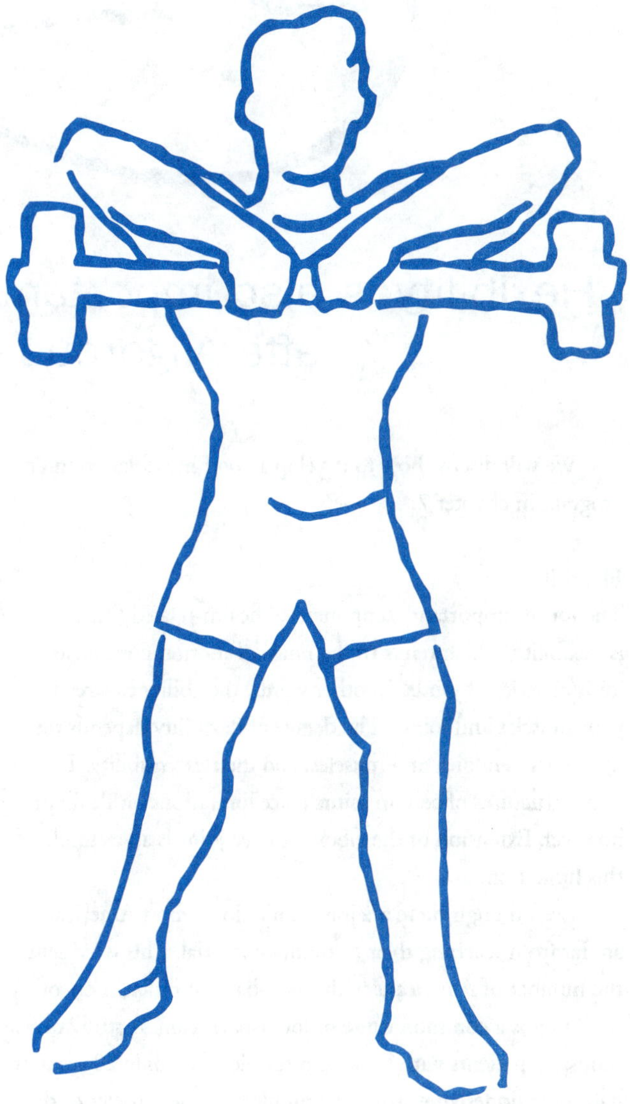

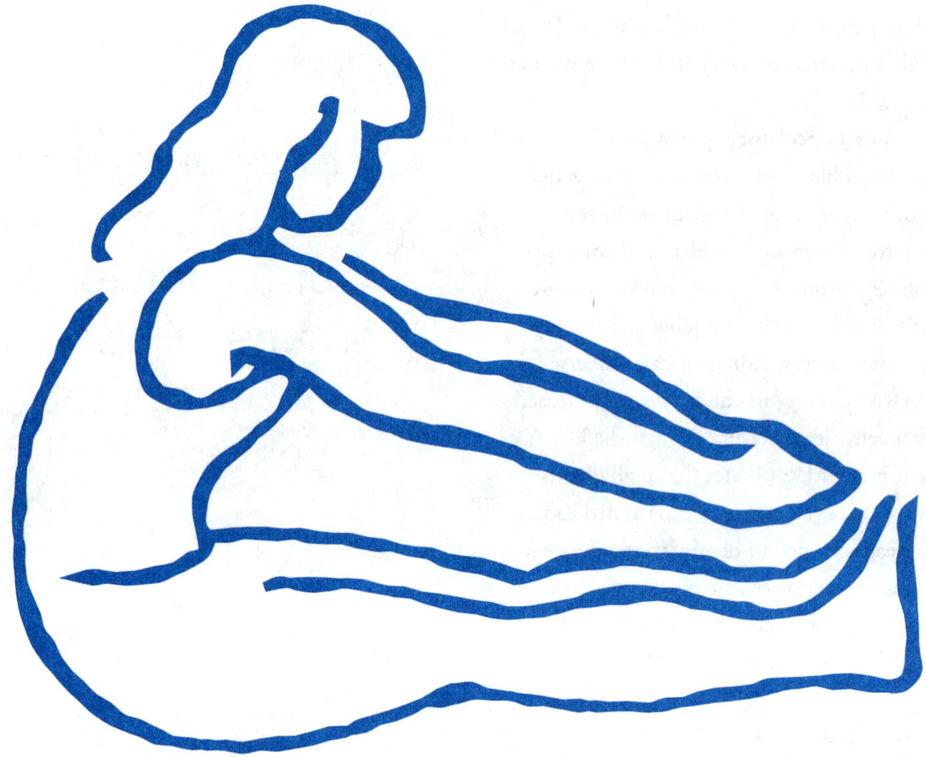

Flexibility is also important in reducing muscle soreness after vigorous physical exertion.

We will discuss how to develop a good muscular endurance program in chapter 7.

Flexibility

The fourth important component of health-related fitness is flexibility, which refers to the range of motion possible at a joint or series of joints. In other words, the ability to stretch your muscles and joints. The degree of flexibility depends on ligaments, tendons, and muscles, and their extensibility. The bony structures of certain joints place limitations on flexibility, however. Extension of the elbow or knee joint is an example of this limitation.

Even though there are joint limitations, most Americans are far from reaching their flexibility potential. This is evident in the number of Americans with lower-back disorders. Loss of flexibility is a common cause of lower-back pain. A study of five thousand patients with back pain revealed that only 20 percent had some underlying structural problem in the muscles of the back of the thigh (hamstring) and lower back such as damaged vertebrae, herniated disc, or arthritis. The remaining 80 percent were diagnosed as being caused by inelastic or weak muscles. The need to develop both flexibility and strength to prevent lower back problems is obvious.

Flexibility is also important in reducing muscle soreness after vigorous physical exertion, whether work or exercise. Flexibility helps reduce the chance of incurring torn ligaments or pulled muscles during activity. In summary, individuals with good flexibility have less postural deviations, less stiffness and soreness of muscles, better skill proficiency, and less chance of injury during movement. A flexibility program is described in chapter 8.

Many Christians in American present an example of poor physical fitness. They are rundown and somewhat pudgy. They eat erratically a grossly unbalanced diet. Some pollute their body's ventilating system with poisonous gases; some drink alcohol; and many sit before the TV 10 to 15 times longer then they spend exercising their bodies.

Are you described in the above paragraph? If so, maybe you have something missing in your life that keeps you from living up to your potential. Being physically fit plays an intrinsic part in developing into the whole person.

[CHAPTER 5]

Developing Cardiovascular Respiratory Fitness

Probably no other component of physical fitness is more important in improving the health and well-being of God's temple than cardiovascular-respiratory (CVR) endurance. CVR endurance means becoming fit in the heart, blood, blood vessels, and lungs. Obtaining fitness in these areas reduces the probability of having a cardiovascular disease such as heart attack, high blood pressure, or stroke. Let's look at the health benefits from developing cardiovascular fitness.

Health Benefits of CVR Fitness

Effects on the Heart

One of the most beneficial long-term effects is an increase in the size and strength of the heart muscle (myocardium) and a high-stroke volume (amount of blood pumped per beat) at all levels of activity. With increased stroke volume, the heart does not have to pump as fast in order to supply the body with a given amount of blood for a particular level of activity. The slower heart rate at all levels of activity, resting and during heavy work, allows the heart more rest between contractions. This slow heart rate is evident in well-trained individuals. Studies done on American Olympic track athletes revealed a resting heart rate in the lower 30s per minute, much slower than for the average American (72 beats per minute for males; 80 beats per minute for females). Simple calculations reveal how much more efficient the heart of a well-trained individual is compared with the average person:

70 beats/minute average American
-40 beats/minute well trained
30 less beats per minute
x 60 minutes in hour
1,800 beats less in one hour
x 24 hours in day
43,000 less beats in one day
x 365 days in year
15,768,000 million beats less in one year

The only time the heart rests is between contractions. From these calculations we can determine that a well-trained heart will rest approximately three months longer than an unconditioned heart in a year's time.

In the well-conditioned individual, the heart rate also

responds more quickly to various workloads and recovers faster to its normal rate. Because of its ability to supply an adequate amount of blood at a lower heart rate, the heart is able to tolerate greater workloads before reaching its maximum rate. For the average person, this can provide a reserve capacity to cope with sudden physical or emotional stresses that accelerate the heart rate. In a well-trained individual, a substantial amount of vigorous activity over a relatively long period of time is required to raise the heart rate to its maximum. For example, let us imagine that Alberto Salizar (former world record holder in the marathon) agreed to run an eight-minute mile with Mr. Average American. If we monitored each person's heart rate during and after the mile run, it would probably reveal that Salizar's heart rate during the run reached approximately 140 beats per minute, whereas the heart rate of Mr. Average American (if he finished) approached 200 beats per minute. Both did the same amount of work (ran an eight-minute mile), but the stress of running had different effects on their hearts. Also, probably within five minutes after the mile run, Salizar's heart rate would recover to its normal resting rate, whereas Mr. Average American's heart rate probably would recover in an hour or more.

> Numerous studies have shown that residual levels of cholesterol and other fatty lipids (such as triglycerides) in the blood can be significantly reduced with vigorous exercise.

Other long-term effects on the heart rate include an increase in the size and elasticity of the coronary arteries and an increase in the size and number of functioning capillaries. Latent ones are opened, and new ones are formed. This increased size of the coronary arteries provides greater blood flow under less resistance and can prevent or delay the closing of these arteries caused by accumulation of fatty deposits on the lining. The greater size and number of capillaries provide the heart with more nourishment and with a better distribution of oxygen for its energy needs, thereby increasing efficiency. They also allow for easier removal of waste products and delay the fatigue that waste-product buildup can cause. To illustrate these findings, an autopsy performed on Clarence De Mar (a distance runner who averaged running nearly 12 miles a day for 50 years), revealed that his coronary arteries were clear of fatty buildup (atherosclerosis) and that his heart muscle did not show any signs of fibrosis (development of scar tissue from lack of circulation) even though he was 70 years old at his death from cancer.

By increasing the capillary beds, regular exercise also develops collateral circulation in the heart. Collateral circulation refers to connection between arteries and veins of the same diameter and between larger and smaller vessels. This is important in continuing or reestablishing circulation when a main vessel is closed off. An autopsy performed on astronaut Ed White (who burned to death in a cabin explosion during a test) showed a complete closing of one major coronary artery from atherosclerosis. Yet, because of a large buildup of collateral circulation, White had been able to function at a high level of physical efficiency.

Effects on the Vascular System

Exercise causes the size and elasticity of the arteries to increase throughout the body as do the size and number of capillaries in the various tissues. Collateral circulation between all major arteries increases, and there is better diffusion between the capillaries and the working tissues. Improved blood flow takes an additional load off the heart. The enlargement and increase in the number of blood vessels decreases resistance to blood flow and lowers an abnormally high blood pressure. The effect also helps blood pressure to return to normal faster following an increase from any cause. By increasing the size and helping to maintain elasticity of the large arteries, hardening of the arteries can be prevented or delayed.

Effects on the Blood

Red blood cells are significantly increased through regular exercise. Studies comparing well-trained with untrained individuals have shown that well-trained individuals have between seven and eight million red blood cells per cubic millimeter of blood, whereas untrained individuals have between five and six million. Because red blood cells combine with oxygen, the well-trained individual is better able to transport more oxygen to the starved cells. Greater oxygen flow to brain cells makes a person think and feel better.

Two other beneficial effects relate to the formation of blood clots and the level of fatty acids in the blood. Exercise affects the clotting time of blood in two ways: The blood coagulates more quickly when it leaves the vascular system, such as from a cut; and the blood plasma activity increases, which breaks up blood clots forming within the blood vessel. This lessens the chance of a blood clot forming in the heart, brain, or other vital organs.

Numerous studies have shown that residual levels of cholesterol and other fatty lipids (such as triglycerides) in the blood can be significantly reduced with vigorous exercise. Reducing cholesterol and triglycerides significantly reduces your chance of atherosclerosis. Vigorous exercise also increases high-density lipoprotein (HDL), which reduces atherosclerosis.

The beneficial effects of regular exercise demonstrate why the incidence of cardiovascular disease has consistently been lower in physically active people than in those who lead more sedentary lives. The effects also explain why an increasing number of doctors are prescribing exercise for patients showing signs of degenerative cardiovascular disease and even patients who are recovering from certain types of heart attacks.

How to Develop Cardiovascular Respiratory Fitness

After realizing the need and understanding the benefits of CVR fitness, the question arises, How can a person develop CVR fitness? Let's look at the intensity, duration, and frequency of exercise.

Intensity

Intensity refers to how stressful an exercise is to the CVR system. Beginners often ask how hard they must exercise in order to develop a training benefit. They want to know at what point in their training they will begin to notice the desirable attributes that accompany CVR conditioning. Everyone wants to know how fast to walk, jog, swim, or exercise for the body to get stronger and improve its health. Actually, I believe they want to know what is the least they have to exercise in order to obtain CVR fitness.

The intensity threshold is directly related to one's present level of CVR condition. This means, the more fit one is, the higher the intensity level must be to improve CVR conditioning. Conversely, the less fit one is, the lower the intensity level has to be to improve CVR condition. The best way to measure this intensity threshold is through determining one's maximum oxygen uptake. This procedure requires the use of specially designed equipment operated by an exercise physiologist. Most individuals do not have the time or money to go through this procedure. Fortunately, exercise physiologists have devised a simpler but less accurate manner in which to determine one's threshold intensity. This procedure does give one a fairly accurate ballpark estimation.

This procedure requires the knowledge of taking one's pulse rate. Use the following formula to determine how fast the heart should beat while exercising in order to produce a training benefit. Examples of persons 20 and 40 years of age with a resting heart rate of 60 beats per minute are used.

20-Year-Old Man		40-Year-Old Man
220		220
-20	age	-40
200	maximum heart rate	180
-60	resting heart rate	-60
140		120
x.70	(threshold intensity)	x.70
98.00		84.00
+60	resting heart rate	+60
158	desired working heart rate	144

Thus a 20 year-old person experienced at exercising with a resting heart rate of 60 must train at 158 heartbeats per minute to receive a training benefit. When the heart rate reaches this threshold level, then the body's physiological functions will become more efficient, the heart will beat more slowly while at rest, blood pressure will achieve normalcy, cholesterol and triglycerides will be utilized for energy, and atherosclerosis will be delayed.

To determine your maximal heart rate, subtract your age from 220. Determine your resting heart rate by first sitting down for fifteen minutes of quiet rest or take it when you first wake up in the morning. At the end of this rest period, count your pulse for one minute. Subtract your resting heart rate from your maximum heart rate. Multiply this difference by 70 percent if you have been exercising consistently. If you have not exercised in months then multiply this difference by 60 percent. Also if you are over 50 years of age, use the 60 percent intensity level, especially if you were inactive in your earlier years. Now add your resting heart rate to get the working heart rate. This is the rate at which you should train.

Ways of exercising to elevate the heartbeat to a desirable threshold intensity include walking briskly, jogging, swimming, bicycle riding, or playing a vigorous game such as tennis or racquetball. To determine the desired intensity or rate of your heartbeat, record your pulse beat immediately after exercising for four or five minutes. If your heart rate is below the desired rate, then speed up your method of exercise. You may need to walk or jog a little faster to cause your heart rate to rise with increased intensity until it reaches a steady state (a condition in which the heart rate can supply enough oxygen to the muscles so they can create enough energy to do the exercise work without an increase in heart rate). If your heart rate is higher than the threshold intensity, you may want to slow down your exercise pace. Slowing down is unnecessary if you desire to increase your CVR fitness. Remember, the higher the intensity, the greater the increase in CVR endurance.

Before beginning a cardiovascular training program, heed

The key to safe exercising is to develop consistency.

these precautions. If you are just beginning an exercise program, or if you have not exercised within the past four weeks, start the program below the suggested threshold rate of 70 or 60 percent. Depending on age and present physical condition, it is advisable to begin at the 40 percent intensity level. Substituting the 40 percent intensity level in the 40-year-old person's example reveals the threshold intensity heart rate to be 108 beats per minute. Slowly allow the CVR system to build itself up to handle the more vigorous stress. Beginning at a low intensity level also helps the muscles, tendons, and ligaments build up their strength to handle the stress of exercise. This alleviates pulled or strained muscles that could occur in exercising. Do not try to do too much in a short time; go slowly and gradually increase your intensity level. You have the rest of your life to obtain your optimum fitness level.

Duration

The duration of an exercise session is important in improving the cardiovascular functions in the body. Recommended times vary from 5 to 30 minutes. From personal experience and research, my conclusion is that the duration of an exercise session should be proportionate to your present level of cardiovascular fitness. If you are highly fit, you should exercise longer. This longer duration increases your cardiovascular fitness to your optimum level. Conversely, if your fitness is low, you should exercise for a shorter period of time or until you are able to slowly, progressively increase your time. As you get stronger, you can safely increase your duration without unduly stressing your cardiovascular system. Research done on duration and its effect on HDL development revealed a significant increase when an exercise session exceeded 30 minutes. Depending on your present fitness level, try to exercise for approximately 30 minutes at your heart rate threshold level.

Frequency

Determining the necessary frequency of exercise is also important. Some of the fitness literature claims that exercising one day each week is ideal in obtaining the optimum level of CVR fitness. In my opinion, if you acquire the urge to exercise once or twice a week, you should go and lie down until that urge passes. It is more harmful to exercise once or twice a week than not to exercise at all. Infrequent exercising can cause stress to the CVR system, which is incapable of handling the severe increase in heart rate, blood pressure, oxygen intake, and respiration that occurs from vigorous exercise.

The key to safe exercising is to develop consistency. Make an effort to exercise at least three times a week, preferably four to six times. Find a specific time of day for exercising (preferably after your working hours) and stick to it. Guard this precious time from any outside interference. Avoid gaps of more than 48 hours between exercise sessions. Research has shown that circulating blood levels of triglyceride and cholesterol, even though reduced by exercise, return to higher levels within 48 hours unless exercise is repeated.

The type of exercise used in these training sessions is relatively unimportant as long as the receding criteria are met. Walking, jogging, skiing, bicycling, swimming, rope skipping, aerobic dancing, roller skating, rowing, and stair climbing are all excellent. Various sport activities that require running also can be beneficial—basketball, racquetball, handball, tennis, and badminton. Variety will keep your interest in the exercise program. Jogging, swimming, skiing, aerobic dancing, and bicycling are perhaps the best all-around activities for CVR conditioning because they require a high percentage of aerobic energy output. Participation in a sport may take longer to gain the same CVR training effects but is satisfactory if that is your choice.

How to Evaluate Your Present Level of CVR Fitness

Before beginning a CVR training program, your present physical condition should be assessed in comparison to established standards of fitness. This will help you to plan the type of program you need. You may even want to repeat this assessment at periodic intervals to chart progress.The best measurement of CVR fitness is maximum oxygen consumption. This is the maximum amount of oxygen the body can consume while working at its higher level of intensity. The body takes oxygen and changes it into energy called *adenosine triphosphate* (ATP). This means a fit person can do more work than an unfit person because of the extra energy created.

Accurate measurement of maximum oxygen consumption requires time-consuming laboratory procedures done by specialists in exercise physiology. Fortunately, valid short-cuts for determining CVR fitness level have been devised. The Cooper one and one-half mile run-walk test and the mile-walk test are probably the simplest to take while providing an accurate measurement of maximum oxygen uptake.

Cooper's One and One-Half Mile Run Test

To evaluate your CVR fitness, run or walk a flat, accurately measured distance of one and one-half miles as fast as possible and record your time with an accurate watch to the nearest second. Compare your fitness with others in your age group (table 5.1).

The one and a half mile test gives a fairly accurate determination of CVR fitness despite some error of determination due to individual differences and motivation to do one's best. All Christians should strive to obtain the excellent to superior rating which would improve their health benefits and show honor to God with their bodies.

Table 5.1 — 1 ½ Mile Test for Men and Women

Fitness Category	13-19		20-29		30-39		40-49		50-59		60+	
	Men	Women	Men	Women	Men	Women	Men	Women	Men	Women	Men	Women
Very Poor	15:31+ (min.)	18:31+	16:01+	19:01+	16:31+	19:31+	17:31+	20:01+	19:01+	20:31+	20:01+	21:01+
O_2 Uptake ML/Kg/min.	<35.0	<25.0	<33.0	<23.6	<31.5	<22.8	<30.2	<21.0	<26.1	<20.2	<20.5	<17.5
Poor	12:11-15:30 (min.)	16:55-18:30	14:01-16:00	18:31-19:00	14:44-16:30	19:01-19:30	15:36-17:30	19:31-20:00	17:01-19:00	20:01-20:30	19:01-20:00	20:31-21:00
O_2 Uptake ML/Kg/min.	35.0-38.3	25.0-30.9	33.0-36.4	23.6-28.9	31.5-35.4	22.8-26.9	30.2-33.5	21.0-24.4	26.1-30.9	20.2-22.7	20.5-26.0	17.52-20.1
Fair	10:49-12:10 (min.)	14:31-16.54	12:01-14:00	15:55-18:30	12:31-14:45	16:31-19:00	13:01-15:35	17:31-19:30	14:31-17:00	19:01-20:00	16:16-19:00	19:31-20:30
O_2 Uptake ML/Kg/min.	38.4-45.1	31.0-34.9	36.5-42.4	29.0-32.9	35.4-40.9	27.0-31.4	33.6-38.9	24.5-28.9	31.0-35.7	22.8-26.9	26.1-32.2	20.2-24.4
Good	9:41-10:48 (min.)	12:30-14:30	10:46-12:00	13:31-15:54	11:01-12:30	14:31-16:30	11:31-13:00	15:56-17:30	12:31-14:30	16:31-19:00	14:00-16:15	17:31-19:30
O_2 Uptake ML/Kg/min.	45.2-50.9	35.0-38.9	42.5-46.4	33.0-36.9	41.0-44.9	31.5-35.6	39.0-43.7	29.0-32.8	35.8-40.9	27.0-31.4	32.2-36.4	24.5-30.2
Excellent	8:37-9:40 (min.)	11:50-12:29	9:45-10:45	12:30-13:30	10:00-11:00	13:00-14:30	10:30-11:30	13:45-15:55	11:00-12:30	14:30-16:30	11:14-13:59	16:30-17:30
O_2 Uptake ML/Kg/min.	51.0-55.9	39.0-41.9	46.5-52.4	37.0-40.9	45.0-49.4	35.7-40.0	43.8-48.0	32.9-36.9	41.0-45.3	31.5-35.7	36.5-44.2	30.3-31.4
Superior	<8:37 (min.)	<11:50	<9:45	<12:30	<10:00	<13:00	<10:30	<13:45	<11:00	<14:30	<11:15	<16:30
O_2 Uptake ML/Kg/min.	>56.0	>42.0	>52.5	>41.0	>49.5	>40.1	>48.1	>37.0	>45.4	>35.8	>44.3	>31.5

Guidelines for CVR Training

Probably the worst thing you can do to begin your CVR program is grab your old tennis shoes, head for the nearest track, and run at top speed around the track. That could cause more harm than good. You must prepare yourself physically before you rush into cardiovascular exercise, or someone may have to rush you to the hospital. Follow these guidelines, and protect yourself from harm and injury.

Get a medical examination, especially if you are over 35 years of age.—The medical examination should consist of a standard stress electrocardiogram (ECG); resting and exercise blood pressure measurements; fasting blood sugar (glucose), cholesterol, triglyceride, and high-density and low-density lipoprotein determinations; and evaluation of any orthopedic problem.

Warm up before exercising.—Before beginning a CVR training program, subject your total body to a proper warm-up. The warm-up is a precaution against unnecessary injuries and muscle soreness. It stimulates the heart and lungs moderately and progressively as well as increases the blood flow and the blood and muscle temperatures gradually. It also prepares you mentally for the approaching strenuous workout.

The following five-minute warm-up routine is recommended. During the first two minutes, do stretching exercises for arms, legs, and back (figs. 5.5—5.7). During the third and fourth minutes, do sit-ups, push-ups, and back raisers (figs. 5.8—5.11). During the final minute, walk or jog slowly. Strive to walk or jog flat-footed as much as possible during the warm-up. This gives the tendons and ligaments in the feet and ankles a chance to stretch gradually, helping to avoid possible irritation from sudden stress.

The time required for warmup varies with each individual. Sweat indicates that the core temperature has increased and more intense conditioning can be done. Keep in mind that cold weather requires longer warmup times.

Cool down after exercising.—Cool-down is a tapering-off period after completion of the main workout and is as important to the body as the warm-up. During the CVR exercise, the large muscles of the legs provide a boost to the circulating blood and help return it to the heart and lungs where the exchange of oxygen and carbon dioxide takes place. As the muscles relax after exertion, blood fills the veins. It is not allowed to flow backward because of the valves in the veins. During exercise the squeezing action of the leg muscles provides about half of the pumping action, while the heart provides the other half. Walking or slow jogging, as in the cool-down, allows the muscle pump to continue to work until the total volume of blood being pumped is decreased to where the heart can handle it without help from the muscles.

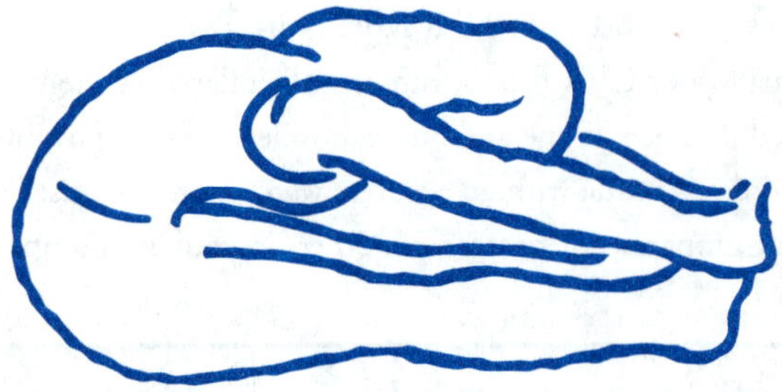

FIG. 5.5
Touch toes; keep legs straight; hold on for eight seconds.

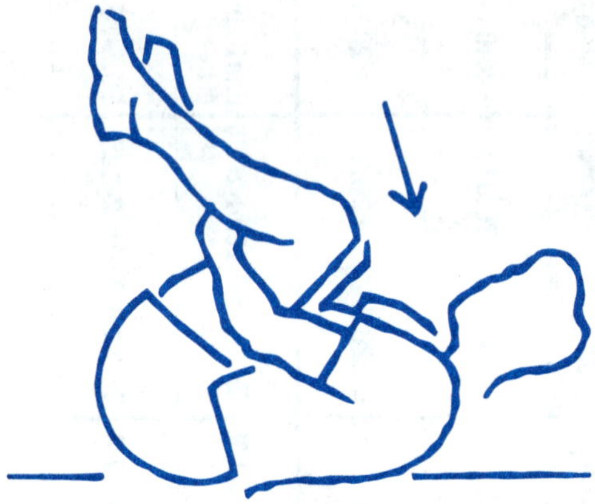

FIG. 5.6
Pull knees to chest.

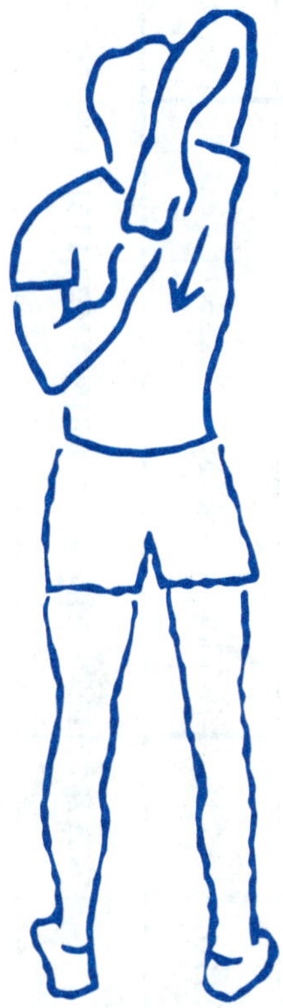

FIG. 5.7
Lower shoulder muscles: Grasp hands behind back; you may need to grasp a towel if unable to grasp hands.

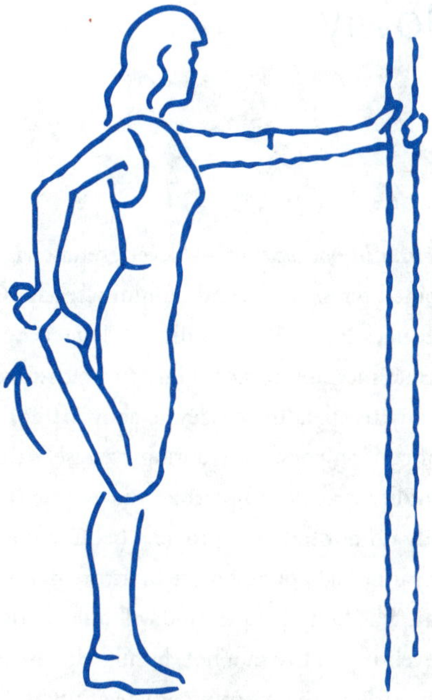

FIG. 5.8
Stand straight; pull heel as close to buttocks as possible.

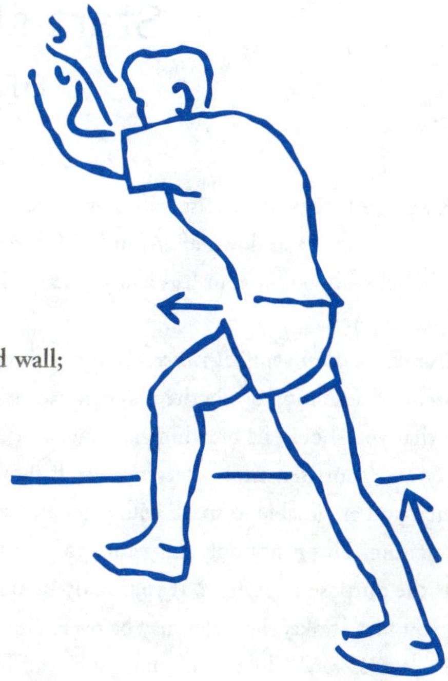

FIG. 5.9
Calf muscles:
Keep heel on floor:
move buttocks toward wall;
exercise both calves.

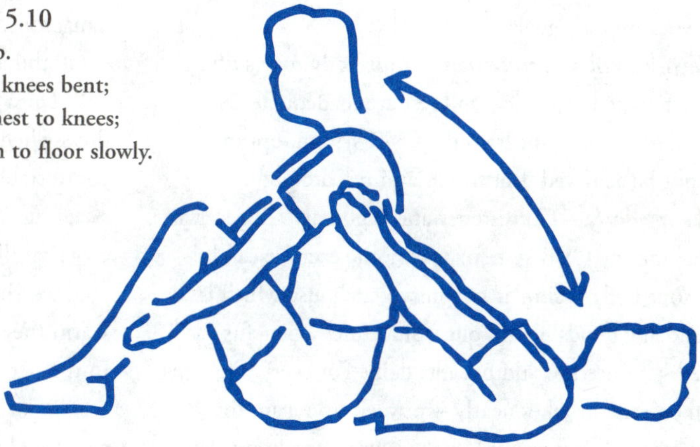

FIG. 5.10
Sit-up.
Keep knees bent;
lift chest to knees;
return to floor slowly.

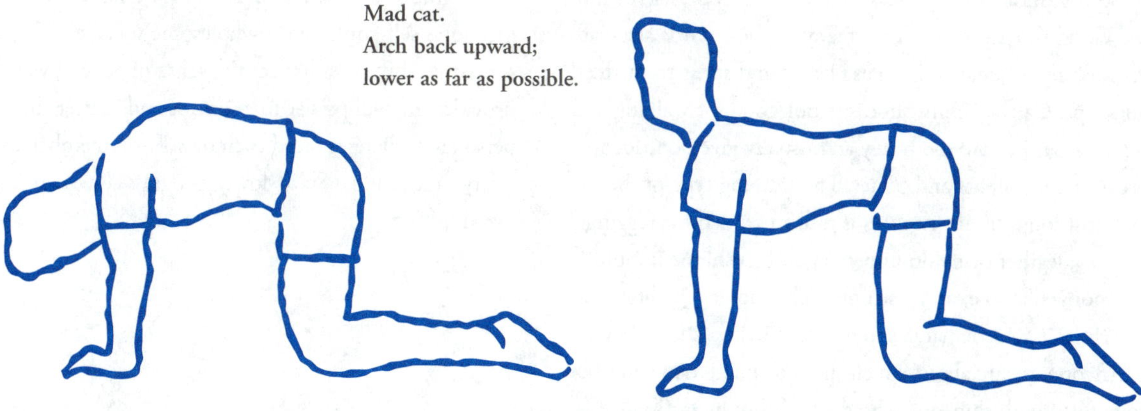

FIG. 5.11
Mad cat.
Arch back upward;
lower as far as possible.

Start slowly, progress slowly, and do not overdo.

Always reduce your exercise pace slowly, never abruptly. Do not stop instantly or sit down after you finish vigorous exercise or the blood will pool in your legs and you can faint from lack of blood to the brain.

Exercise within your tolerance.—Do not push yourself to the extent of becoming overly tired. When exercising, a general rule is that you should be breathing at a rate which allows you to carry on a short-sentenced conversation. It should not be at a level that you are unable to speak with someone with whom you are exercising. This is not only dangerous to your health but also defeats the purpose of exercise. If your body does not feel strong when you first awake, then you may be overtraining.

Progress slowly.—In exercise, hurrying your fitness development does not work; it merely invites trouble, such as muscle and joint injuries. You do not have to be first in everything you do. Take your time in your development of fitness. Gradually work up to your exercise goals.

Get adequate rest and nutrition.—Your body may suffer from chronic fatigue if nutrition and rest are inadequate. No matter how hard or long you train the CVR system, optimal results will not be achieved if nutrition and rest are poor.

Exercise regularly.—Consistency and regularity are necessary for strengthening the CVR system. Spasmodic exercise can be dangerous. Your body is similar to a busy warehouse which is constantly moving goods in and out. Your exercise benefits cannot be stored; you need to add benefits daily. For every one week you cease to exercise, it takes nearly two weeks to regain the previous fitness level. Just as food intake is used up almost daily, so are the benefits of exercise unless they are replenished with more exercise.

Wear proper shoes.—A faulty pair of exercise shoes can erase your good intentions to exercise as well as cause foot, leg, or hip injuries. Good shoes can eliminate many of the hazards associated with walking or jogging, such as blisters and stress to the feet, legs, and hips. Canvas tennis shoes are not good for walking and jogging because they are too heavy and usually give poor foot support to the ligaments and bones. The training type of shoe used by most long-distant runners is recommended for jogging. These have a leather or nylon upper; a good, cushioned, multi-layered, spongelike sole; and a strong heel counter. Quality is the key here. Exercise participants should buy the best shoes they can afford. Anyone unsure about which shoes to purchase would be wise to consult with someone who does a lot of long-distance running.

Exercise cautiously in hot weather.—Never exercise vigorously when a combined temperature and humidity reach 165 or above (that is, 85 degrees F and 80% humidity). Exercising over this recommended rate increases susceptibility to heat stroke. Never allow your body temperature to elevate above 105° F. The best method of cooling your body during exercise is through evaporation. If humidity is above 80 percent, the evaporative processes of the body do not function properly because the humid atmosphere cannot accept any more moisture that would come from the body. The body temperature will quickly rise above the danger level. If you live in a hot, humid climate, you may have to exercise early in the morning or late at night. Wear clothes that allow your body to cool itself by evaporation. Never wear a sweatsuit or rubberized suit that promotes sweating. Do not try to lose weight by sweating it off. Not only is this dangerous, but you will also gain the weight back when you drink fluids.

Dress appropriately in cold conditions.—Most people overdress when they exercise in cold temperatures. Dress to feel comfortably warm during the exercise period without profuse sweating. Usually one or two layers of light clothing, a knit cap covering the head and ears, and knit gloves are sufficient. In very cold weather, a ski mask can be worn to protect the face and warm the air as it goes into the lungs. Always run with the wind in the latter stage of your exercise. The chill factor is increased when you run into the wind. If you run against the wind after sweating has increased, the chilling effects of the wind will be magnified.

Regular, systemic CVR exercise is an important key to a happy life, as it promotes physical, mental, psychological, and social fitness. It provides an outlet for emotional tensions and promotes self-confidence, wholesome social activity, and good sportsmanship. It enhances the sense of general well-being that provides the will power to confront and master the difficult personal challenges faced each day. But remember to heed these safety precautions: Start slowly, progress slowly, and do not overdo.

[CHAPTER 6]

IMPROVING BODY COMPOSITION

In the good old days, before progress lured us off the farm and made us affluent and fat, we had strong muscles and simple diets. When the cow was in the barn and the manure on the fields, the meat was pure and the vegetables organic. Before the advent of giant agribusiness, wheat was rich enough to make bread the staff of life. The protein content of bread was 18 to 20 percent in 1886, whereas it was 9 to 12 percent in 1995. In those days we were poor in things; and food distribution, processing, and preserving were not all they could be. But the 45 percent of the American population who lived and ate on the farms were well furnished with natural vitamins and minerals.

Affluence turned our diet rich and our bodies soft. By the 1990s the average American was annually consuming 130 pounds of fat, 250 pounds of meat and poultry, 120 pounds of refined and processed sugars, and 485 twelve-ounce bottles or cans of soda per year. The Standard American Diet (SAD) has become increasingly dominated by highly refined carbohydrates and fast foods. Only 20 percent of our calories (compared to 40% in 1900) comes from fresh fruit, vegetables, and whole grains. Because most of our food is raised with the aid of chemical fertilizers and pesticides, we ingest an unknown quantity of poisons, in addition to a smorgasbord of perhaps as many as 1,800 chemicals (which averages out to five pounds in a year's time) that are routinely added to processed food to color, preserve, and flavor.

Unfortunately, nutrition doesn't sell. "All people want is Coke™ and potato chips," are the words of biochemist Arthur Odell, former director of special projects, General Mills research division.

Americans are now seeing the results of improper nutrition. Forty percent of Americans are overweight, and 18 percent of North American men and 28 percent of North American women are obese. One out of 10 Americans is more than one hundred pounds overweight. Americans outweigh every country in the world in excess fat.

Among children, the incidence of obesity is reported to be about 15 percent. At one year of age, infants are now 50 percent heavier than they were a generation ago. However, the reported weight gain among women between pregnancies appears to be no higher than that among nonpregnant women of the same age.

Who Is Fat?

Because obesity has been defined as a condition in which there is an excess of body fat, its diagnosis must depend on methods of estimating body fat. Possibly the simplest test for fatness is to stand naked in front of a mirror and closely examine your body. If you look fat, then you are fat. Another simple way is to compare your height and weight to norms set up by insurance companies (see table 6.1). These charts are not always reliable, however; for these tables have been devised on desirable weights, not actual weights. These desirable weights are derived from people showing the lowest mortality rates, and such individuals happen to be below the average weight. Another weakness in these charts can be shown by the example of the fat-determination studies done on the Dallas Cowboy football team. Running back Herschel Walker was determined to have 2 percent body fat, which is classified as excellent; yet the height-weight tables revealed that he was 20 pounds overweight. Strong individuals with much muscle development can appear fatter

Table 6.1
BODY MASS INDEX (BMI)

HEIGHT	19	20	21	22	23	24	25	26	27	28	29	30	35	40
	WEIGHT (POUNDS)													
4'10"	91	96	100	105	110	115	119	124	129	134	138	143	167	191
4'11"	94	99	104	109	114	119	124	128	133	138	143	148	173	198
5'0"	97	102	107	112	118	123	128	133	138	143	148	153	179	204
5'1"	100	106	111	116	122	127	132	137	143	148	153	158	185	211
5'2"	104	109	115	120	126	131	136	142	147	153	158	164	191	218
5'3"	107	113	118	124	130	135	141	146	152	158	163	169	197	225
5'4"	110	116	122	128	134	140	145	151	157	163	169	174	204	232
5'5"	114	120	126	132	138	144	150	156	162	168	174	180	210	240
5'6"	118	124	130	136	142	148	155	161	167	173	179	186	216	247
5'7"	121	127	134	140	146	153	159	166	172	178	185	191	223	255
5'8"	125	131	138	144	151	158	164	171	177	184	190	197	230	262
5'9"	128	135	142	149	155	162	169	176	182	189	196	203	236	270
5'10"	132	139	146	153	160	167	174	181	188	195	202	207	243	278
5'11"	136	143	150	157	165	172	179	186	193	200	208	215	250	286
6'0"	140	147	154	162	169	177	184	191	199	206	213	221	258	294
6'1"	144	151	159	166	174	182	189	197	204	212	219	227	265	302
6'2"	148	155	163	171	179	186	194	202	210	218	225	233	272	311
6'3"	152	160	168	176	184	192	200	208	216	224	232	240	279	319
6'4"	156	164	172	180	189	197	205	213	221	230	238	246	287	328
								OVERWEIGHT					OBESE	

Source: World Health Organization

than they actually are. Also, fat people will look at these charts and automatically determine that they have large frames, when they actually may have small frames. Tables 6.1 and 6.2 can help you determine your frame size and true weight.

Frame size is determined from wrist circumference, which should be measured with a tape measure at the smallest point above the two bones which protrude on each side. Pull the tape measure as tight as possible.

Another method of estimating fatness is by measuring the thickness of fatfold with a skinfold caliper. Because much of the body fat is just under the skin and overlaying muscles, the thickness of a pinch of skin and fat can be used as an indicator of total body fatness. Most physical education departments at colleges and church recreation ministers are skilled in determining percentage of body fatness with skinfold measurements. Contact one of these professionals in your area to determine how fat you really are.

Body mass index (BMI) is a convenient way of assessing body composition. BMI is calculated by dividing your weight in Kg by your height in meters squared. You can use that formula or consult table 6.1. Find your height; move across to your weight, then up to your BMI.

Overweight for men is usually considered 15–20 percent body fatness. Obesity for men is body fatness that is greater than 20 percent. Being overweight for women is considered 25–30 percent body fatness. We should strive to keep our total percentage of body fat below 15 percent for men and 20 percent for women. We need to lose that excess body fat that causes spiritual, physical, mental, and emotional havoc to God's temple. Probably the most practical criterion for evaluating fatness is the length of our belt. Remember the longer the belt, the shorter the life (see table 6.3).

The questions: How do I lose weight? and What can I eat? are answered in chapters 10–16.

Table 6.2
Determination of Relative Frame Size of the Human Body
Wrist Circumference

Sex	Small Frame Inches	Medium Frame Inches	Large Frame Inches
Male	6½" or less	6½ – 7½"	7½" or more
Female	5½" or less	5½" – 6"	6" or more

Table 6.3
Fatness Rating Scale

Classification	Men	Women
Very lean	0–10	0–12
Lean	11–14	13–19
Marginal	15–17	20–24
Fat	18–19	25–29
Obese	20 plus	30 plus

[CHAPTER 7]

Developing Strength and Muscular Endurance

"Strengthen the weak hands, and make firm the feeble knees" (Isa. 35:3, RSV). The prophet Isaiah knew the value of a strong body. Yet many Christians, when hearing the term *muscular,* are immediately turned off to exercise. Senior adults think they are going to break a bone or injure themselves if they lift weights. Women think they will become musclebound and lose their femininity. Others don't want to lift weight for fear of becoming so sore that even their hair seems to hurt the day after exercise.

Each of these excuses is invalid if weight training is done properly. Research has shown that muscles will atrophy (degenerate) if they are not constantly used and strengthened. Senior adults should never just sit in a rocking chair, for their muscles will deteriorate along with their mobility. Research now shows that weight training causes electrical activity from the nerves to stimulate the growth and strength of bones. This can help prevent osteoporosis (softening of bones), a prevalent disease among senior adults.

Research has proven that muscular endurance training, if done properly, will not cause bulging muscles in women. In fact, these endurance exercises will actually enhance a woman's appearance. Toning up muscles can reduce the circumference of the upper arms, thighs, and buttocks.

For those who fear soreness, weight training—if done on a gradual progression, with proper warmup and stretching—will not cause severe soreness. The problem that causes the greatest amount of soreness is that individuals try to lift too much, too many times, and too often.

Don't use these excuses about weight training, for many health benefits are received when one has good strength in all six hundred plus muscles. Let us analyze some of the benefits received from strength training.

Postural Defects

One of the most important health benefits from muscular training is the rehabilitation of postural defects. As people age, their muscles weaken from disuse, causing the skeleton system to deviate from its natural alignment. In many instances, shoulders slump and rotate forward, stomach muscles weaken, and the abdomen protrudes outward. Sometimes the pelvis rotates forward, causing severe lower back pain. Also, the muscles in the hips, legs, and feet weaken, causing the skeletal structure to fall

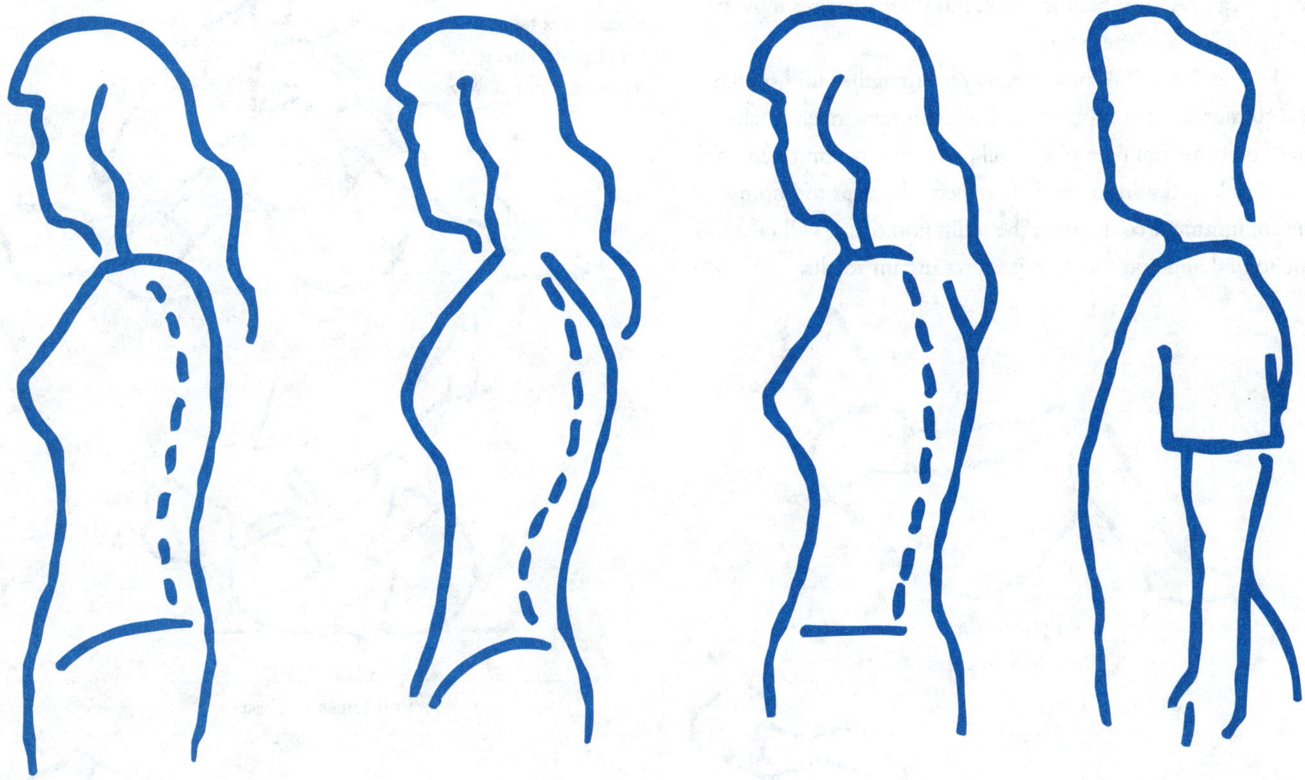

FIG. 7.1
Pelvic positions: (a) normal, (b) downward pelvic tilt, (c) backward pelvic tilt, (d) ptosis and lordosis.

from its natural position, which places pressure on nerves. Therefore, many suffer needlessly from postural deviations that can be prevented through proper muscular exercises. Most postural deviations are caused by weak muscles that are unable to support the skeletal system properly. On the other hand some postural deviations are caused by stronger muscles overpulling weaker muscles. For example, in children (especially young girls 11–14 years old) the muscles on their right side may be stronger than those on the left. This can cause their spine to be pulled to the right side, causing the shifting vertebrae to pinch the spinal nerves. This condition, called *scoliosis,* can lead to paralysis.

Lower-Back Pain

Lower-back pain ranks second to headache as the most common pain in the United States. About 80 percent of the adult population in this country has experienced lower-back pain. And half of these will experience a second episode of back pain.

Lower-back pain has many causes. One textbook lists 103 causes. One medical expert states that 90 percent of all patients with lower-back pain suffer muscular strain or tearing and accompanying ligament and tendon damage. The remaining 10 percent suffer from congenital (present at birth) defects in the spine, infections, arthritis, or disc problems.

A sedentary lifestyle, with help from automated technology, has contributed significantly to lower-back pain. Working at a desk job under the stress and strain of a competitive office situation can cause tension, which causes the muscles to remain contracted, causing discomfort.

Many medical authorities believe that emotions, anxiety, tension, and depression are significant factors in at least 80 percent of back problems. These cause the biological fight-or-flight mechanism to pour adrenaline into the system, and people become tense and strung out with no release. The end result is backache.

Another cause of lower-back pain is being overweight. Tremendous stress is borne by muscles and bones carrying extra pounds. Most fat accumulates around the stomach and pelvis. This extra weight causes the pelvis to rotate forward, thus placing extra stress on the vertebrae of the lower back. This condition is known as lordosis or swayback.

The cure for lower-back pain lies in therapeutic exercise, including stretching and strengthening routines. For the back that aches because of insufficient activity and loss of muscle tone, appropriate exercise may be the cure. In severe cases, including those resulting from acute injury or surgery, muscle-building exercises can restore a painless back. But these exercises must be repeated daily year after year.

Figures 7.2 to 7.8 show exercises to strengthen and stretch the 140 muscles that support the back. But remember, it takes what no doctor can prescribe—will power and commitment. You must decide you want to get better, then take steps to improve. The commitment comes with the realization that it will take time to heal and you should not expect instant results.

FIG. 7.2
Sit-up.
Keep knees bent;
lift chest to knees;
return to floor slowly.

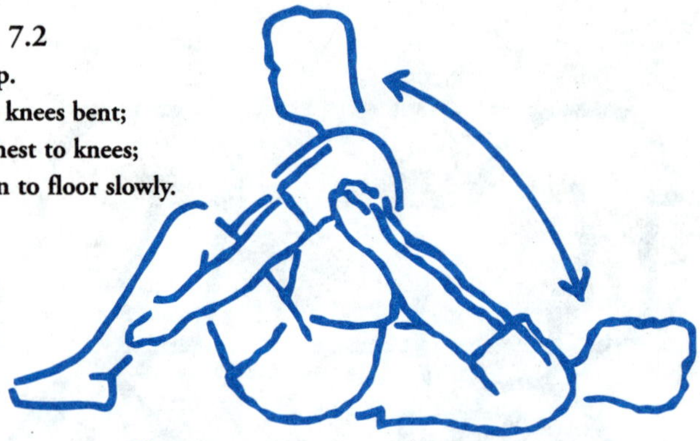

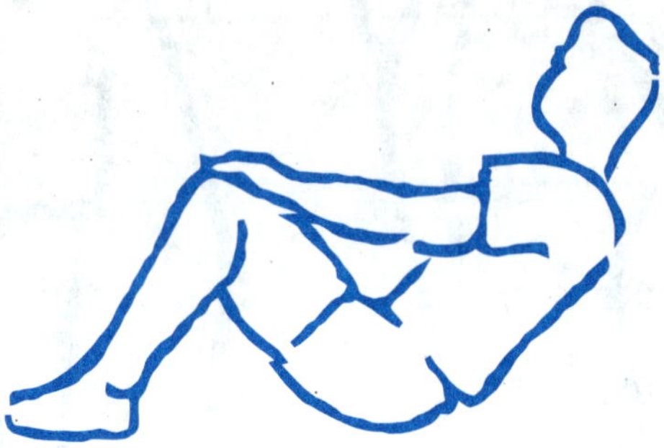

FIG. 7.3.A
Pull chest to knees.

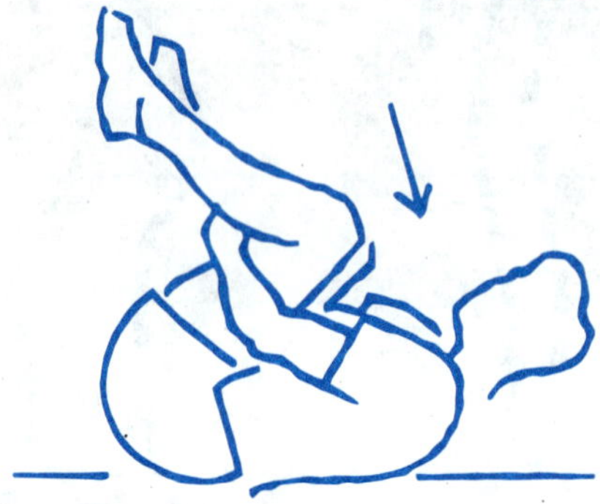

FIG. 7.3B
Pull knees to chest.

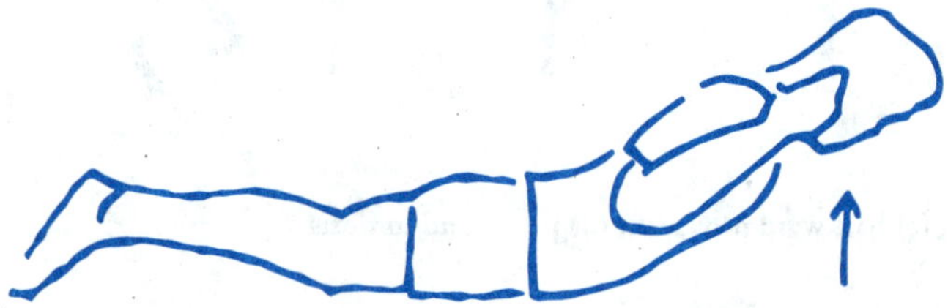

FIG. 7.4
Raise trunk as high as possible; keep feet on floor.

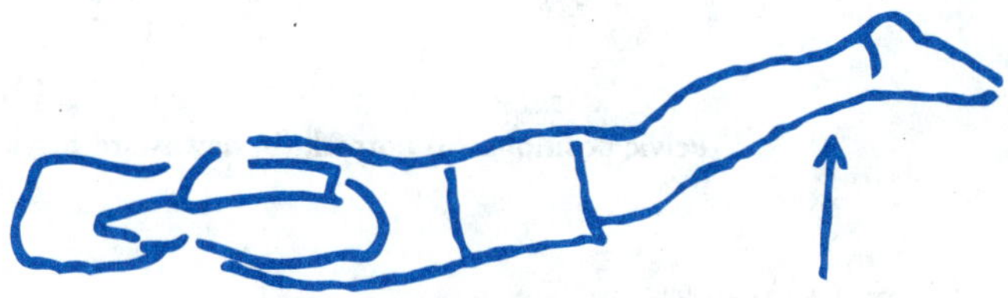

FIG. 7.5
Raise legs as high as possible; keep chin on floor.

FIG. 7.6
Mad cat.
Arch back upward;
lower as far as possible.

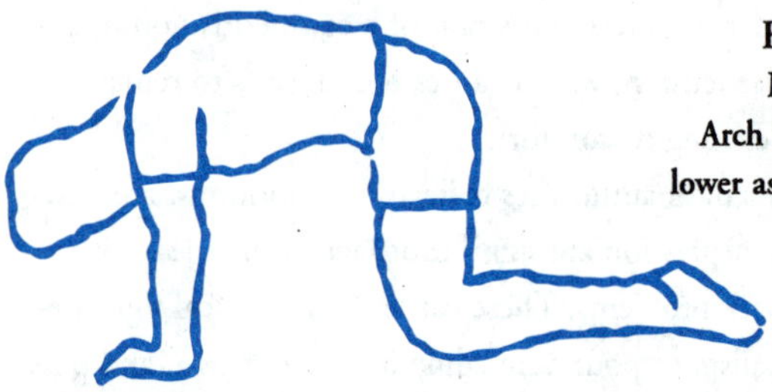

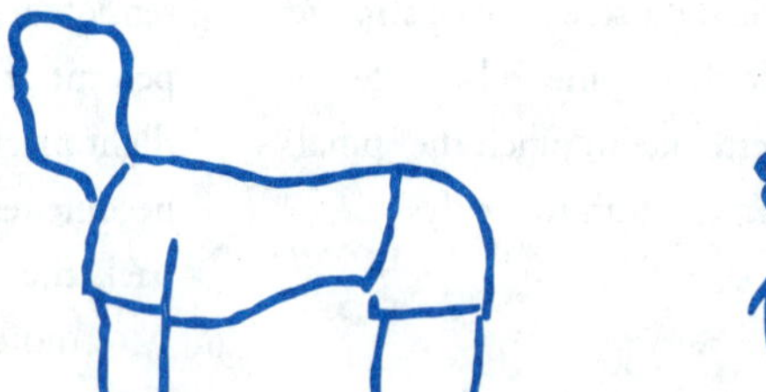

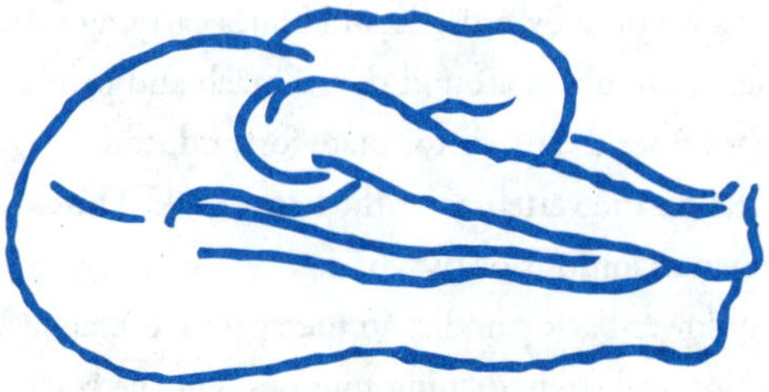

FIG. 7.7
Touch toes; keep legs straight; hold on for eight seconds.

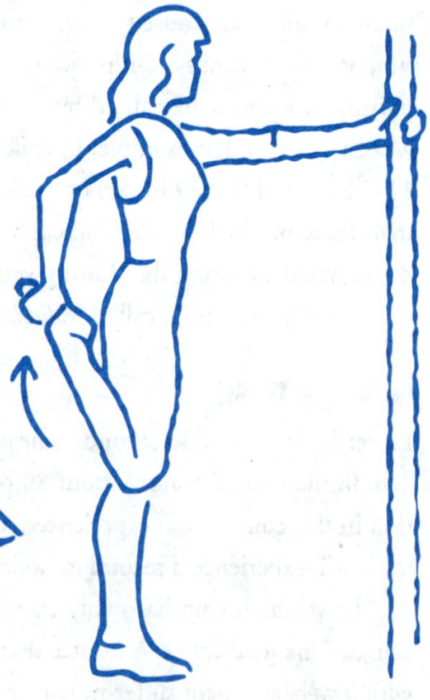

FIG. 7.8
Stand straight; pull heel as close to buttocks as possible.

Neck Joint Disorders

Forward head.—Forward head (fig.7.9) often occurs when the muscles in the back of the neck are stretched and weakened, usually because of habitual malposition of the head. Correcting this condition involves aligning the head properly with the chin tucked so that the lower jaw is basically in line with the ground and the chin is not tipped when the head is drawn back. This requires reorientation of the head and neck so that the individual knows how it feels to hold the head correctly. The head should be held so that the earlobe is in line with the center of the shoulder. The exercises in figures 7.10–7.12 should be beneficial in correcting forward head.

Cervical lordosis.—Cervical lordosis (fig. 7.13) may result from an attempt to compensate for other spinal curves occurring lower in the spinal column. Back neck muscles are often tight and contracted so the head is tilted well back and the chin is tipped upward. As in forward head, reeducation of the antagonistic muscles is necessary so that the lower jaw is held in line with the ground. To correct cervical lordosis and forward head, the proper head position must be learned by exercising in front of a mirror to recognize the correct position. The exercise in figure 7.14 should correct cervical lordosis.

Head tilt or twist.—Looking at the head from the front or back, the head may appear tilted directly to the side and/or with a concomitant twisting of the head and neck (fig. 7.15). In either case, the individual must learn the proper position. Sometimes deviations in the position of the head and neck are compensatory for the postural deviation located below this area. Correction of the head position involves strengthening and shortening the muscles opposite the head tilt, and stretching the muscles toward the head tilt. The exercise in figure 7.16 helps eliminate this deviation.

Many musculoskeletal disorders occur from weakened muscles such as scoliosis, kyphosis (humpback), hip, knee, and foot problems. If you suffer from one of these abnormalities, correction and prevention are discussed in detail in several books.

Developing a Weight-Training Program

A basic weight-training program should strengthen all the major muscle groups in a balanced manner. One should never strengthen one part of the body without strengthening other parts equally. Muscle imbalances can cause postural deviations or joint injuries. A knowledge of the proper lifting and breathing techniques is mandatory in order to improve the strength of God's temple. Proper use of weights will increase not only strength and endurance but also flexibility and power.

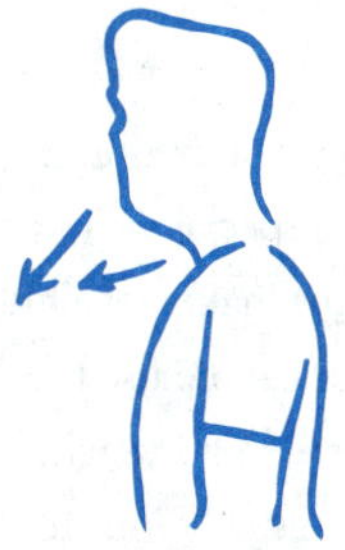

FIG. 7.9
Forward head

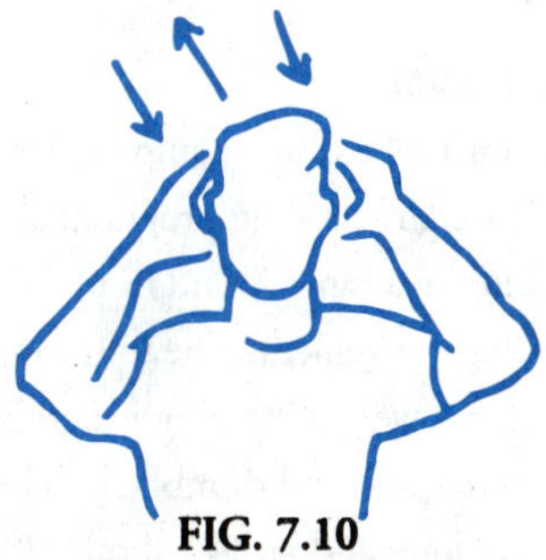

FIG. 7.10
Pull forward with arms; push backward with head.

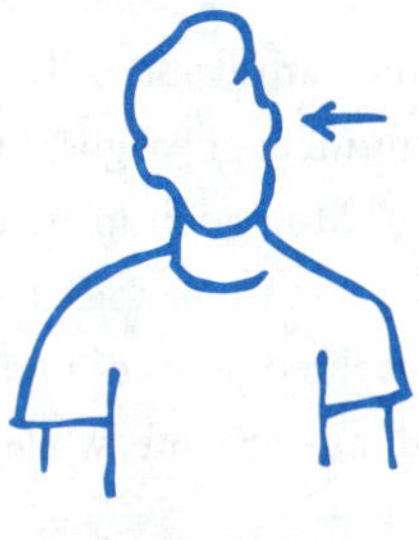

FIG. 7.11
Roll head to side as far as possible.

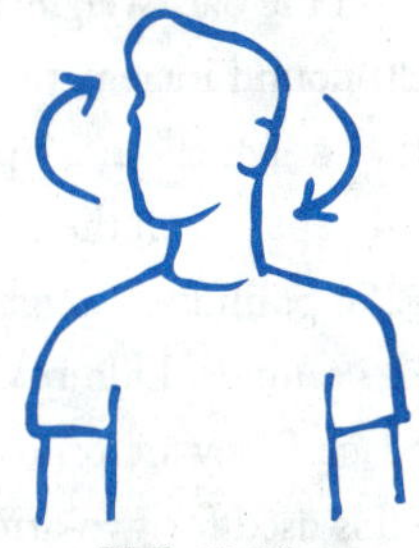

FIG. 7.12
Roll head in all directions.

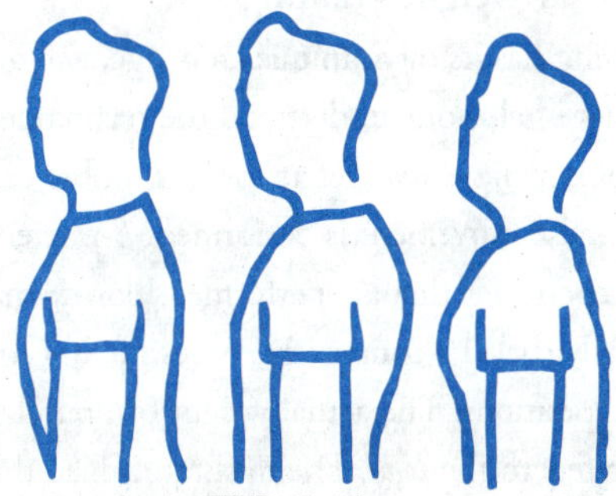

FIG. 7.13
Cervical lordosis. Notice the abnormal curve in back of neck. a. Normal, b. Forward head, c. Cervical Lordosis

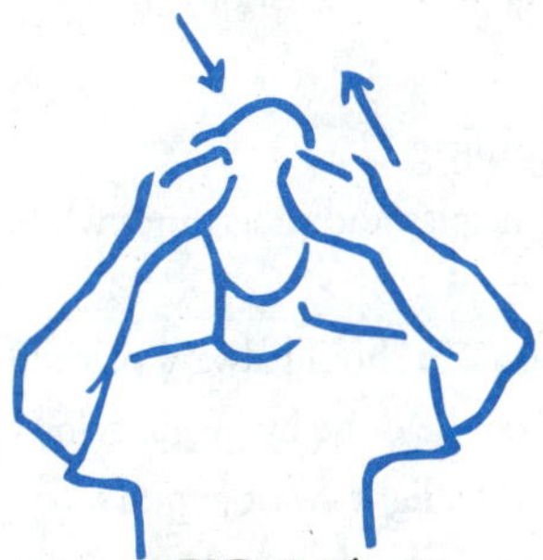

FIG. 7.14
Push backward with arms; push forward with head.

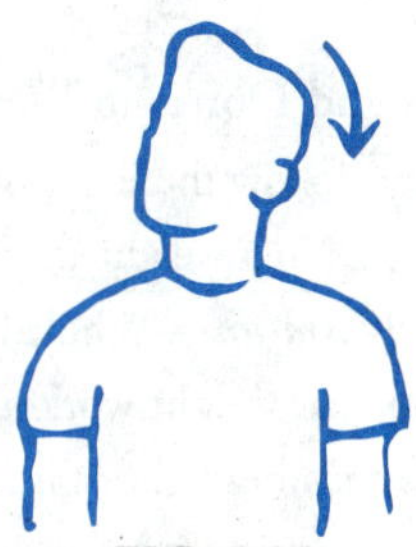

FIG. 7.15
Head tilt

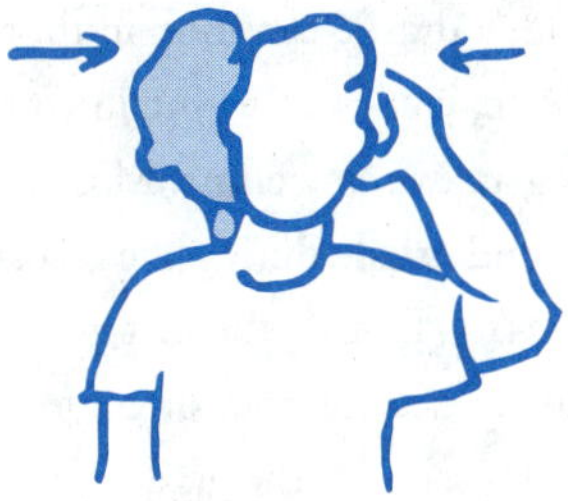

FIG. 7.16
Push sideways with arms; push opposite direction with head.

Equipment

It doesn't take much equipment or money to get started in a good weight-training program, although using special weight-training machines found in private health clubs makes weight-training convenient. The following equipment can be used to develop a weight-training program at home: steel bar, weight plates, collars, and dumbbells. The steel bar is usually four to six feet long and weighs about 20 pounds. It has collars at each end which function as protective locks to secure the weight plates on the bar. Weight plates usually come in 2.5-, 5-, 10-, and 20-pound increments. Normally, the barbell and collars together weigh about 25 pounds. The number of weighted plates needed depends on the type of program. Most adult men need 175–250 pounds of weight for the bar; most women need 75–125 pounds. Dumbbells are end-weighted plates of varying poundage. They are primarily used with one-arm lifts while the barbell is used for two-arm lifts.

Basic Terms in Weight Training

Weight training has its own unique language, and a knowledge of this language helps one understand the techniques of the activity. The term *repetitions* refers to the number of times a complete exercise movement is performed. *Sets* refers to the number of repetitions that are performed. For example, if a person lifts a barbell 10 consecutive times, he has completed 1 set of 10 repetitions. The actual weight or poundage used for an exercise refers to the *load.* The maximum load that can be lifted a given number of times is called *repetitions maximum* (RM). For example, 10 RM is the greatest weight that can be lifted 10 times.

Do's and Don'ts in Weight Training

Always follow these important principles and procedures while engaging in a weight-training program.

Warm-up.—Whole body warm-up should always precede the regular weight workout. This can be done by jogging slowly or performing light calisthenics until a light sweat appears.

Breathing.—Never hold your breath when performing an extreme effort to overcome heavy resistance. When you hold your breath, it causes the glottis (covering over windpipe) to close. This creates a drastic elevation in thoracic and abdominal pressure. Therefore, you must maintain an open glottis by breathing during an extreme effort. Most weight trainees inhale during exertion and exhale during the relaxation phase.

Starting loads.—During the first week of training, use lightweight loads to develop the correct form for each exercise and prepare the muscles for the gradual increase in resistance. Lift only the load that can be controlled through a complete range of motion without deviations from the correct form.

Form.—Never sacrifice correct form to lift a heavy weight. Correct form is essential in developing one's body symmetrically and protecting a person from injury.

Range of motion.—Failure to perform each exercise movement through the complete range of motion will result in only partial development of the primary movers with a corresponding loss of flexibility in the antagonist muscles. This will cause muscleboundness.

Frequency of workout.—Normally, a person should exercise at least three times per week with a day of rest after each workout. You can work out daily if your exercise routine is alternated between upper- and lower-body exercises. For the beginner a 30- to 45-minute workout should be sufficient. You may want to lengthen it as strength, endurance, and experience are gained.

Number of repetitions for strength.—Between four and six repetitions should be used to develop strength. If you cannot perform an exercise at least four repetitions, then decrease your weight resistance. If you can perform more than six repetitions, then add approximately 10 pounds to your total weight resistance. Try to increase gradually until you can do at least three sets per workout period.

Number of repetitions for muscular endurance.—If you desire primarily to gain muscular endurance, then do three sets of 10–20 repetitions.

Safety Precautions

Improper techniques of lifting can result in injury to yourself or to a training partner. The following hints should be observed:

1. Do not lift more than you can handle with good form. The amount lifted is not important but rather how well each exercise is performed.
2. Never lift a barbell without collars secured tightly around the weight plates.
3. Make sure the plates are balanced on the barbell.
4. Use chalk or a towel to avoid wet hands caused by perspiration.
5. Always use a spotter when lifting heavy weights to keep from incurring serious injury.
6. Always keep your head up and back straight when lifting. Severe damage can occur to the intervertebral discs of the spinal column if you try lifting with your back bent.
7. Always warm up before lifting.
8. Use rubber-soled shoes to avoid slipping, and wear cotton clothing to absorb perspiration.

Basic Weight Training Movements

Muscle contraction causes the body to move in various planes. To strengthen a muscle at a particular joint, you need to know what movement that muscle will cause when it contracts. Kinesiologists (those who study human movement) have given certain terms to describe this joint movement. Learning five of these terms will aid understanding the muscular training program. All movement terms are made in reference to the human body standing erect, arms hanging to the sides with the palms of the hand turned outward. The five basic movements (fig 7.17) are as follows:

Flexion.—Bending or decreasing the angle between two bones, for example, bringing the forearm toward the shoulder.

Extension.—Increasing the angle between two bones, for example, returning the forearm to its original straight position.

Abduction.—Moving the bone away from the midline of the body that is drawn to divide the body into right and left halves, for example, raising the arm out to the side of the body.

Adduction.—Moving the bone toward the midline of the body, for example, returning the arm to the side.

Circumduction.—Moving in all planes, for example, rotating the arms in circles.

The following muscular training program is designed to strengthen the basic movements at the major joints in your body. Each exercise is only one example of how to strengthen a certain movement. Many exercises can be used. You might even be creative and design some preferred exercises to strengthen the desired movement.

Remember to warm up properly and to do some stretching exercises before you begin strenuous work. Begin your program by lifting light weights, especially the first three weeks of training. This will reduce much of the soreness that usually accompanies muscular training. Keep a workout record on a chart to help accurately regulate your workouts. Avoid doing the same exercise in three consecutive sets. Do one set that works the upper body, then follow this with an exercise that works the lower body. This will eliminate some of the muscular fatigue associated with weight training.

The muscles at these major movements at each joint must be strengthened equally. If a muscle imbalance occurs either from strengthening one group more or failure to strengthen the muscles at all, then postural deviations are probable. Do strength exercises for each of these movements. If muscle endurance is your goal, then perform 1–20 repetitions of each exercise. If strength is your goal, then perform 4–6 repetitions of each exercise. The muscular system is an important component of physical fitness that we, as Christians, must develop in order to build God's temple as it was originally designed (see figs. 7.18 to 7.49).

FIG. 7.17
Main movements by the body

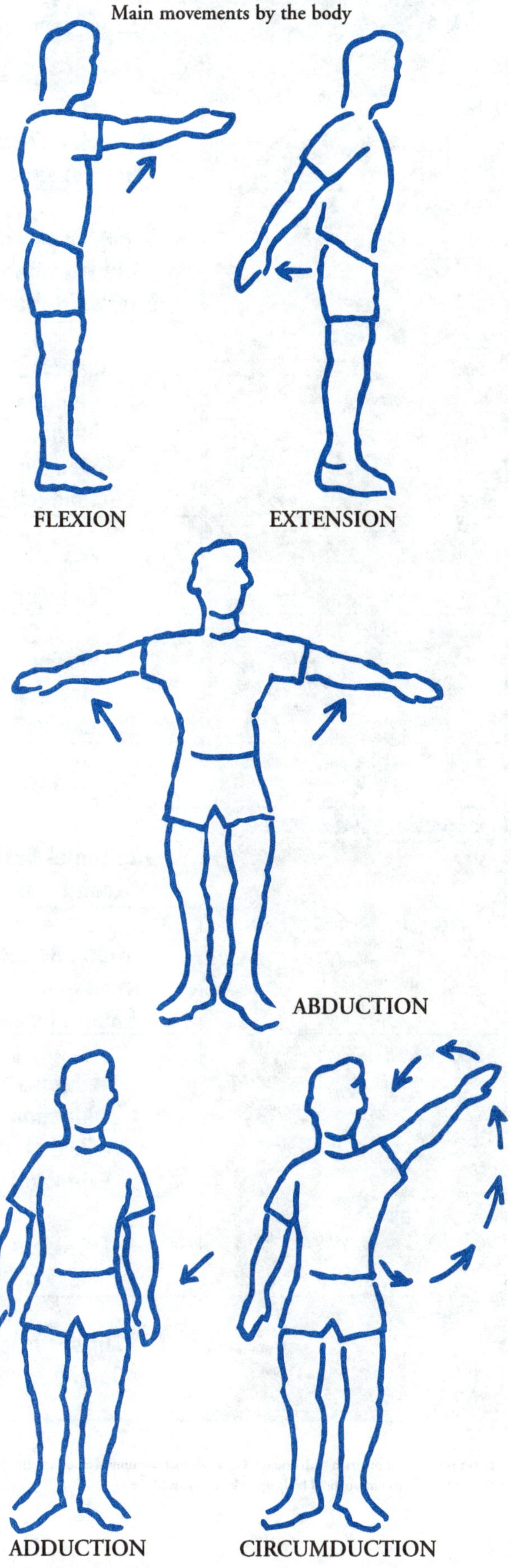

Table 7.1 Basic Weight Training Program

	Exercise	Starting Load	Repetitions	Sets
Neck[1]				
	Neck flexion	5 pounds	10–20	1 to 3
	Neck extension	5 pounds	10–20	1 to 3
Shoulder Girdle				
	Shoulder elevation	25 pounds	10–20	1 to 3
	Forward rotation	25 pounds	10–20	1 to 3
	Backward rotation	25 pounds	10–20	1 to 3
Shoulder Joint				
	Abduction	10 pounds	10–20	1 to 3
	Adduction[2]	10 pounds	10–20	1 to 3
	Flexion	20 pounds	10–20	1 to 3
	Extension	20 pounds	10–20	1 to 3
	Circumduction	10 pounds	10–20	1 to 3
Elbow Joint				
	Flexion	25 pounds	10–20	1 to 3
	Extension	25 pounds	10–20	1 to 3
Wrist Joint				
	Flexion	10 pounds	10–20	1 to 3
	Extension	10 pounds	10–20	1 to 3
	Circumduction	10 pounds	10-20	1 to 3
Finger and Hand Joints				
	Finger flexion	Squeeze ball	20–30	1 to 3
Upper Trunk Exercises				
	Horizontal flexion	20 pounds	10–20	1 to 3
	Horizontal extension	20 pounds	10–20	1 to 3
Lower Trunk Exercises				
	Trunk flexion	10 pounds	20–30	1 to 3
	Trunk extension	10 pounds	20–30	1 to 3
	Lateral flexion	10 pounds	20–30	1 to 3
Hip Joint				
	Abduction	Squeeze for 5 sec.	10–20	1 to 3
	Adduction	5 pounds	10–20	1 to 3
	Flexion	5 pounds	10–20	1 to 3
	Extension	5 pounds	10–20	1 to 3
Knee Joint				
	Extension	10 pounds	10–20	1 to 3
	Flexion	10 pounds	10–20	1 to 3
Ankle Joint				
	Plantar flexion	50 pounds	10–20	1 to 3
	Dorsi flexion	5 pounds	10–20	1 to 3

1 Begin your weight program with one set. Gradually increase until able to perform three sets.
2 If unable to do a chin-up, hold body up as long as possible.

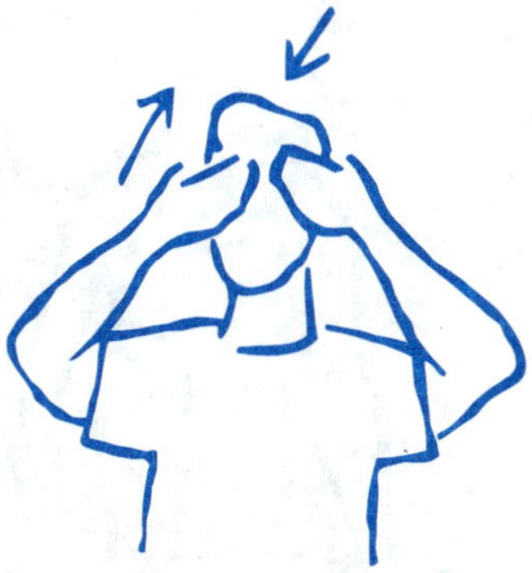

FIG. 7.18
Neck flexion: Push backward with hands; resist with head.

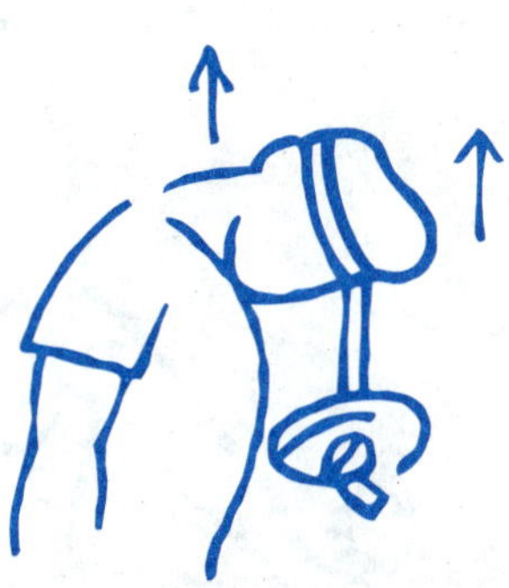

FIG. 7.19
Neck extension:
Raise and lower head as far as possible.

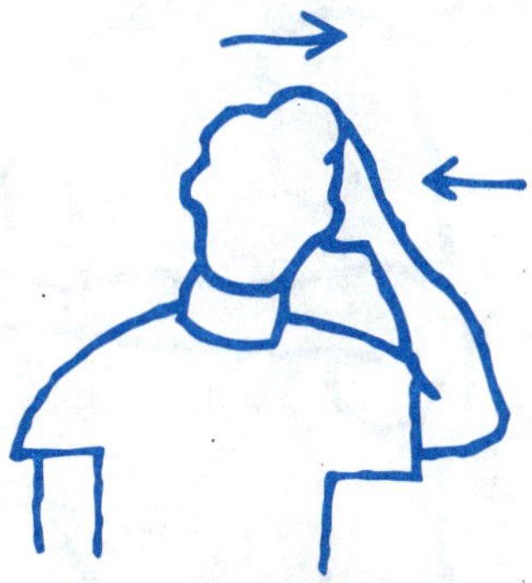

FIG. 7.20
Neck abduction:
Press with hands; resist with head.

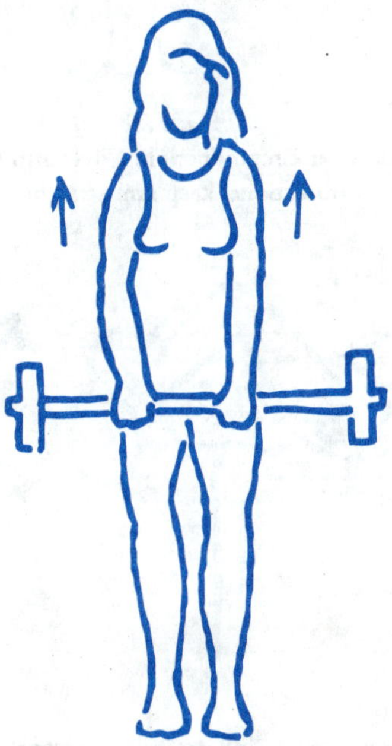

FIG. 7.21
Shoulder girdle elevation:
Keep arms straight; raise shoulder up; relax shoulder; repeat up-and-down movement.

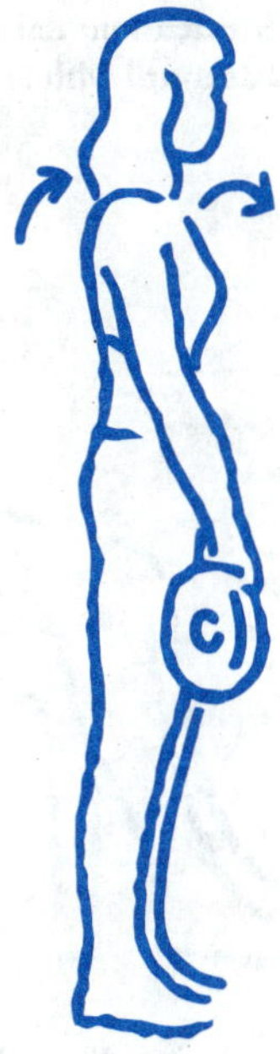

FIG. 7.22
Shoulder girdle forward rotation:
Keep arms straight; rotate shoulders forward as far as possible.

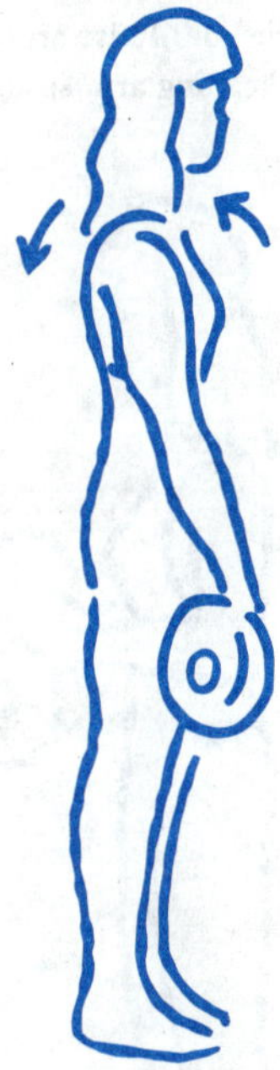

FIG. 7.23
Shoulder girdle backward rotation:
rotate shoulders backward;
keep arms straight.

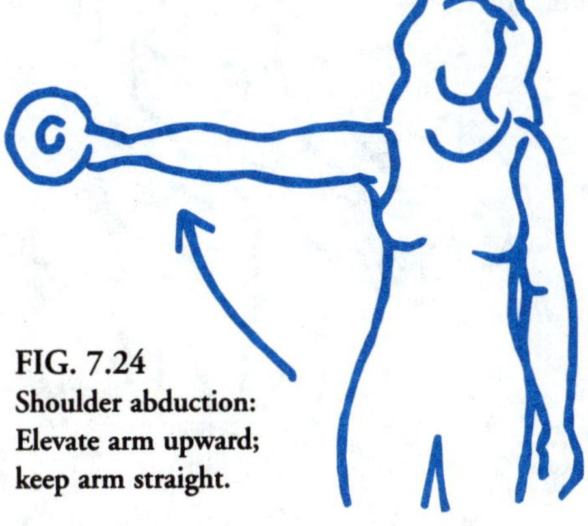

FIG. 7.24
Shoulder abduction:
Elevate arm upward;
keep arm straight.

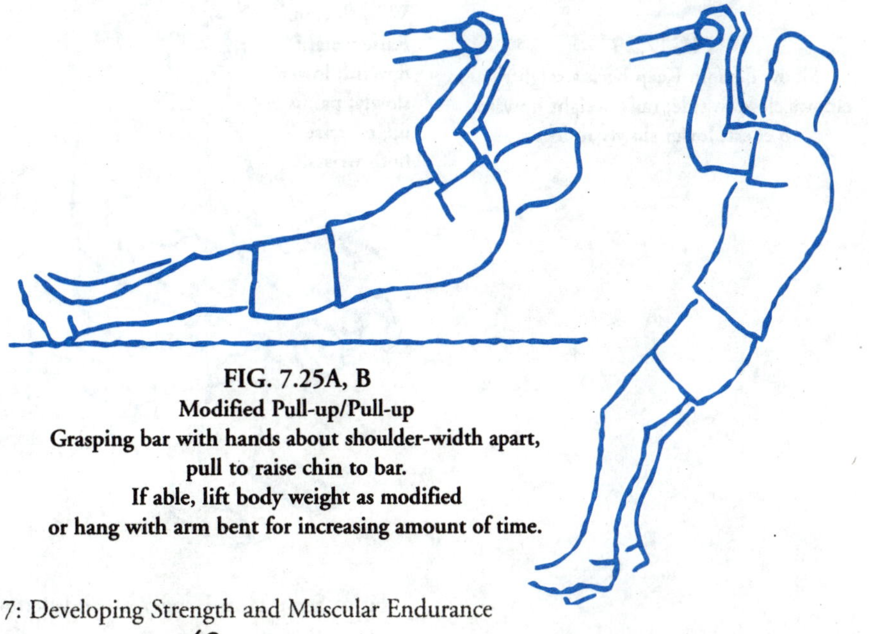

FIG. 7.25A, B
Modified Pull-up/Pull-up
Grasping bar with hands about shoulder-width apart, pull to raise chin to bar.
If able, lift body weight as modified or hang with arm bent for increasing amount of time.

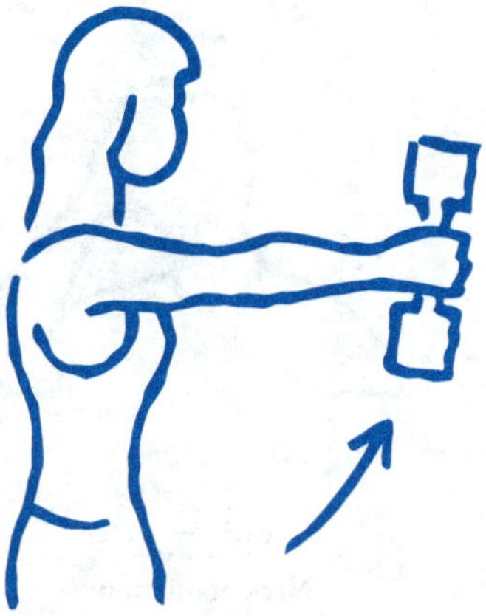

FIG. 7.26
Shoulder flexion: Raise arm upward while keeping arm straight.

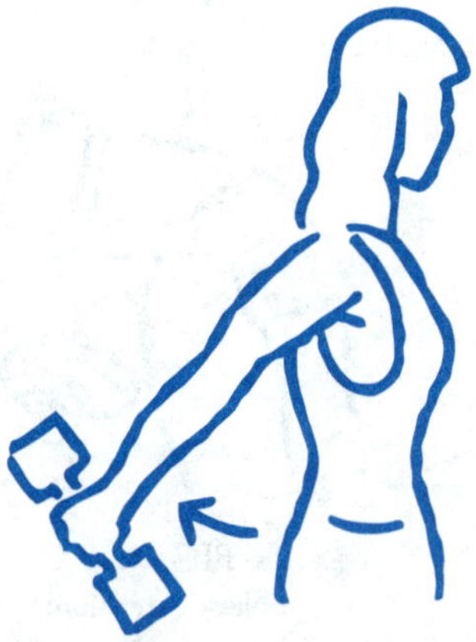

FIG. 7.27
Shoulder extension: Raise arm upward and backward with arm straight.

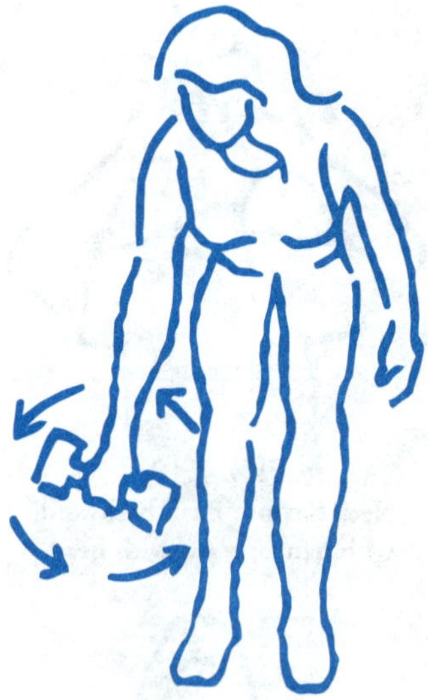

FIG. 7.28
Shoulder circumduction: Circle arm in all directions; keep arm straight.

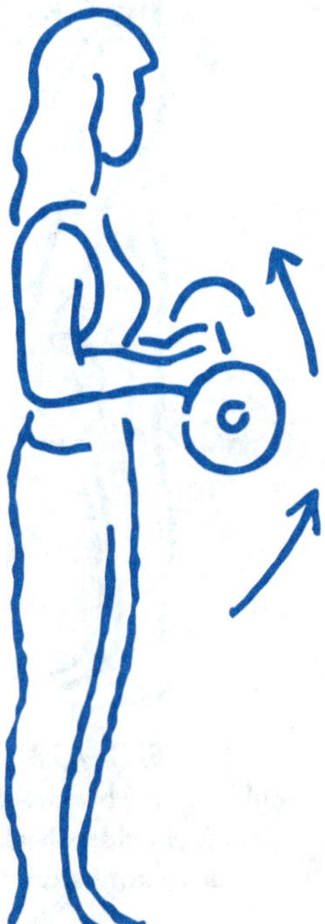

FIG. 7.29
Elbow flexion: Keep back straight; elbows close to side; raise weight upward to chest; lower slowly to legs.

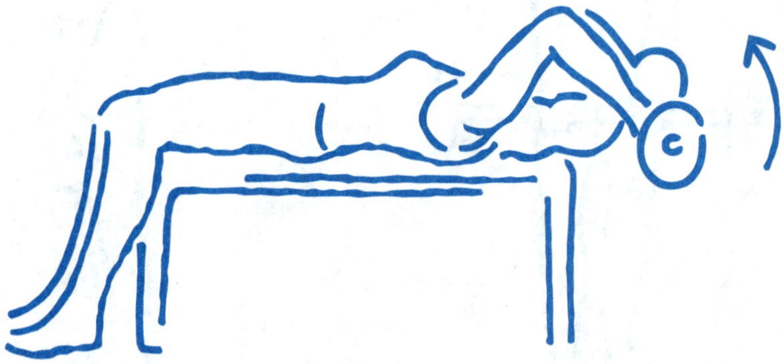

FIG. 7.30
Elbow extension: Keep elbows over ears; straighten arms to full extension; lower slowly.

FIG. 7.31
Wrist flexion: Raise weight upward; lower slowly; palms up; exercise both wrists.

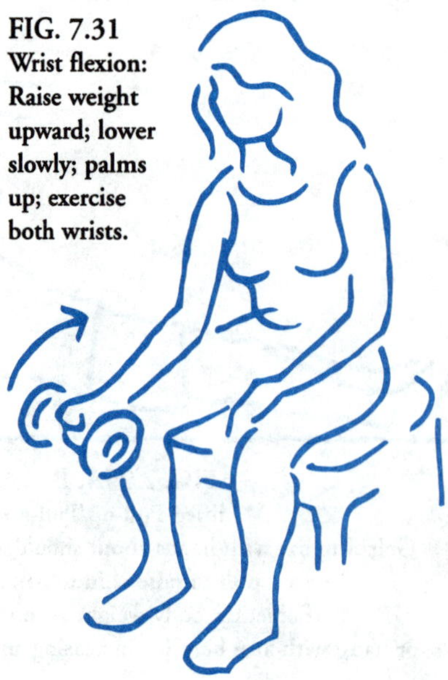

FIG. 7.32
Wrist extension: Reverse grip and extend wrist; lower slowly; exercise both wrists.

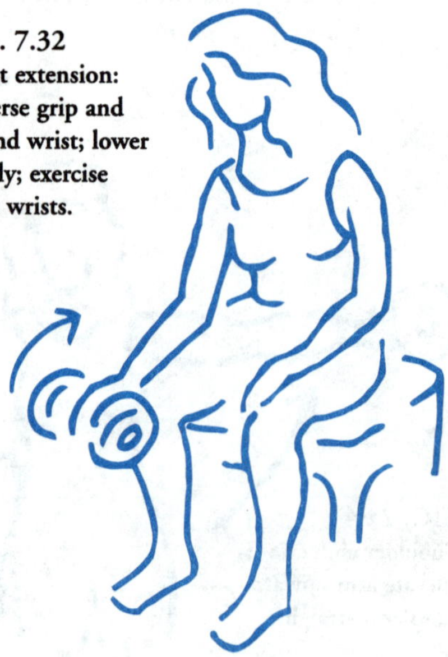

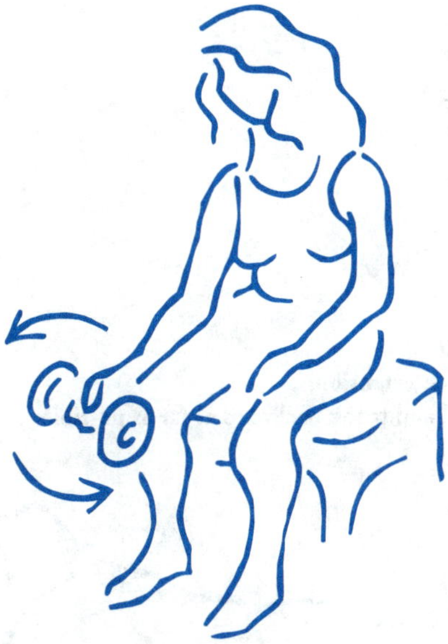

FIG. 7.33
Wrist circumduction:
twist wrist in all directions;
exercise both wrists.

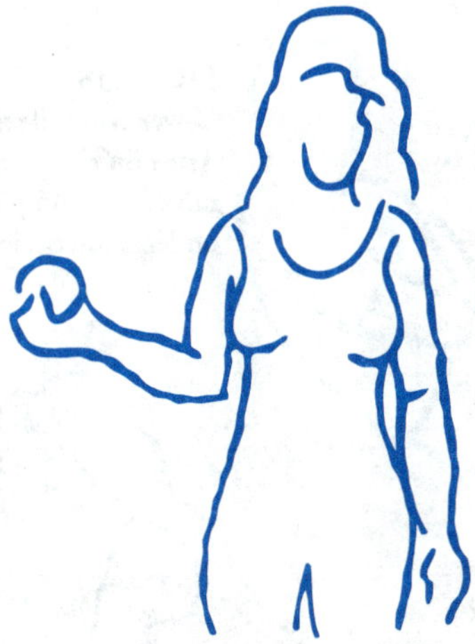

FIG. 7.34
Finger flexion: Squeeze ball tightly;
exercise both hands.

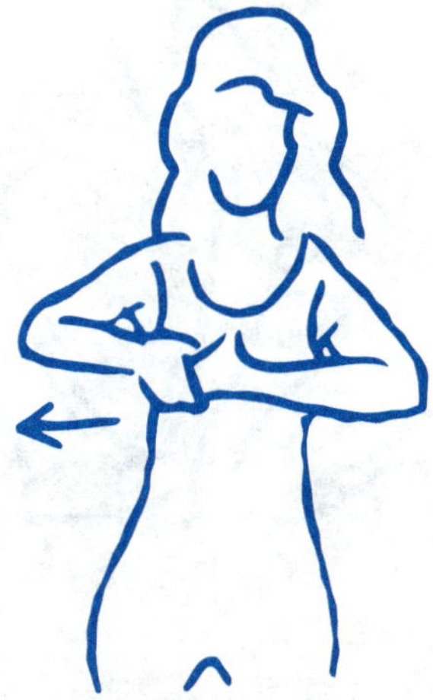

FIG. 7.35
Finger extension:
Push outwardly with fingers; resist with other hand; exercise both hands.

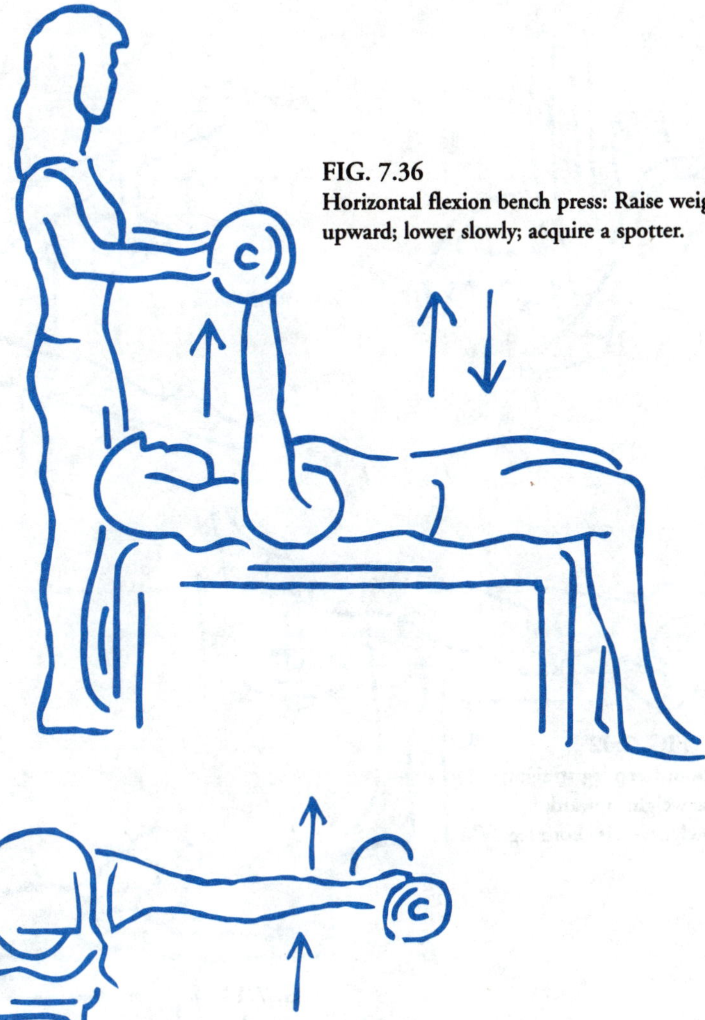

FIG. 7.36
Horizontal flexion bench press: Raise weight upward; lower slowly; acquire a spotter.

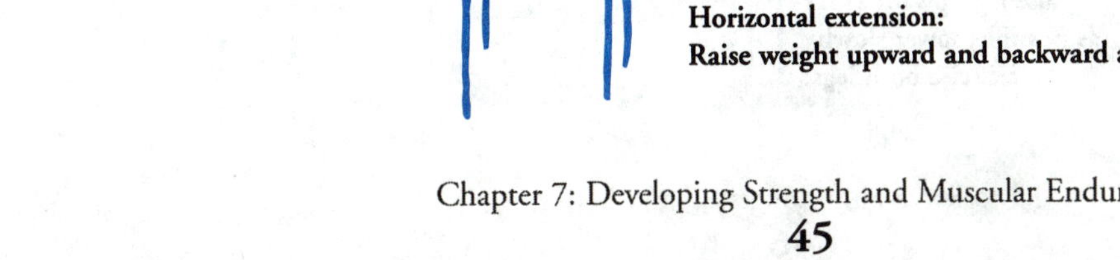

FIG. 7.37
Horizontal extension:
Raise weight upward and backward as far as possible; lower slowly.

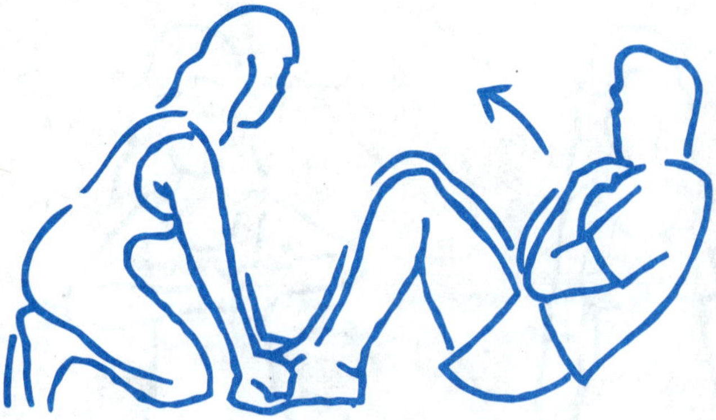

FIG. 7.38
Lower trunk flexion sit-up:
Arms on chest; legs bent; raise head and place chest on legs; lower slowly.

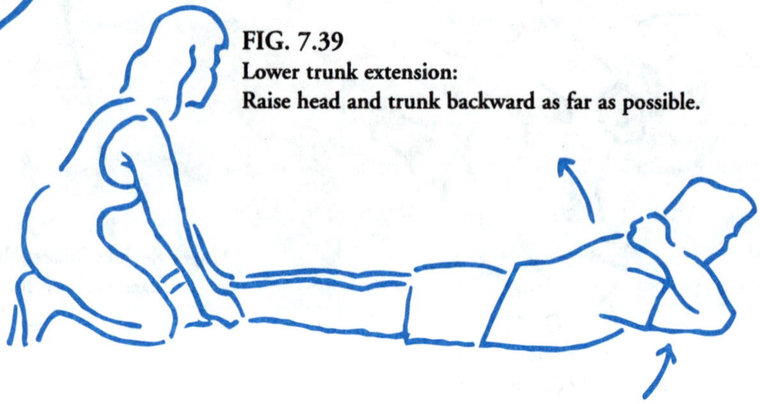

FIG. 7.39
Lower trunk extension:
Raise head and trunk backward as far as possible.

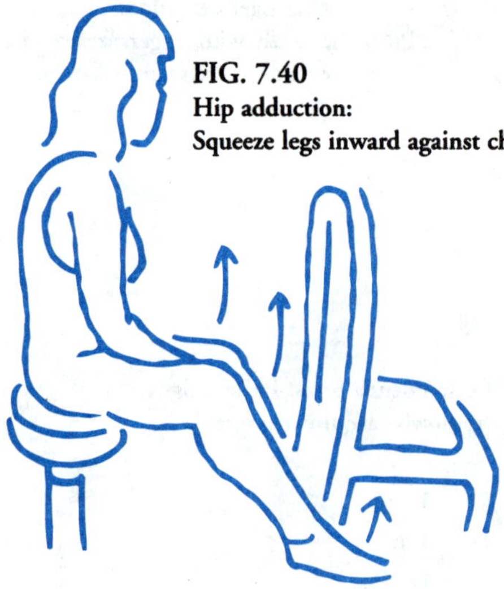

FIG. 7.40
Hip adduction:
Squeeze legs inward against chair.

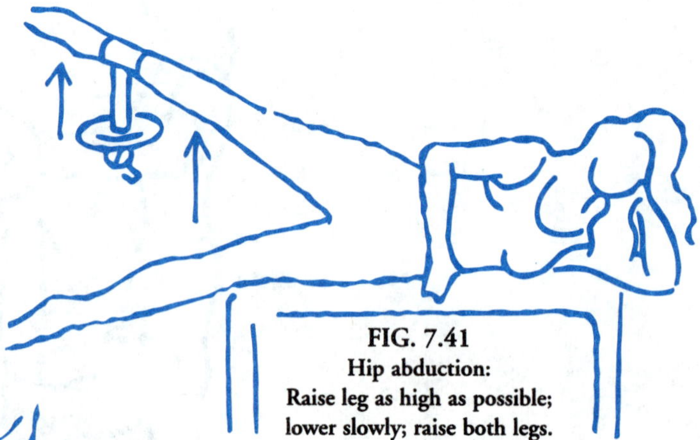

FIG. 7.41
Hip abduction:
Raise leg as high as possible; lower slowly; raise both legs.

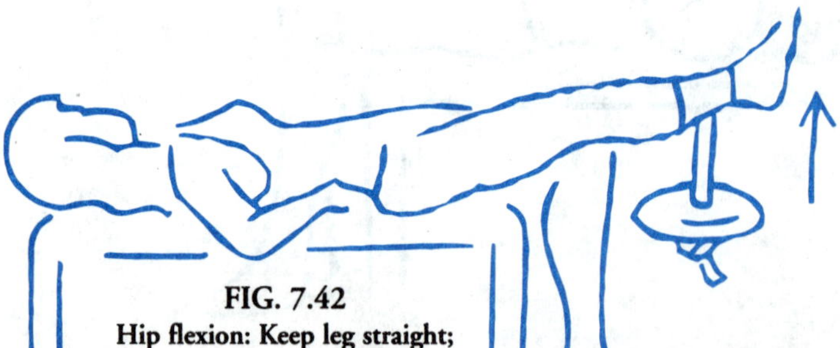

FIG. 7.42
Hip flexion: Keep leg straight; raise weight upward; lower slowly; exercise both legs.

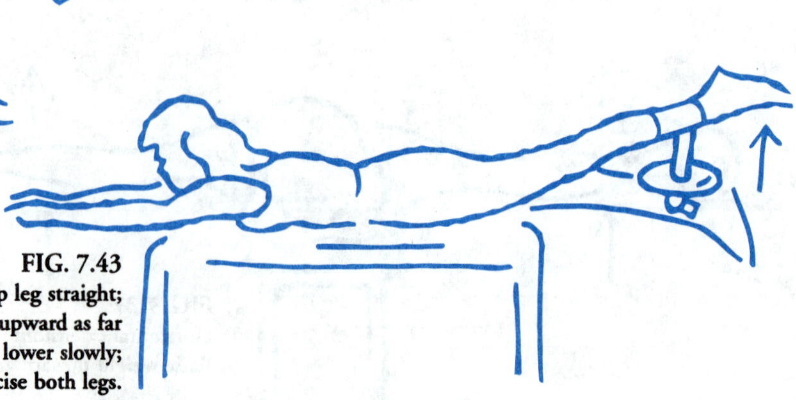

FIG. 7.43
Hip extension: Keep leg straight; raise leg upward as far as possible; lower slowly; exercise both legs.

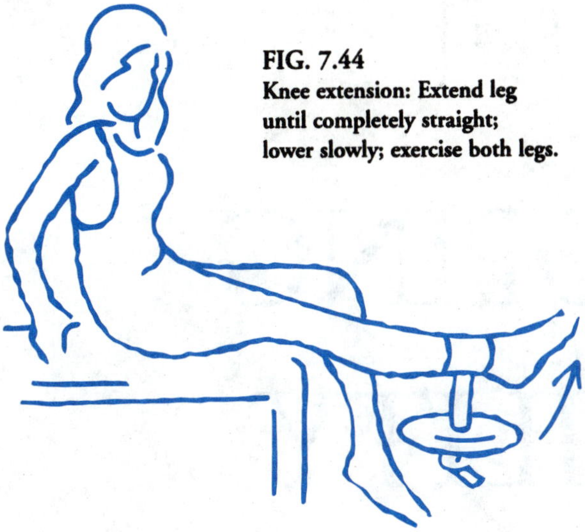

FIG. 7.44
Knee extension: Extend leg until completely straight; lower slowly; exercise both legs.

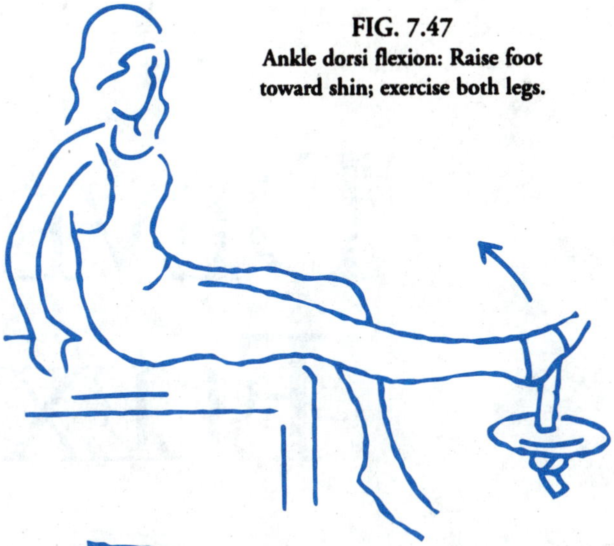

FIG. 7.47
Ankle dorsi flexion: Raise foot toward shin; exercise both legs.

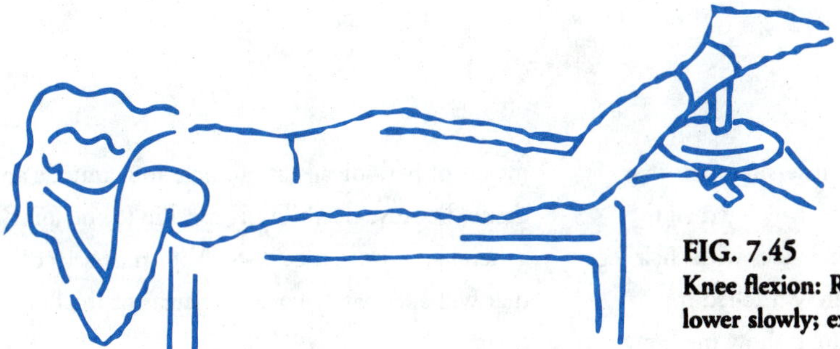

FIG. 7.45
Knee flexion: Raise leg upward; lower slowly; exercise both legs.

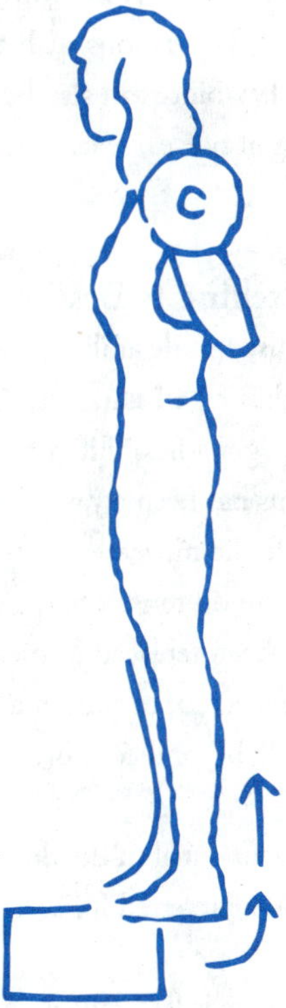

FIG. 7.46
Ankle plantar flexion: Raise and lower toes as far as possible.

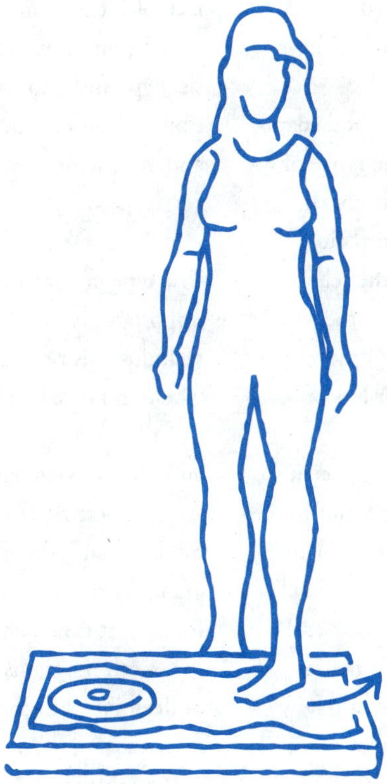

FIG. 7.48
Ankle abduction: Turn foot outward; pull weight toward foot; exercise both feet.

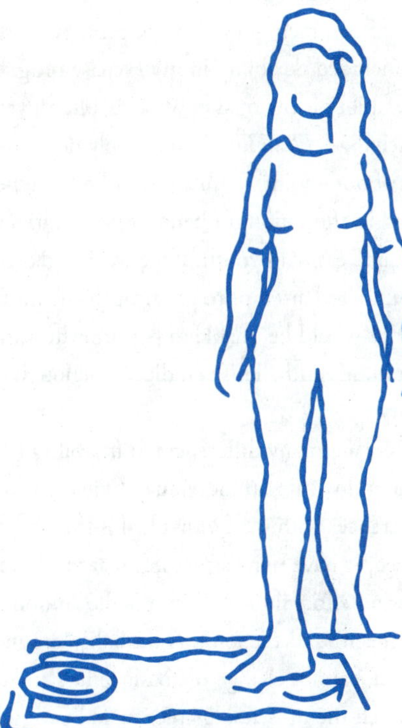

FIG. 7.49
Ankle adduction: foot inward; pull weight toward foot; exercise both feet.

[CHAPTER 8]

Developing Flexibility

Several years ago I attended a physical-fitness seminar that was conducted by an elderly man who challenged all the participants to stand up and touch their toes with their legs straight. To my surprise my fingers barely reached my ankles. I was embarrassed to let this older man show me how inflexible I had become. He also stated that if we couldn't touch our toes with our legs straight we had greatly increased our chances of contracting lower-back pain. Since that time, I have always included flexibility in my exercise program.

Flexibility is the quality of being pliant, versatile, and adaptable to change. *Flexibility* is commonly defined as the range of motion about a joint. With age, our bodies tend to become restricted in the actions of bending, stretching, and reaching, which came easily in youth. If we were to return to the school playground and attempt to go through the motions of the past, most of us would be unable to perform the antics and movements of our youth. This is indication enough of our loss of flexibility.

There are many differences in flexibility from one person to the next and within an individual. One contributing factor to the differences within an individual is the type of joint structure. Some people have bone structures that yield greater flexibility. Another potential limiting factor is the amount of muscle and fatty tissue around the joint. A flexibility program, no matter how good, cannot change the basic joint structure. It can, however, stretch the muscles, ligaments, and connective tissue that surround the joint structure.

A muscle sheath that is seldom stretched beyond its normal resting length can easily become so shortened that range of motion is limited. In a flexibility program you must devise a safe means of periodically stretching your muscle and connective tissue. Because flexibility is specific to the joint involved, no one general exercise can be used. You must select flexibility exercises that will adequately cover the areas of the body needing the exercise.

Flexibility is an important aspect of physical fitness, and the lack of it can create many health disorders. Anyone with a stiff spinal column is susceptible to postural deviations such as lordosis, kyphosis, and scoliosis. Lack of flexibility can also be responsible for muscle injury, compression of nerves, severe headaches, and even some forms of arthritis.

What Type of Stretching Is Best?

The type of stretching movements used in flexibility programs is important. An understanding of ballistic and static stretching techniques is necessary before you begin a flexibility program. The trend in safe flexibility programs has been away from ballistic or bouncing-type stretches, where the movement is suddenly and forcefully ended by an abrupt pull on muscle and connective tissue. These types of stretches have been replaced in preference by slow, static stretches, where the resistance of the stretch is gradually developed to a joint slightly beyond comfort and held for a short time before it is released.

Both programs appear to be about equal in the development of flexibility, but the static approach is preferred for several reasons.

• Injuries are reduced because there is less danger of tearing the connective tissue when the force is gradually applied and held.

• Slow, static stretching seems to cause far less muscle

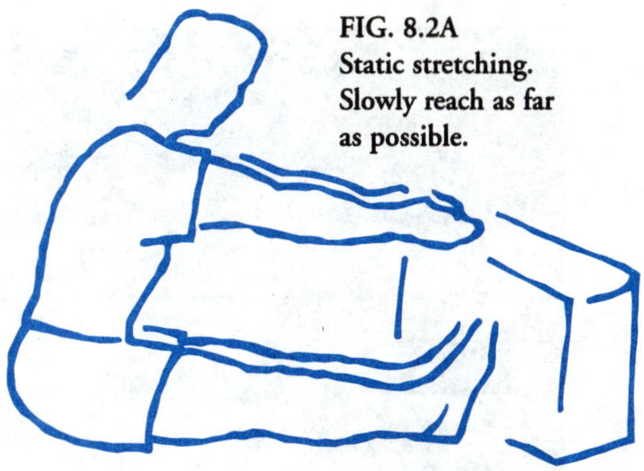

FIG. 8.2A
Static stretching. Slowly reach as far as possible.

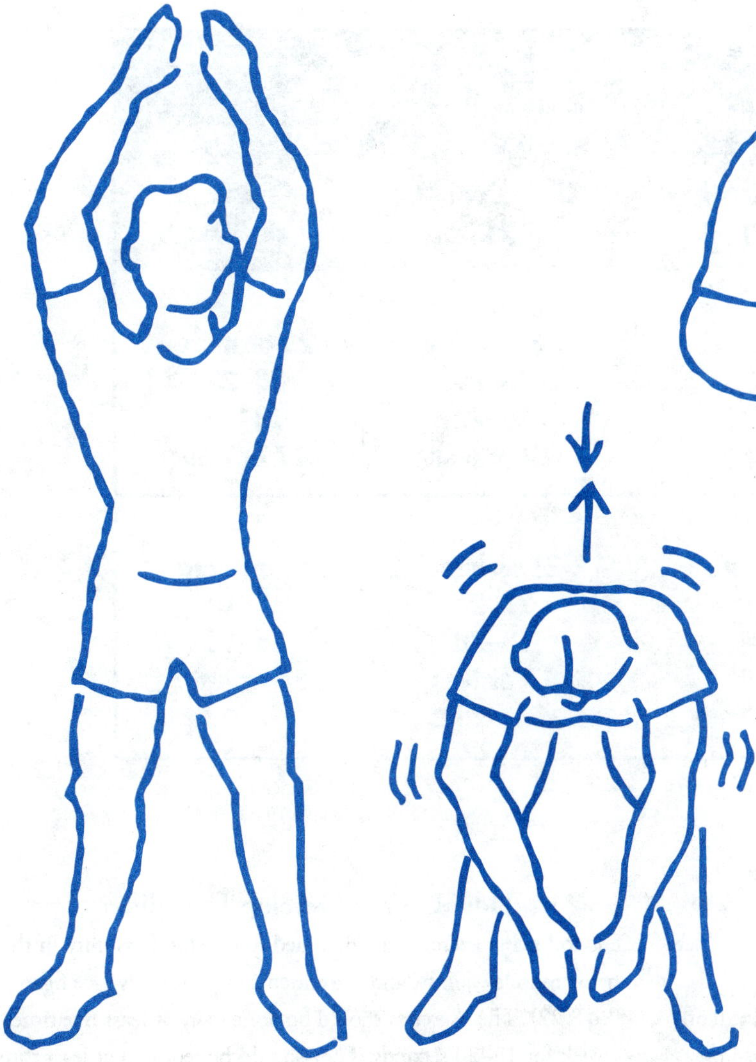

FIG. 8.2B
Ballastic stretching; bouncing to reach the floor.

soreness than the bouncing-type stretch. In fact, a good way to relieve muscle soreness is by using the slow, gradual static stretch.

• The stretch receptors (muscle spindles and golgi tendon organs) located in the muscles and joints are stimulated by stretching movements. These stretch receptors protect the muscles and joints from overstretching and injuring themselves.

Using fast, jerky, bouncy movements causes the muscles you are attempting to stretch to contract at the same time. This not only reduces the effectiveness of stretching but also causes muscle soreness. When a slow, sustained stretch is used, the stretch receptors cause the muscles to relax and lengthen and thus aid in obtaining increased flexibility.

How Flexible Are You?

Every Christian should be able to answer the above question, for it is important to develop flexibility in all your muscles to prevent God's temple from deteriorating. Flexibility is not a general factor but is specific to each muscle joint. No single test, therefore, can measure the flexibility of all the major joints of the body. The following flexibility tests were chosen to represent the major areas of the body that must remain flexible if good health is desired. Find a partner and determine your flexibility in these important areas.

Lower Back and Hamstrings

The sit-and-reach test (fig. 8.3) measures flexibility of the lower back and hamstring muscles (back of upper leg).

1. Sit on the floor with knees together and feet flat against a bench or box with a yardstick on top.

2. While a partner holds the knees straight, bend forward and extend both arms and hands as far as possible.

3. Measure the distance on the yardstick from the fingertips of both hands together to the edge of the bench. If the fingers do not reach the edge, the distance is expressed as a negative score; if they reach beyond the edge, it is expressed as positive score (table 8.1). Place the edge of the bench at the "10 inches" marker on the ruler.

Table 8.1
Flexibility Classifications

Classification	Sit & Reach (in.)	Shoulder Lift (in.)	Trunk Extension
MEN			
Excellent	7 or more	26 or more	23 or more
Good	4–6	23–25	20–22
Average	1–3	20–22	18–19
Poor	0	19 or less	17 or less
WOMEN			
Excellent	8 or more	25 or more	20 or more
Good	5–7	21–24	17–19
Average	2–4	18–20	15–16
Poor	0–1	17 or less	14 or less

Shoulder Joint and Shoulder Girdle

The shoulder lift test (fig.8.4) measures flexibility of the shoulder joint and shoulder girdle.

1. Lie on the floor. Touch your chin to the floor and extend your arms forward directly in front of your shoulders, grasping the stick at exactly shoulder width apart.

2. Hold the stick horizontally with both hands. Keep your elbows and wrists straight. Watch for bending of the wrist.

3. Raise your arms upward as far as possible while keeping your chin on the floor. Measure the distance in inches from the bottom of the stick to the floor (table 8.1)

Trunk

The trunk extension test (fig.8.5) measures flexibility of the trunk.

1. Lie on the floor with a partner holding down your buttocks and legs.

2. With fingers interlocked behind your neck, raise your chest and head off the floor as far as possible. Measure the distance in inches from the floor to your chin.

Being inflexible in these areas is often a warning signal for lower-back problems or tension headaches. If your muscles in these areas are tight and tense, then in all probability your muscles may spasm and cause severe pain. Always maintain good flexibility in these body areas.

How Do You Develop Flexibility?

The following exercises are designed to develop flexibility in the major muscles, joints, and movements of your body (see figs. 8.6–8.22). The exercises should be done daily at least five times a week for 15–20 seconds. They should be repeated at least three times. Stretching should never proceed to the point of actual pain and subsequent soreness. There will usually be some discomfort (moderately miserable), but any aftereffects should be noted and given time to repair. Start out easy and slow; do not bounce when you stretch. The following guidelines are recommended.

1. Stretch gently and gradually to prevent soreness and damage to the tissues. Do not bounce.

2. Exercises that do not cause a muscle to lengthen beyond normal may maintain flexibility but will not increase flexibility. The overload principle also applies to flexibility. To increase flexibility, stretch the muscle beyond its normal length.

3. Perform exercises for each muscle group or joint in which flexibility is desired. Do not skip one group. Maintain a balanced program for all muscle groups.

4. Perform flexibility exercises before and after a cardiovascular-respiratory or strength workout to prevent strains, reduce soreness, and stretch muscles that may have been shortened by the workout. Always perform flexibility exercises both before and after other forms of physical activity.

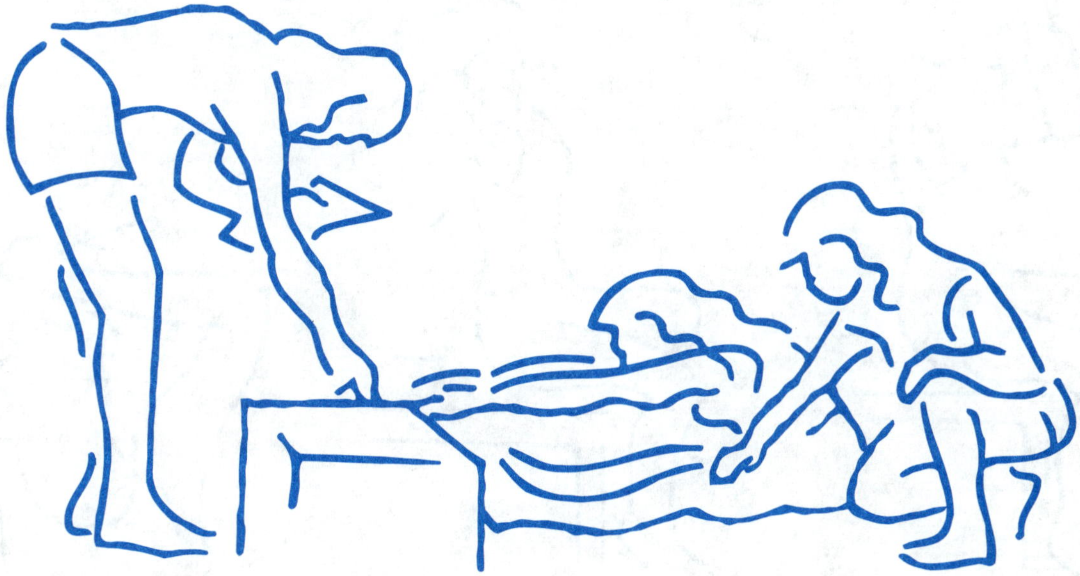

FIG. 8.3
Sit-and-Reach Test

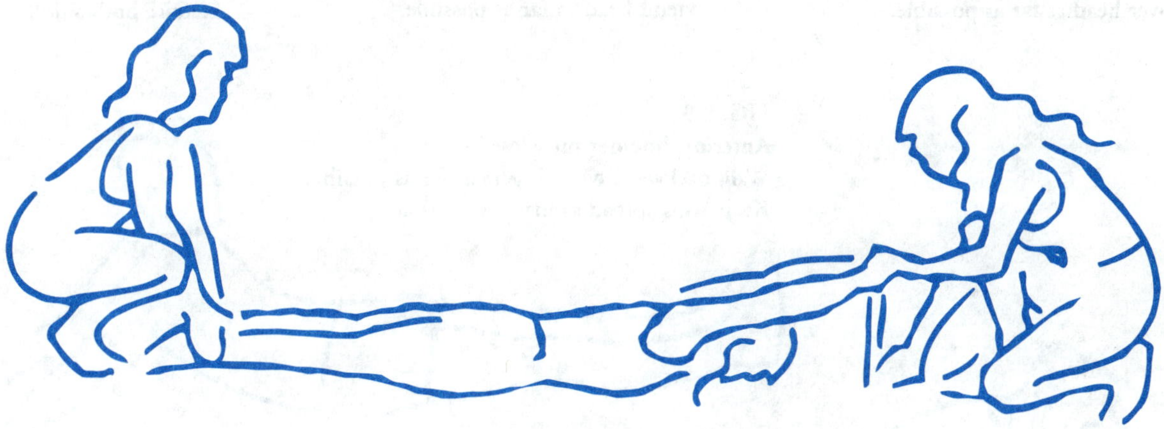

FIG. 8.4
Shoulder Lift Test

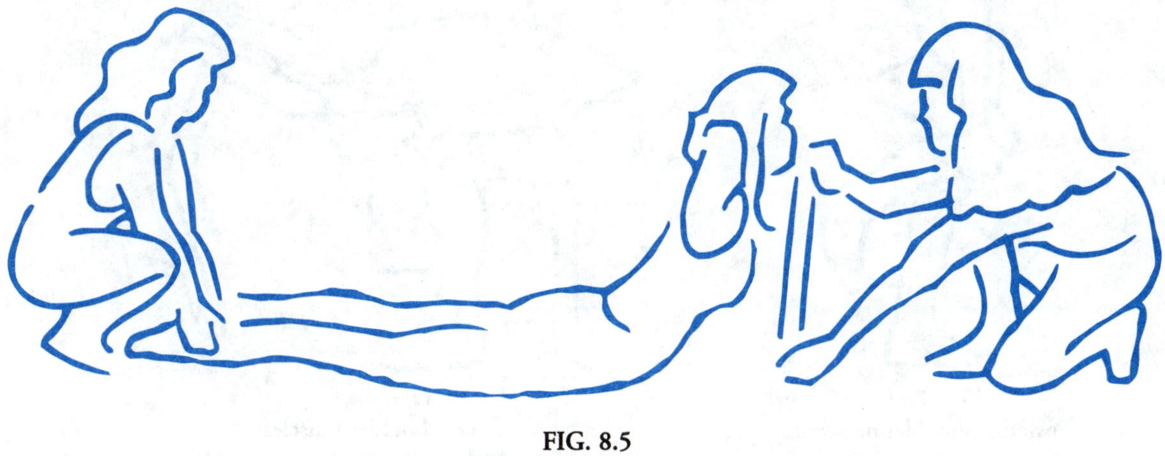

FIG. 8.5
Trunk Extension Test

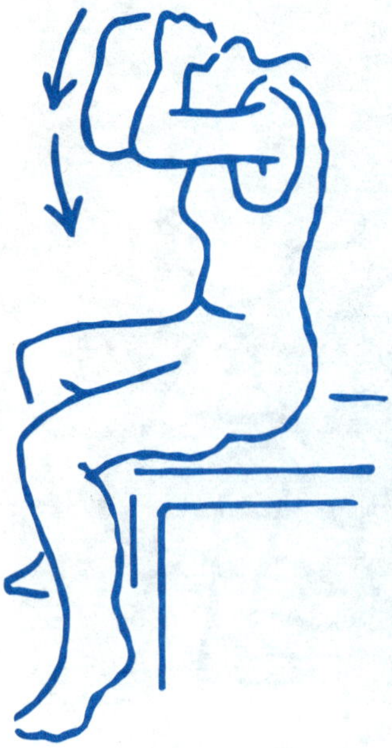

FIG. 8.6
Posterior neck muscles:
Apply light pressure with hands;
lower head as far as possible.

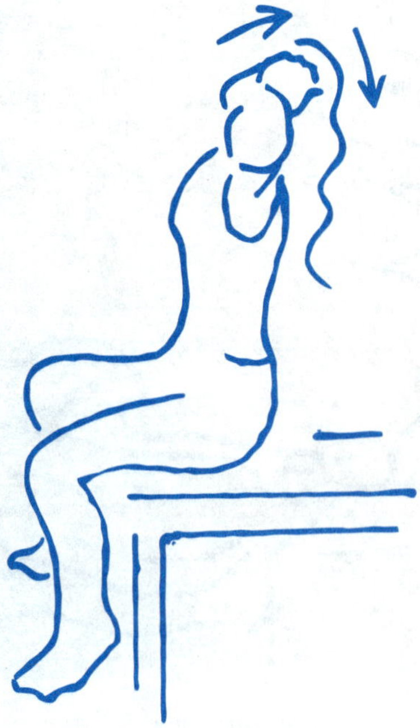

FIG. 8.7
Anterior neck muscles:
Apply light pressure with hands;
extend head as far as possible.

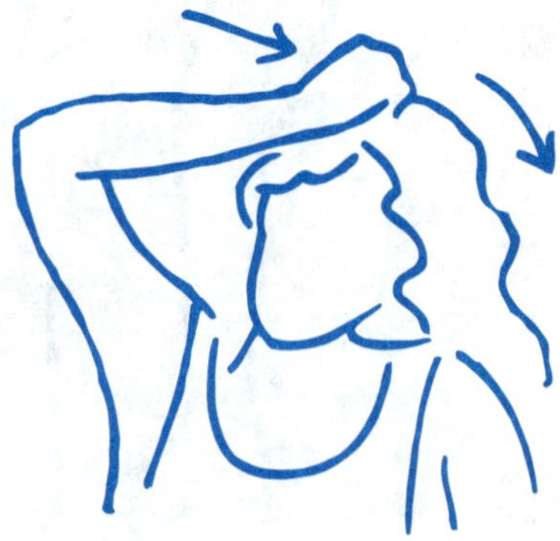

FIG. 8.8
Lateral neck muscles:
Apply light pressure to head;
lower head to side as far as possible;
exercise both sides.

FIG. 8.9
Anterior shoulder muscles:
Walk backward with fingers as far as possible.
Keep arms spread as little as possible.

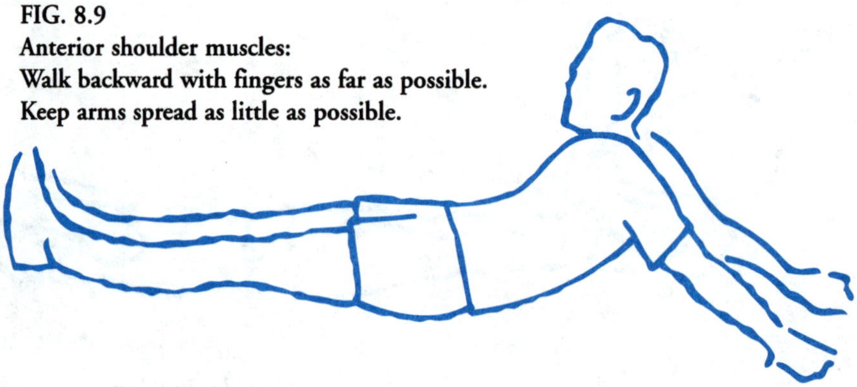

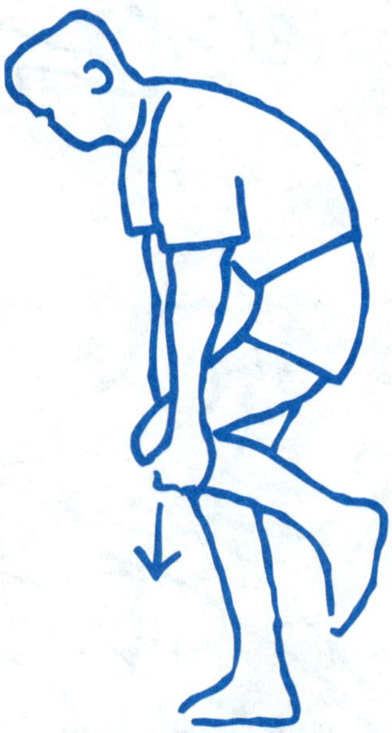

FIG. 8.10
Posterior shoulder muscles:
Push down on hands with knee.

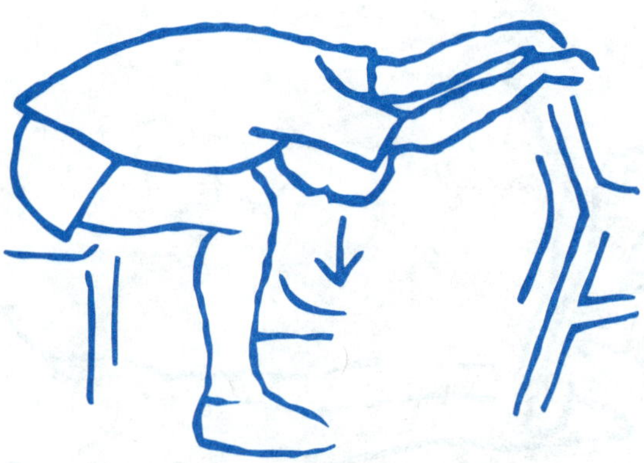

FIG. 8.11
Upper shoulder muscles:
Lower body to floor as far as possible.

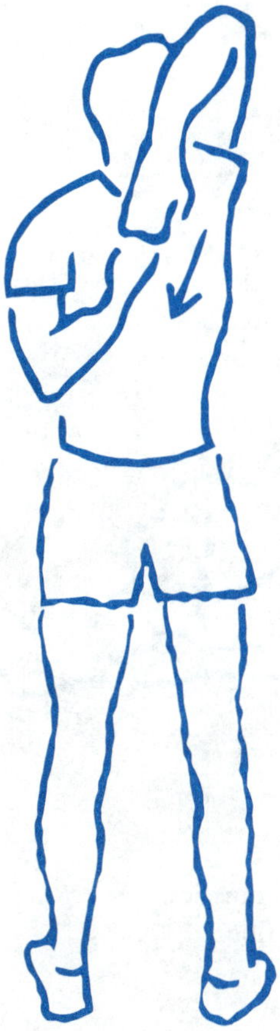

FIG. 8.12
Lower shoulder muscles:
Grasp hands behind back;
you may need to grasp
a towel if unable
to grasp hands.

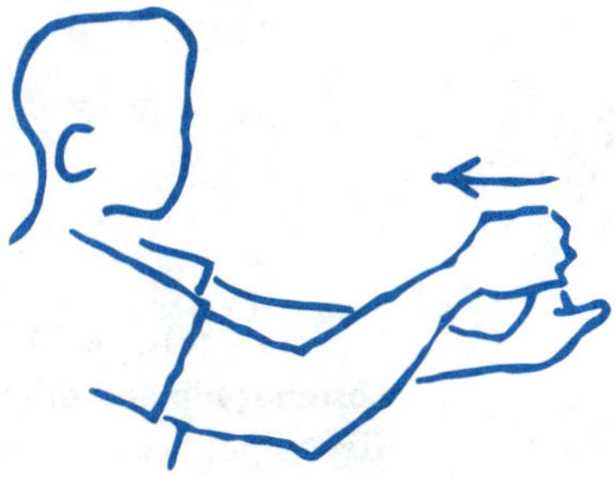

FIG. 8.14
Wrist and finger extension:
Pull backward on fingers;
exercise both wrists.

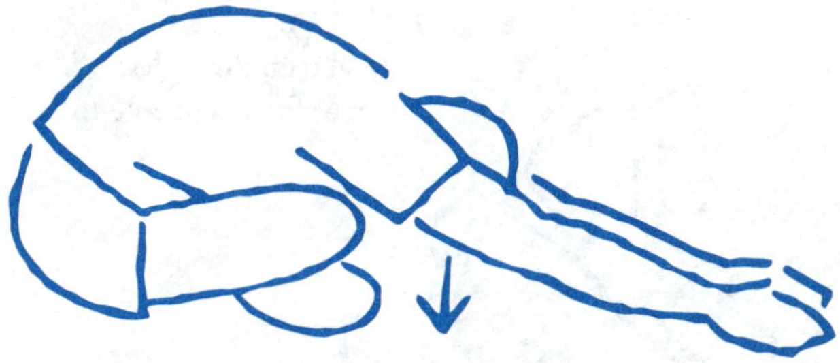

FIG. 8.15
Upper trunk muscles:
Reach forward; try to place forehead on floor.

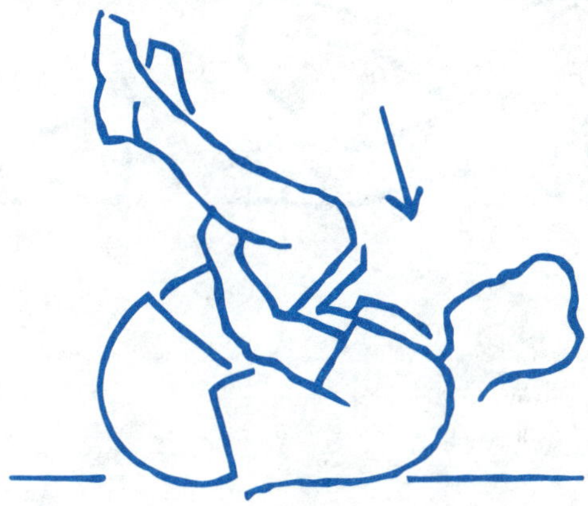

FIG. 8.16
Lower trunk muscles:
Try to touch toes behind head; keep legs straight.
Alternate to exercise (below):
Try to touch toes behind head; keep legs straight.

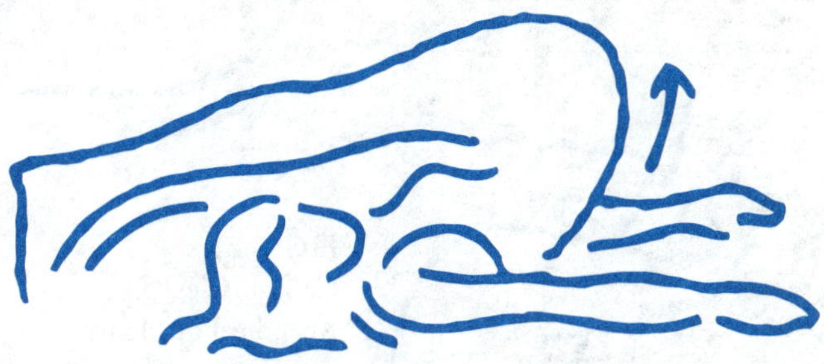

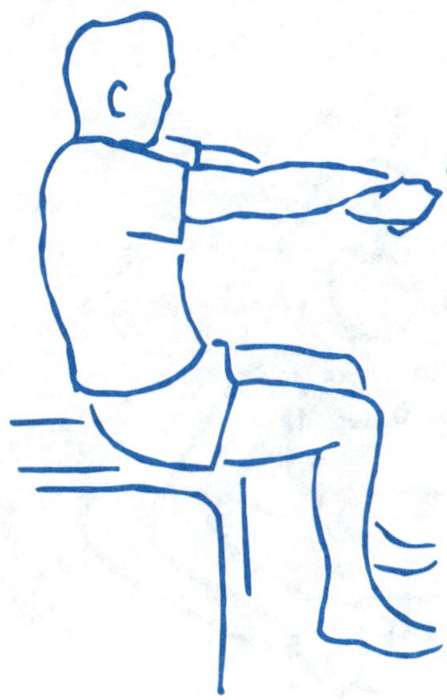

FIG. 8.13
Pronation and supination of arms:
Twist to both sides.

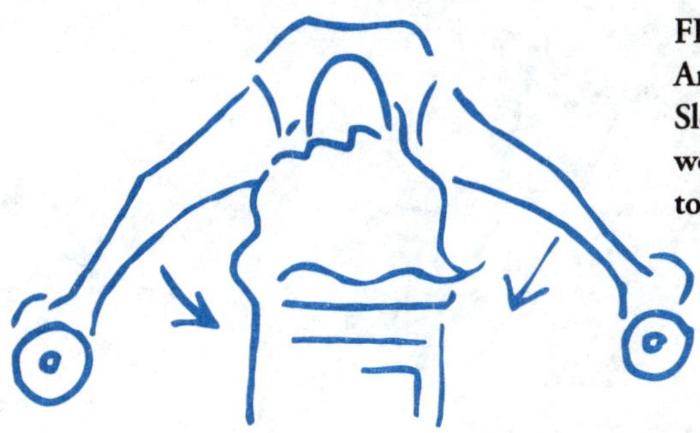

FIG. 8.17
Anterior trunk muscles:
Slowly allow the
weight to pull arms
toward floor.

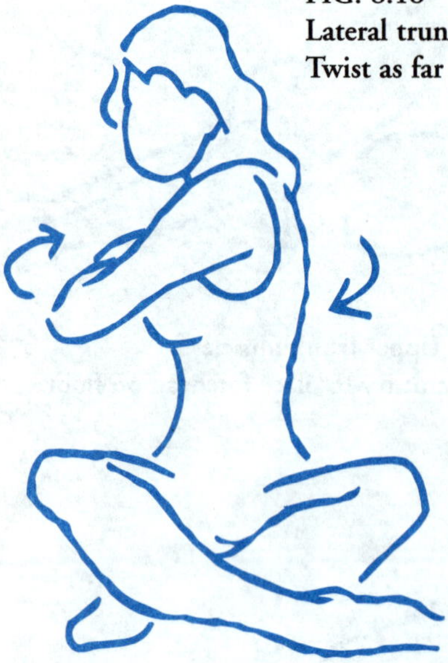

FIG. 8.18
Lateral trunk muscles:
Twist as far as possible to both sides.

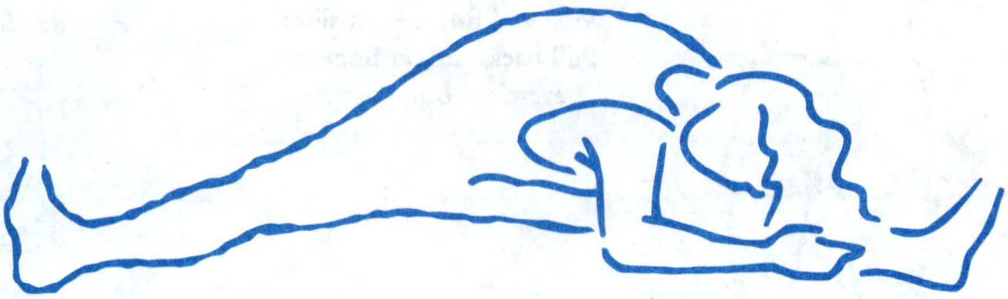

FIG. 8.19
Posterior hip and thigh muscles:
Try to put head on both knees;
try to place chest on floor in front.

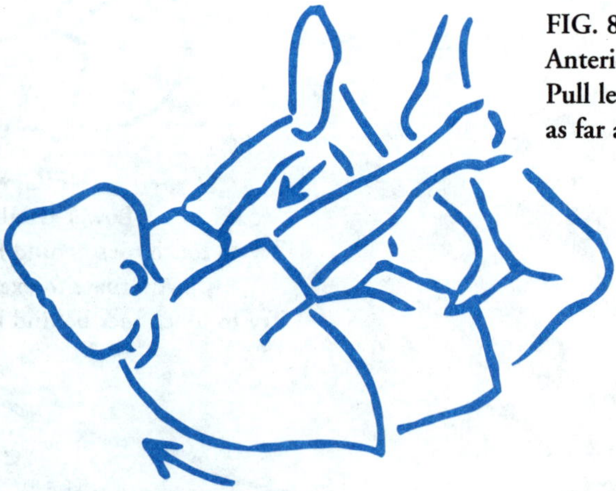

FIG. 8.20
Anterior hip and thigh muscles:
Pull legs and chest off floor
as far as possible.

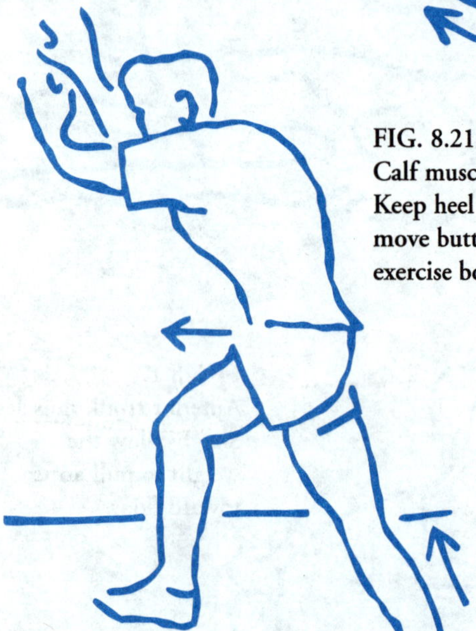

FIG. 8.21
Calf muscles:
Keep heel on floor:
move buttocks toward wall;
exercise both calves.

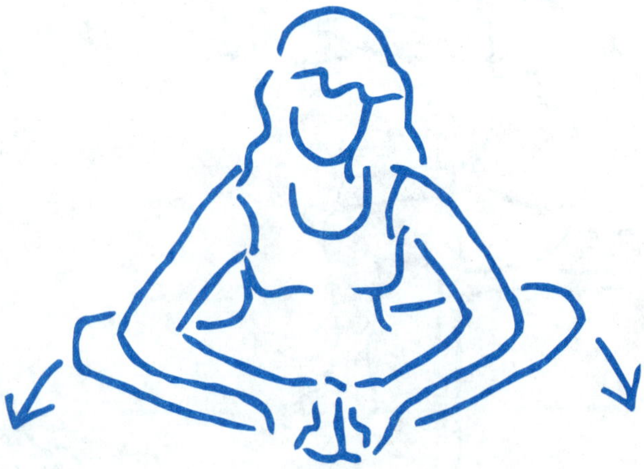

FIG. 8.22
Groin muscles: Push down on legs with elbows.

[CHAPTER 9]

Coping with Stress

Stress has been called the fastest growing disease in the Western world. It first afflicts infants abruptly faced with learning to adjust to life outside the womb. Each progressive stage toward adulthood brings accompanying stresses, frustration, loneliness, difficult personal relationships, and challenging crises. Although there appears to be no cure for whatever causes psychological and physical harm, which also influences us spiritually, there are positive ways to cope with stress. We can learn to use stress beneficially as we grow to maturity.

Everybody experiences stress, but no one can define it. Stress creates upset stomachs, splitting headaches, intense grief, excessive drinking, and violent arguments. Stress dulls memories, cripples thinking, weakens bodies, upsets plans, stirs up emotions, and reduces efficiency. But stress also motivates people to work, encourages us to keep going when life gets difficult, spurs us to action in the midst of crises, helps us to mature, and, at times, makes life exciting.

Hans Selye, a biologist, described stress as essentially the wear and tear of living. Each person experiences stress differently, but every day each of us experiences physical and emotional wear and tear from the pressures of life.

As a cell physiologist, I define *stress* as anything that upsets the homeostasis of the cell. *Homeostasis* can be defined as the normal resting state needed for proper cell metabolism. For example, the cell can better perform its inner metabolic reactions when the pH (acid-alkaline balance) is 7.3, and the temperature is 98.6 degrees. Therefore, stress can be defined as anything that upsets this normal resting state.

Selye says that stress can be divided into two types—eustress and distress. *Eustress*, from the Greek *eu* meaning good, can be defined as good stress. Obviously, *distress* means bad stress. Good stress is responsible for the exhilaration felt by an athlete before competition or by a business person before an important presentation. On a smaller scale, stress also keeps us enthusiastic about everyday activities.

Stress can be further divided into being either physiological or psychological. Some examples of good physiological stress are proper exercise, good nutrition, good sleeping habits, and enjoyable hobbies. Bad physiological stress might be represented by smoking, excessive drinking, inactivity, and poor nutrition. Whereas good psychological stress might be determined as love for others, kindness toward others, and worshiping God, bad psychological stress could be seen as jealousy, hatred towards others, and coveting material gains.

According to Selye, stress is not simply nervous tension or something to be avoided or always unpleasant. Parachute jumping, playing tennis, or watching an emotional television program can all be stressful; but these are stresses we often seek out and enjoy. When it motivates us to action, stress can be good; but when it places our bodies under prolonged physical and emotional pressure, the things that might be stimulating and enjoyable become destructive and unpleasant.

Selye believes that just as unused muscles or organs become slack and inefficient, inactivity deprives our bodies and minds of an innate urge to create. He recommends that we be exposed to as many positive stresses as we can handle. As long as we stay within our optimal stress level, our mind and body will be at peak performance.

Trouble starts when too much negative stress occurs, such as

Stress will attack our weakest organ and cause severe damage to our health.

pressures at work or school or friction at home. Even good stress can be a problem if there is too much or if we cannot handle it well. If a promotion generates panic, we need to recognize our individual responses to too much stress and not push beyond our endurance. The body sends out warning signals telling us that our system is overloaded, and we experience changes in sleep patterns, appetite, sexual desire, or mood.

Stress will attack our weakest organ and cause severe damage to our health. For example, 8–10 million Americans suffer from ulcers. In fact, Tagamet, a drug that helps cure stress and ulcers is one of the most widely prescribed drugs in America. People who suffer from ulcers are usually highly competitive, go-getter men, women, and children. They feel pressure from the world around them, but they experience a lot of inner pressure as well. They have an inner drive to succeed and to get ahead. Whenever they accomplish a particular goal, they set their aspirations higher and continue pushing. This keeps the body under such a constant state of physical alertness that the stomach lining begins to bleed and becomes irritated by the increased production of acids. This is the start of an ulcer. The biggest producer of ulcers is stress that cannot be controlled. A person under such stress cannot predict what will happen or make things happen.

Stress not only can bring on ulcers but can also affect the heart. Two cardiologists divided potential heart-attack victims into two broad categories, Type A and Type B. Type A personalities are ambitious, aggressive, self-demanding, competitive, and strive for success. They are driven by the clock. In contrast, Type B personalities are more casual. They are less competitive, less worried about time, and are not unnecessarily preoccupied with achievement. Perhaps no one fits these categories completely, but most of us tend to fall into one of these classifications.

Their research found that persons with Type A personalities were seven times more likely to have a heart attack than Type B individuals. Even if they did not smoke or exercise and had normal blood pressure with no family history of coronary disease, Type A people were more likely to have coronary attacks.

Stress has also been linked to migraine headaches, arthritis, backaches, and high blood pressure. Some researchers believe that stress can cause certain forms of cancer.

Yet another classification of personality goes beyond Type A or Type B. Type D personality seems to indicate individuals who have an increased risk of serious disease. A Type D personality is one that is hostile and unforgiving toward others. Such persons do not consider the long-term consequence of any action. Their way is the only way and is to be carried out at the expense of others. Couple this with a spirit of grudges and holding on to blame, and a Type D becomes a prime candidate for serious illness.

In a study of 450 adult cancer patients, Lawrence LeShan found three prominent characteristics of stress. Most patients experienced termination of a close personal relationship immediately prior to the disease; about half the patients had trouble expressing hostility, and about a third showed tension over death of their parents.

We probably cannot conclude from this and similar research that stress alone causes cancer, heart attacks, or other physical symptoms; but we do know that stress is a key factor in illness; and diseases not caused by stress alone may be influenced by life's pressures. Stress places the body on alert and makes it more susceptible to disease.

In his study of more than 5,000 patients, Holmes discovered that disease often follows any event that requires us to adapt or to change our reactions in some way. He devised a test to measure the influence of change by assigning points to those events that require the greatest adaptation to change. Table 9.1 shows these stressors and the points assigned to their degree of stress.

Every reader should check all the items in table 9.1 that have applied to them during the last year. Add up the points to get a total life change unit score. According to Holmes' research, a score less than 150 indicates only one chance in three that you will have a serious change in health during the next two years. A score between 150 and 300 points indicates your chances rise to about 50–50. A score over 300 points indicates an 80 percent chance for a major health change (disease, surgery, accident, mental illness, etc.) within the next two years.

How Do You Overcome Stress?

Most medical authorities recommend four ways to cope with stress: develop a positive mental attitude, practice good nutrition, get proper exercise, and get proper rest and relaxation.

Develop a Positive Mental Attitude

Understanding stress is the best way to become free from its negative aspects. As with most problem solving, we must first become aware of our particular source of stress before we can

Table 9.1 — The Stress of Adjusting to Change

Event	Life Change Points	Event	Life Change Points
Death of spouse	100	Immediate family member seriously ill	30
Divorce/breakup of family	73	Son or daughter leaving home	29
Loss of job/setback in your career	70	Beginning a new friendship/relationship	29
Serious communication problem with spouse	69	Trouble with in-laws	29
Marital separation	65	Outstanding personal achievement	28
Death of immediate family member	65	Conflict with close friend	27
Personal injury or illness	63	Holiday away	26
Unemployment of spouse	60	Serious restriction of social life	25
Being physically abused by your spouse	59	Problem with children	24
Immediate family member attempts suicide	55	Onset of prolonged ill health requiring doctor's treatment	23
Getting into debt beyond means of repayment	51	Increase in family arguments	22
Beginning of heavy drinking by immediate family member	46	Addition of new resident in the home	21
Change of lifestyle; move to new community	43	Demanding relationship outside nuclear family	18
Pregnancy	40	Spouse introduces stresses from joy to home	18
Miscarriage	40	Single parenting/spouse unavailable	17
Difficulties in sexual relationship	39	New job in same line of work	17
Serious illness or injury requires hospitalization	39	Remodeling of home	16
New job in new line of work	38	Development of new friendship	16
Change in financial state	38	Buildup of tedious household chores	15
Death of close friend	37	No privacy in living arrangements	15
Increased arguments with spouse	37	Change in sleeping habits	16
Severing intimate relationship/friendship	35	Change in appetite/eating habits	15
Abortion (voluntarily induced)	32	Vacation at home	15
Immediate family member sent to jail	32	Christmas	12
Divorce within extended family	32	Lent	12
Purchase of house, mortgage over $100,000	31	Easter	12
New problem related to use of alcohol or drugs	30	Minor violation of law	11
Foreclosure of mortgage or loan	30		
Spouse begins or stops work	30		

Reprinted from *Clergy Self-Care: Finding a Balance for Effective Ministry* by Roy M. Oswald (AL125) with permission from the Alban Institute, Inc., 7315 Wisconsin Ave., Suite 1250W, Bethesda, Maryland 20814-3211.

reduce or alleviate it.

Try to develop an "I can handle it" attitude. Once you do that, you will find that the expectation of coping successfully goes a long way toward actually doing it.

We should also establish priorities to put our problems in perspective. If we feel overworked and that there are not enough hours in a day, we should set schedules based on a clear sense of what can be realistically achieved. This is significant, because only irritation and frustration accompany trying to accomplish things without first assessing our capabilities and planning accordingly. I have seen many Christians mishandle stress because they were unable to budget their time to deal with the complexity of life.

Remember, whether the stress is in your personal or professional life, you will always have some degree of conflict and pressure. Those who realize that complete harmony is more an ideal than a reality will be able to accept stressful feelings. Nothing is wrong with feeling angry or frustrated if it is properly expressed. In dealing with feelings, though, we must communicate with those around us. Do not be afraid to let people know when you need their help or support; do not expect them to be mind readers. A little communication does a lot for interpersonal relationships, and many people find that talking about problems helps to solve them.

Almost any emotional upset can trigger the body's stress response and the accompanying physical effects. When you feel yourself becoming tense, slow down and try to be rational. You may find that some of the things that are most annoying or frustrating are just not worth getting worked up over. To stay happy and healthy, remember that worrying over things that cannot be controlled prevents dealing effectively with the things that can be controlled. If you want to be happy and healthy and are willing to work toward it, then chances are you will be.

> Everyone needs sleep time but also time for just relaxing . . .

As Christians, we need to learn to cast our burdens on our Creator and expect that He will sustain and help us, just as the Bible promises. Then the stresses of life will help us grow. They are no longer obstacles to be overcome but steps that enable us to grow to maturity. The positive mental attitude for Christians is found in Philippians 4:13, "I can do all things through Christ which strengthenth me" (KJV). Add to the force of Philippians 4:13 the focus of Philippians 3:13-14 to get a handle on stress—forgetting what is behind you and reaching for what is in front of you and pressing on the high calling of Jesus Christ.

Practice Good Nutrition

Eating properly improves overall general health, but under stressful conditions it is even more important. Often tensions and nervous problems are symptoms of poor eating habits.

When stress is compounded by hectic schedules, people tend to consume convenience or overrefined foods that lack significant nutritional benefits. No one should skip meals no matter how busy the schedule. Those foods richest in protein, vitamins, and minerals should always be part of the diet. Good nutrition helps your immune system stay viable and strong. While stressful circumstances can lower the body's defenses to infection and disease, good nutrition—even in the midst of stress—will increase the body's chances of defeating many diseases.

Get Proper Exercise

Exercise is an ideal way to channel frustration and energy. People in good physical condition can withstand periods of stress—including overwork, quarrels, and depression—better than people who are not in good physical condition.

Exercise relieves neuromuscular tension. Job stress causes muscles to tighten and shorten. Muscle contraction places stress on the nerves that serve them and results in neuromuscular tension. Tension can be relieved by participating in vigorous exercise. After strenuous exercise or hard physical labor, muscles are relaxed, and tensions leave the body. Exercise tends to break the vicious stress cycle which begins with each new day. So while setting lifestyle priorities, include daily time (preferably after work) for favorite activities such as tennis, racquetball, jogging, bicycling, swimming, or walking. Regardless of the time of day, exercise helps moderate the effects of stress.

Get Proper Rest and Relaxation

The final prescription for coping with stress is to allow time for adequate rest and relaxation. Everyone needs sleep time but also time for just relaxing, time to write an overdue letter, or time to put up one's feet and daydream.

Research has shown that the best way to relax muscles and nerves is through a progressive relaxation program. This program consists of lying on a firm mat on the floor in a dimly lighted room with soft music playing. Lie flat on your back with arms to your side, close your eyes, take deep breaths, and allow your mind to relax all your muscles.

After you have achieved silence in your nerves and muscles, you are ready progressively to relax each group of muscles in your body. Begin by contracting all the muscles in your legs and arms for five seconds. After the five seconds, allow your mind to concentrate on relaxing those muscles. After achieving relaxation in your upper and lower extremities, contract the muscles in your jaw, eyes, and forehead for five seconds. Then achieve complete relaxation in your head muscles. After achieving relaxation in the head muscles, concentrate on relaxing the whole body for about five minutes. Don't allow any movement to occur to any part of your body. After approximately five minutes, arise, stretch your muscles, and experience how much better you feel.

Achieving complete neuromuscular silence in the nerves and muscles helps eliminate harmful stress. This tension-reducing program has proven successful in reducing stress and tension in hyperactive children. Clearly the words of Isaiah 26:3 still hold: "He will keep in perfect peace all those who trust in him, whose thought turn often to the Lord" (TLB).

References

Selye, Hans. *The Stress of Life.* New York: McGraw-Hill, 1976.

[CHAPTER 10]

EAT NUTRITIONALLY

For years little attention has been given to nutrition and health. Health scientists are legitimately concerned. For example, only in recent years has clinical nutrition been included as a subject in some medical schools.

Despite this lack of attention to nutrition, health professionals, as well as the general public, have been aware that water and food are second only to air in being central to life. As we become more aware of just how important water and food are to health, nutrition is coming into its own as a field of study central to our health and well-being.

Nutrition is of such broad influence that it is defined as all the interactions between food and the body. Nutrition is concerned with the way food is produced, with any changes that occur in it before it is eaten, and with the way the body uses food until it is either built into body tissues or excreted. This includes the study of digestion, absorption, and transportation of nutrients to and from cells and the way in which nutrients are used within the many types of cells.

A nutrient is a substance in food that is used by the body for normal growth, reproduction, and health maintenance. Nutrients are the basic materials from which the body is constructed and by which it is fueled and regulated.

Unfortunately, most Christians do not instinctively eat foods that contain the nutrients they need. This is understandable because deciding which foods are the most beneficial to eat is a challenge. Many contradictory views are presented in our media. How can anyone know what is accurate? For example, you may read different points of view on whether nutrition affects such conditions as cancer or heart disease. Or, you may read that eating certain foods will enhance the performance of an athlete. Sorting out which information is valid and applicable to you is difficult.

This chapter is based on careful scientific investigation. There are still many gaps in the knowledge base in nutrition, and we will endeavor to point out the limits of what is known.

Chemical Elements in the Human Body

The human body is made of elements that must be obtained mainly from nutrients. It is possible to learn what substances are important for maintaining the body by analyzing what it contains.

There are 105 elements (chemicals) found on earth. When a body is analyzed, 27 of these substances can be identified. Oxygen accounts for 65 percent of the body's weight, carbon for 18 percent, hydrogen for 10 percent, and nitrogen for 3 percent. The remaining 4 percent of the body's weight is all the other elements together.

The body can use some of these elements only when they are consumed in chemically combined compounds. For example, hydrogen does nothing useful for the body if it is available in the form of a gas, but the body readily makes use of various compounds that contain it. If hydrogen is combined with oxygen, carbon, and other elements into specific structures such as water, carbohydrates, fats, proteins, and vitamins, the body can incorporate the hydrogen. Therefore, the body's need is not for the hydrogen per se but rather for certain compounds that contain it.

Essential Elements: The Nutrients

Humans require close to 45 specific substances that must be taken into the body. These substances are called the essential nutrients, for they are necessary for bodily functions. The nutrients are distinguished from thousands of nonessential substances that are also found in food. The nonessentials substances can either be produced within the body or are not needed by it.

The nutrients are grouped into six classes: water, carbohydrates, lipids, proteins, vitamins, and minerals. The classes of nutrients needed in the largest amounts are water, carbohydrates, lipids, and protein; for this reason they are called macronutrients. Vitamins and minerals, which are needed in small amounts, are micronutrients.

. . . deciding which foods are the most beneficial to eat is a challenge.

Three Basic Purposes of Nutrients

Nutrients have three functions in the human body: They form body structures. They provide energy. They serve as regulators of body processes.

Structure.—The expression, "You are what you eat," succinctly expresses the truth, for your body consists of materials that were created from nutrients that you or your mother, while pregnant with you, consumed. These nutrients were biochemically reconstructed to form your unique body.

Of course, this is not to say that you can completely determine what you become by what you eat. The limits of your body's physical potential are determined by your genetic makeup. The degree to which you achieve that potential is influenced substantially by nutrition.

For example, if your genes contain instructions for developing long bones, you have a chance of being taller than others whose genes do not carry that genetic information. But if you receive far less than the level of nutrients you should have as you grow, your chances of dunking a basketball may be bleak.

Similarly, if a baby is seriously deprived of adequate nutrients during periods of rapid brain growth both before and after birth, brain size may be smaller than normal. For the body to be able to generate the full extent of well-organized cells, tissues, organs, and systems for which it has the potential, it must have the appropriate level of nutrients.

Energy.—Another vital function of nutrients is to provide energy. Without energy production, life ceases. Our cell's first primary function is to produce energy.

Energy is measured in a unit of heat called a kilocalorie, which will be abbreviated in this book as kcal. (The term *calorie* is in popular use, although this usage is not technically correct, since a calorie is only 1/1,000 as large as a kilocalorie.) A kilocalorie is defined as the amount of heat needed to raise the temperature of 1 kilogram of water 1 degree Celsius—a measure of energy.

Carbohydrates, lipids, and proteins are nutrients that provide energy. These nutrients are available both from food and from your own body stores of these substances. These energy nutrients do not provide equal numbers of calories. Carbohydrates and proteins each have the potential to produce 4 cal per gram, and fat produces 9. Alcohol, which is variously classified as a nutrient or a drug, furnishes 7 cal per gram.

Regulation.—The third most important function that nutrients perform is regulation of body processes. The biochemical reactions that take place in our cells, which is called "metabolism," do not occur in random fashion; they are intricately controlled. Proteins, vitamins, and minerals are the chief nutrient regulators.

For example, many of the vitamins and minerals participate in the series of reactions needed to generate energy, although they themselves are not energy sources. If these nutrients are missing or inadequate, the body will not be as efficient a producer of energy. The result is tiredness, listlessness, limited growth, and poor health.

A listing of the essential nutrients in each of the main categories is shown in table 10.1. The nutrients listed are absolutely essential for human growth and maintenance of life. Some nutrients are present in a wide variety of foods, so there is little likelihood of a deficiency occurring. On the other hand, some are distributed in a limited number of foods and will be present in less than optimal amounts if the variety in the diet is limited. There are, however, an infinite number of ways in which foods can be combined to provide an adequate amount of these nutrients.

A comparison of the nutrient composition of five representative foods is listed in table 10.2 on page 61. From this table it is evident that water, carbohydrates, lipids, and proteins constitute 98 percent of the weight of food; and vitamins and minerals constitute an extremely small portion. However, these small amounts are enough to make the difference between a healthy, well-functioning body and one with nutritional inadequacies. Nutrients that have been identified as "problem nutrients," or those most likely to be consumed in less than recommended amounts in the United States, are indicated in table 10.1.

Although each of the essential nutrients is needed for normal body functions, the amount needed bears no relationship to the nutrient's importance. For instance, the nutritional needs of an adult man vary from 1/4,000,000 of an ounce of cobalamin (Vitamin B_{12}) to 56 grams (2 ounces) of protein.

A deficiency of a nutrient needed in extremely small amounts may cause more severe symptoms more rapidly than a deficiency of one needed in much larger amounts. For instance, iron deficiency is much more common than calcium deficiency, yet the requirement for calcium is 80 times the requirement for iron. Besides being the result of inadequate intake, nutrient deficiencies can result from increased needs, decreased absorption, or depressed use of a nutrient.

Table 10.1
Essential Nutrients as Classified in 1995

CARBOHYDRATES	MINERALS	VITAMINS
Glucose	Calcium[1]	FAT-SOLUBLE
	Phosphorous	A (retinal)[1]
FAT OR LIPID	Sodium[2]	D[3]
Linoleic Acid	Potassium	E (tocopherol)
	Sulfur	K
PROTEIN	Choline	WATER-SOLUBLE
	Magnesium[2]	Thiamin
AMINO ACIDS	Iron[1]	Riboflavin
Leucine	Selenium	Niacin
Isoleucine	Zinc[2]	Biotin
Lysine	Manganese	Folacin[2]
Methionine	Copper	Vitamin B6[1]
Phenylalanine	Cobalt	Vitamin B12[1]
Threonine	Molybdenum	Pantothenic Acid
Tryptophan	Iodine[3]	Vitamin C
Valine	Chromium	
Histidine	Vanadium	WATER
Nonessential Nitrogen	Tin	
	Nickel	
	Silicon	

[1] Most likely a problem in U.S.
[2] Potential problems.
[3] Previous problems; they have been corrected.

Table 10.2
Approximate Composition of Some Representative Foods

	Whole Milk %	Bread %	Carrots %	Chicken %	Bananas %
Water	87.0	35.8	88.2	69.0	74.0
Carbohydrates	5.0	50.4	8.4	0.0	24.0
Lipid	3.5	3.2	0.2	8.0	0.9
Protein	3.7	8.7	1.1	19.0	0.9
Minerals	0.7	1.1	1.9	1.0	1.0
Vitamins	0.1	0.1	0.1	0.1	0.1

One important factor in the development of deficiencies is how quickly body reserves are depleted in terms of dietary deficiency. This time varies from a few hours in the case of labile amino acids (easily mobilized protein reserves), which the body has virtually no capacity to store, to about 60 days for many water-soluble vitamins, to seven years for calcium. The major site of storage differs with the nutrient. For example the liver stores iron, vitamin A, and carbohydrates; the adrenal gland stores vitamin C; and bone stores calcium. For some nutrients there is no storage site. In these cases, deficiency symptoms will become evident as soon as individual cells have become depleted of the nutrient (see table 10.3).

Table 10.3
Extent of Body Reserves of Nutrients

Nutrient	Time Required to Deplete Reserves	Nutrient	Time Required to Deplete Reserves
Amino Acids	Few Hours	Niacin	60–180 days
Carbohydrate	13 hours	Riboflavin	60–180 days
Sodium	2–3 days	Iron	125 days (women)
Water	4 days		750 days (men)
Fat	20–40 days	Iodine	1,000 days
Thiamin	30–60 days	Vitamin A	90–365 days
Vitamin C	60–120 days	Calcium	2,500 days

Too Little or Too Much of a Nutrient

Every nutrient has a beneficial range of intake. To go either below or above that range can result in disaster. Both undernutrition and overnutrition are forms of malnutrition.

Too Little

If all or some of the nutrients are totally missing, the body will stop growing, fail to thrive, be more susceptible to infection, be incapable of reproduction, and eventually die. On the other hand, if all of the nutrients are present but are generally available in less-than-adequate amounts, the obvious consequences will be less severe. In children, for example, stunted growth is likely along with increased susceptibility to infection. In adults, low body weight, poor work capacity, and increased susceptibility to infection are likely.

If just one nutrient is restricted to low levels while the others are adequate, a more specific effect is likely to be apparent. For example, if your body did not get enough vitamin A over a period of years, you might begin to have reduced visual acuity at night (night blindness). Worse than that, eye damage (so serious as eventually to cause permanent blindness) could result. Although it would be unusual to see this vitamin A deficiency in people in America, thousands of people in developing countries become blind each year because of poor nutrition.

Too Much

The old saying, "If a little is good for you, then a lot must be better," does not apply in nutrition. For example, if vitamin A is consumed in much higher-than-recommended amounts for a period of many months, toxicity symptoms such as headache, nausea, and vomiting can occur. High doses can result in elevated pressure of the fluid surrounding the central nervous system, sometimes causing the condition to be mistaken for a brain tumor.

In recent years the danger of taking excessive amounts of nutrients has become more apparent. This is because concentrated nutrients can be produced inexpensively in the laboratory as pills, powders, or liquids; and many people consume overdoses thinking more is better. Although nutrient toxicities have resulted once in a while from a person eating too much food that is high in a particular nutrient, nutrient overdoses are caused much more frequently by the indiscriminate use of nutritional supplements.

An example of the danger of supplement overdose involves vitamin B_6, a nutrient formerly thought to be safe at high levels of intake. Now it is known that when vitamin B_6 is consumed for long periods of time in amounts that are hundreds or more times the recommended intake, it can cause nerve problems that make both large and small muscle control difficult. For example, reports describe people who were unable to walk unassisted and typists who complained of impaired typing skills.

This is not to say that using vitamin supplements is always

dangerous. In some situations they are beneficial if used properly, as in pregnancy. We will discuss this in detail in chapter 14.

What Are the Recommended Daily Allowances (RDAs)?

A committee funded by the U.S. government publishes recommendations concerning appropriate nutrient intake for Americans. These are called Recommended Daily Allowances (RDA). First published in 1943, RDAs have been revised nine times. The number of nutrients tabulated has grown considerably over the years. In the 1943 edition, RDAs were given only for calories; protein; vitamins A, D, B_1, B_2 , and C; niacin; calcium; and iron. By contrast, the 1980 edition gives recommended daily allowances for calories; protein; vitamins A, D, E, B_1, B_2, B_6, B_{12}, and C; niacin; folacin; calcium; phosphorous; magnesium; zinc; iodine; and iron, as well as ranges of estimated safe and adequate daily dietary intakes (recommended) of vitamin K; biotin; pantothenic acid; molybdenum; selenium; chromium; copper; manganese; fluoride; and the electrolytes sodium, potassium, and chloride. The complete 1989 RDAs are reproduced in table 10.4.

The RDA has been much misunderstood by Americans. Many do not like Uncle Sam telling them exactly what they should eat. This is not the committee's intention, and the RDAs are not commandments. The following facts will help put the RDA in perspective:

1. They are funded by the government.
2. The group that recommends them is composed of scientists such as nutritionists, biochemists, physiologists and medical specialists.
3. They are based on the latest scientific evidence and are revised about every five years to keep them up-to-date.
4. They are based on the concept that there is a range within which most healthy persons' intakes of nutrients probably should fall. But it should be noted that individual needs differ (figure 10.4).
5. They are for healthy persons only. A point of interest: medical problems alter nutrient needs. People who are recovering from infection, surgery, and wounds may need higher levels of nutrients.

The U.S. RDA

Many food products have nutrition information on their labels that refers to the "U.S. RDA." The U.S. RDA is different from the recommended dietary allowances, although it was derived from them. The U.S. RDA provides a standard that was designed for use in nutrition labeling, and the term applies to healthy people of various ages.

Table 10.4 shows the U.S. RDA. This standard was developed so that people would be able to see at a glance what relative levels of nutrients a serving of food contains, expressed as a percentage of the standard. The U.S. RDA standards were set to include the highest recommended level of intake for most nutrients on the RDA table for anybody from four years old through adulthood, except pregnant and lactating women.

First published in 1943, RDAs have been revised nine times.

Therefore, if a nutrition label states that a serving of canned corn provides 6 percent of the U.S. RDA for riboflavin, it means that four-year-olds through adults, except pregnant and lactating women, will get at least 6 percent of their RDA for riboflavin from a serving. The nutrition label must specify what serving size was analyzed.

Best Way to Receive Nutrients: Food Pyramid Recommendation

Translating the RDA guidelines into daily meal plans takes time and training. Accordingly, nutritionists and home economists in the U.S.D.A. have translated the scientific recommendations into specifications of the kinds and amounts of food needed for good nutrition. These translations, known as daily food guides, provide an easy way to make good food choices.

Scientists are not aware of any one perfect food that can supply all the RDAs. To meet all our nutritional needs, we must eat a variety of foods so that we can consume the 45 known nutrients in their proper amounts. This may best be represented by the food pyramid introduced in 1992 by the U.S. Department of Agriculture. The food pyramid replaces the four-food-group pie chart used since the early 1950s. The pyramid recommends 6–11 servings of grains and cereals, 3–5 servings of vegetables, and 2–4 servings of meats, fish, poultry, dried beans, eggs, and nuts; fats, oils, and sweets are to be eaten sparingly (see page 167).

Many foods don't fit into any of the first three layers of the pyramid. Consider butter, margarine, cream, sour cream, salad dressing, mayonnaise, jam, jelly, broth, coffee, tea, alcoholic beverages, synthetic products, and others. These items are grouped into a miscellaneous category. Some of them do contribute some nutrients to the day's intake. However, either they are not foods, their nutrient content is not significant in enough of the nutrients characteristic of a food group, or their nutrient content has been greatly diluted by fat, sugar, or water.

Table 10.4
Recommended Dietary Allowances (RDA)
National Academy of Sciences

The Recommended Dietary Allowances (RDA) are a set of nutrient standards established by the Committee on Dietary Allowances. The RDA are the average daily intakes of energy and nutrients considered adequate to meet the needs of most healthy people in the United States under usual environmental stresses. They were designed for the maintenance of good nutrition. People are urged to base their diets on a variety of common foods in order to obtain other nutrients for which human requirements have been less well defined.

Age (yr)	Weight (kg)	Weight (lb)	Height (cm)	Height (inches)	(kcal) Energy	(g) Protein	(ug RE) Vitamin A	(ug) Vitamin D	(mg TE) Vitamin E	(ug) Vitamin K	(mg) Vitamin C	(mg) Thiamin	(mg) Riboflavin	(mg NE) Niacin	(mg) Vitamin B6	(ug) Folate	(ug) Vitamin B12	(mg) Calcium	(mg) Phosphorus	(mg) Magnesium	(mg) Iron	(mg) Zinc	(ug) Iodine	(ug) Selenium
Infants																								
0.0–0.5	6	13	60	24	650	13	385	7.5	3	5	30	0.3	0.4	5	0.3	25	0.3	400	300	40	6	5	40	10
0.5–1.0	7	20	71	28	850	14	375	10	4	10	35	0.4	0.5	6	0.6	35	0.5	600	500	60	10	5	50	15
Children																								
1–3	13	29	90	35	1300	16	400	10	6	15	40	0.7	0.8	9	1.0	50	0.7	800	800	80	10	10	70	20
4–6	20	44	112	44	1800	24	500	10	7	20	45	0.9	1.1	12	1.1	75	1.0	800	800	120	10	10	90	20
7–10	28	62	132	52	2000	28	700	10	7	30	45	1.0	1.2	13	1.4	100	1.4	800	800	170	10	10	120	30
Males																								
11–14	45	99	157	62	2500	45	1000	10	10	45	50	1.3	1.5	17	1.7	150	2.0	1200	1200	270	12	15	150	40
15–18	66	145	176	69	3000	59	1000	10	10	65	60	1.5	1.8	20	2.0	200	2.0	1200	1200	400	12	15	150	50
19–24	72	160	177	70	2900	58	1000	10	10	70	60	1.5	1.7	19	2.0	200	2.0	1200	1200	350	10	15	150	70
25–50	79	174	176	70	2900	63	1000	5	10	80	60	1.5	1.7	19	2.0	200	2.0	800	800	350	10	15	150	70
51+	77	170	173	68	2300	63	1000	5	10	80	60	1.2	1.4	15	2.0	200	2.0	800	800	350	10	15	150	70
Females																								
11–14	46	101	157	62	2200	46	800	10	8	45	50	1.1	1.3	15	1.4	150	2.0	1200	1200	280	15	12	150	45
15–18	55	120	163	64	2200	44	800	10	8	55	60	1.1	1.3	15	1.5	180	2.0	1200	1200	300	15	12	150	50
19–24	58	128	164	65	2200	46	800	10	8	60	60	1.1	1.3	15	1.6	180	2.0	1200	1200	280	15	12	150	55
25–50	63	138	163	64	2200	50	800	5	8	65	60	1.1	1.3	15	1.6	180	2.0	800	800	280	15	12	150	55
51+	65	143	160	63	1900	50	800	5	8	65	60	1.0	1.2	13	1.6	180	2.0	800	800	280	10	12	150	55
Pregnant					+300	60	800	10	10	65	70	1.5	1.6	17	2.2	400	2.2	1200	1200	320	30	15	175	65
Lactating																								
1st 6 mo.					+500	65	1300	10	12	65	95	1.6	1.8	20	2.1	280	2.6	1200	1200	355	15	19	200	75
2nd 6 mo.					+500	62	1200	10	11	65	90	1.6	1.7	20	2.1	260	2.6	1200	1200	340	15	16	200	75

Table 10.5
Recommended Numbers of Servings from the Food Pyramid

Food Group	Serving/Day (Adults)	Sample Foods and Serving Size	Main Nutrient Contributions
Milk and Milk Products	2[1]	1 c (8 oz) milk; 1 c yogurt; 1½ c cottage cheese; 2 c ice cream; 1 c milk pudding; 1–2 oz. cheese	Calcium, Protein Riboflavin, Zinc Vitamin B_{12}[2]
Fruits and Vegetables	4[3]	½ c fruit, vegetable, or juice; 1 medium apple, orange, banana, or peach	Vitamin A[4] Vitamin C[4] Folacin
Grains (Whole-grain and enriched bread and cereal products)	4[5]	1 slice bread; ½ c cooked cereal or 1 c (1 oz) ready-to-eat cereal; ½ hamburger bun or hot dog bun or English muffin; ½ c cooked rice, grits, macaroni or spaghetti; 2 tbsp. flour; 6 saltines; 1 6-inch tortilla	Additional amts. of Niacin, Iron, Thiamin[6] in whole grains, fiber, Zinc
Meat and Meat alternatives	2	2–3 oz. cooked meat, fish, or chicken; ¼ c tuna; 2 eggs; 4 tbsp. peanut butter; 1 c cooked legumes; ½ c nuts	Protein, Iron, Riboflavin, Niacin, Zinc, Vitamin B, Thiamin

1 For children up to 9, 2–3c; for children 9–12, 3–4 c; for teenagers and pregnant women, 3–4 c; for nursing mothers, 4 c. or more; for women past 50, 3–5 c.
2 Vitamin B is contributed only by foods that come from animals.
3 One should be rich in Vitamin C; at least one every other day should be rich in Vitamin A.
4 Dark green and deep orange vegetables are especially reliable vitamin A sources; other fruits and vegetables are not. For Vitamin C, citrus fruits, green leafy vegetables, and selected other fruits and vegetables are superior sources.
5 Enriched or, preferably, whole-grain products only. Whole grains include wheat, oats, barley, rye, bulgur.
6 One serving is not a significant source of one of these nutrients, but if the recommended four or more servings are eaten, they contribute significant quantities to the diet. This group also contributes most of the complex carbohydrates of the diet. Whole-grain products are highly recommended in place of refined enriched products.

Foods can also fulfill psychological needs. Moods and emotions, for example, can affect eating behaviors.

The Modified Four Food Group Plan

Recently, the USDA introduced the modified four food group plan. Since the four food group plan was originally devised, many more nutrients have been discovered and studied. A test of the plan as real people apply it shows that a person can follow all its guidelines and still fail to meet the day's needs for some of the nutrients, especially vitamin B_6, magnesium, zinc, and vitamin E. Iron is also a problem, as it has been from the beginning.

Below is a modification of the four food group plan devised to solve these problems. It recommends:

1. Two servings of milk and milk products (as before).
2. Two servings of meat, fish, or poultry (serving size 3 ounces, not 2–3 ounces).
3. Two servings of legumes and/or nuts (serving size ¾ cup), to provide more of the vitamin B_6, magnesium, zinc, vitamin E, and iron.
4. Four servings of fruits and vegetables.
5. Four servings of whole-grain products for more of those same nutrients. Enriched products are not acceptable.
6. One serving of fat or oil (vitamin E).

Most solutions of food based on this plan would supply 100 percent of the recommended amounts of all nutrients for men and all except iron for women. This plan would miss providing a woman's full recommended amount of iron by only 10 percent. Because this plan is high in calories, it restricts the user's freedom to choose luxury items such as desserts or other sweets. But this disadvantage is outweighed by the advantage of a virtual guarantee of diet adequacy.

What Shapes Our Eating Behaviors?

Before we can take a closer look at how to change our eating behaviors, we must direct our attention toward what shapes our eating behavior.

Physiological Influences

Certainly hunger is the signal that our body needs fuel for energy, growth, repair, and maintenance. Physiological needs vary with factors such as age, sex, metabolic rate, health status, level of physical activity, pregnancy, lactation, hormonal secretions, use of drugs, and disabilities. Illness, diseases, and related treatments may physiologically influence eating, though not always appropriately. These factors may alter the number of calories or the specific nutrients needed.

Psychological Influences

Foods can also fulfill psychological needs. Moods and emotions, for example, can affect eating behaviors. Children are told that foods will make them feel better. Still wanting to feel better, adults eat to relieve tension, boredom, and depression. Food is also used as a reward in our society. Children who are quiet or well-behaved may be given a candy bar. Likewise, adults who have completed a difficult task may be rewarded with a dinner in their favorite restaurant. Additionally, some foods are eaten to fulfill the need for self-esteem. For example, we might order steak, lobster, or snails at a restaurant to impress others with our knowledge, money, or good taste. Even serious eating disorders such as anorexia nervosa, bulimia, or obesity can develop from fulfilling psychological needs with the overindulgence or deprivation of food.

Environmental Influences

Various environmental influences affect our food choices, including exposure to food-related customs and traditions, ethnic factors, religious factors, parental and peer influence, and merchandising and marketing techniques. Let's look at each of these factors.

Food-related customs and traditions.—Each person associates particular foods with customs and traditions. Thanksgiving dinner, for instance, may always include turkey. Birthdays mean having cake and ice cream. Breakfast on the weekends may always involve pancakes and fresh fruit. Food association based on tradition or custom becomes integrated into our eating behaviors and is often passed from one generation to the next.

Ethnic factors.—Ethnic background strongly shapes our eating behavior. For instance, beans and corn are often associated with Mexico, rice with China, tomato sauce and pasta with Italy, beef and potatoes with England, and pastry with France. Individual preferences often result from early exposure to these foods at home. Today we can experience many different ethnic foods through cookbook recipes, international restaurants, food festivals, and friends from different ethnic backgrounds.

Religious factors.—Religious background may also influence what people eat. For example, individuals who belong to the orthodox Jewish faith abstain from eating pork and shellfish, and members of Seventh-Day Adventist faith observe a vegetarian diet. As Christians, whatever we eat or drink, we should do it to show honor and glory to God (see 1 Cor. 10:31).

Parental and peer influence.—Until we leave home, our parents usually influence what we eat, when we eat, and how much we eat. Parents are not only responsible for our early exposure to foods but also for our psychological responses to food. During adolescence, peers become a powerful influence over our eating behavior. Whether we choose to bring a lunch from home or buy a lunch at school often depends on what our friends do. Certainly society's alcohol consumption is directly related to that of peers.

Merchandising and marketing techniques.—The food industry is highly competitive, and billions of dollars are spent each year to market old food products. Research may be done to see if a new food product is acceptable to consumers. As a product evolves, consumers test it for taste, smell, texture, and other sensory perceptions. Suggestions are then incorporated into the development of the final product. Once the test market approves, packaging and marketing begin.

Advertising is a powerful tool to influence potential consumers. Consider these advertising budgets for 1996:

Nabisco Cookies	$45 million
Mars Candy	$150 million
Coca-Cola	$355 million
McDonalds	$595 million

A large portion of the advertising budget for many products is devoted to television. This is not surprising, since the average American watches 25 hours of television per week. In supermarkets, marketing strategies are at work in the placement and display of products. For example, children's cereals are always placed at their eye level. Food packaging may tout "fat free" or "natural" ingredients. Some have added natural sounding names in an effort to entice health-conscious buyers.

Both the affordability and the availability of foods affect whether we use them. The price of food may limit our ability to purchase it. Buying items in the supermarket to make meals from scratch is usually cheaper than buying more convenient, prepackaged items; and eating out may cost between 3 and 10 times as much as preparing the same meal at home. Even so, more than one in every three food dollars is spent eating out. Less than one fourth of all lunch meals are eaten at home. As consumers, we must constantly weigh the value of our time against the extra cost of convenience. Furthermore, convenience may also have nutritional costs to consider.

How Can You Change Your Eating Habits?

Although personal and social factors must be taken into consideration when we attempt to change our eating behavior, commitment is based first on making ourselves accountable for our food choices. Many times we convince ourselves and others that someone or something beyond our control makes us act the way we do. For example, one student who lived in a dorm and ate in the dorm cafeteria said that he was gaining weight because most of the cafeteria food was fried. Many housewives remark that, although they want to eat lower-fat meals, their families would rebel against any change. They feel defeated before they try any changes. Although these are difficult situations, each of us can take control of what we eat.

With self-discipline and God's help, we can change our lifestyle and choose the proper foods.

A major step in taking responsibility for ourselves is to realize we make choices that impact our physical, mental, social, and spiritual well-being. If you are not moving toward your nutritional goals, you have the power, the right, and the responsibility to choose differently. Realizing that you have a choice can help you plan your strategy for change. Consider Paul's words: "For God has not given us a spirit of timidity, but of power and love and discipline" (2 Tim. 1:7). With self-discipline and God's help we can change our lifestyle and choose the proper foods.

U.S. Dietary Guidelines

This basic set of dietary guidelines developed from increasing public interest in nutrition and health beginning in the 1960s and the resulting Senate investigations in the 1970s of hunger and nutrition in the U.S. They are based on a growing concern about chronic health problems in an aging population and a rapidly changing food environment. The initial U.S. Dietary Goals of 1977 were revised somewhat in 1985 and 1990. These seven statements emphasize health promotion through risk reduction. Of course, no guideline can guarantee health, and people differ in their food needs. But these general statements can lead persons to evaluate their food habits and move toward basic improvements.

Eat a variety of foods.—About 45 different known nutrients and probably additional as yet unknown factors are needed to maintain health. No single food can supply all the essential nutrients in the amounts needed. Thus the greater the variety of foods used, the less likely a person is to develop either a deficiency or an excess of any single nutrient. One way to ensure variety, and with it a balanced diet, is to select foods each day from all the major food groups.

Increasing the use of less-refined, complex carbohydrates will help increase dietary fiber.

Maintain healthy weight.—Excessive fat is associated with some chronic disorders such as hypertension, heart disease, diabetes, cancer, and low back pain. The ideal body weight, however, must be determined individually; for many factors are involved, such as body composition, body metabolism, genetics, and physical activity.

Choose a diet low in fat, saturated fat, and cholesterol.—Americans as a population have traditionally consumed a high-fat diet. In many peoples, excess fat leads to high levels of blood fats and cholesterol carried in lipoprotein compounds. Elevated serum levels of these fats and cholesterol are associated with a higher risk of coronary heart disease. Americans are wise to cut down on fats in general, using them only in moderation.

Choose a diet with plenty of vegetables, fruits, and grain products.—Complex carbohydrate foods (starches) are better fuel sources for energy than are simple carbohydrates (sugars) and fats. Starches also contain many essential nutrients and calories needed for energy. With an increased use of processed and refined foods, most Christians in this country have a diet that is relatively low in dietary fiber. Increasing the use of less refined complex carbohydrates will help increase dietary fiber. Evidence exists that certain types of dietary fiber may help control chronic bowel diseases, contribute to improved blood glucose management for persons with diabetes millitus, and bind dietary lipids such as cholesterol. Starches, especially forms with more dietary fiber, may therefore be sustained for some of the fats and sugars as energy sources.

Use sugar only in moderation.—The major health hazard from eating too much sugar is tooth decay (dental caries). Contrary to popular opinion, however, too much sugar does not in itself cause diabetes. It may contribute to the cause, and it does contribute to poor control of diabetes in persons who have inherited the disease. Most Americans consume a relatively large amount of sugar, over 120 pounds per person per year. Much of this sugar occurs in processed food products. Again moderation is the key.

Use salt and sodium only in moderation.—Excessive sodium (more than 3,000 mg per day) is not healthy for anyone and certainly not for persons who have high blood pressure. In general, since many processed food products contain considerable sodium or salt and since most Americans eat more sodium than they need, it is wise to limit the use of these products, especially salty ones, and reduce added salt in food preparation. These practices will lower individual salt tastes, which are learned habits and not biologic necessities. There is ample sodium as a natural mineral in foods to meet usual needs.

If you drink alcohol, do so in moderation.—Alcohol offers no physiological benefits to the cell. It can contribute to chronic liver disease, throat and neck cancers, heart disease, and brain damage. Alcoholic beverages tend to be high in calories and low in nutrients which can lead to obesity. If you must drink alcohol, moderation is the key.

[CHAPTER 11]

UNDERSTANDING THE CARBOHYDRATES

In recent years, carbohydrates have earned a rather schizophrenic reputation. One commonly held belief is that they are fattening; many weight-reduction diets in the popular press include only limited amounts of high-carbohydrate foods. On the other hand, athletes (who are also concerned about controlling body weight) are counseled about the benefits of a high-carbohydrate diet.

Part of the confusion may come from the inaccurate belief held by some people that carbohydrates are especially high in calories. Other problems may arise from the fact that there are several types of carbohydrates. Sugars, starches, and fiber are all forms of carbohydrates; and each has somewhat different characteristics and functions. General statements about carbohydrates are often inaccurate because they may not be true of all forms.

Carbohydrates are a major source of food energy for most people. Americans obtain approximately half of their energy requirements from carbohydrates. Since carbohydrates are generally an inexpensive source of food energy, the consumption of carbohydrates is conversely related to income. In poorer countries, 80 to 90 percent of people's food energy may come from carbohydrates.

As a whole, the human body derives most of its energy needs from plant carbohydrates, the most abundant organic substance on earth. By means of photosynthesis, all green plants convert carbon dioxide and water, with the assistance of sunlight and chlorophyll, into carbohydrate and oxygen. Plant carbohydrate exists in two forms: the woody structure or cellulose, and the plant's sugar and starch storages. The relative amount of sugar and starch stored in plant foods depends on the plant's maturity (as in the ripeness of a fruit) and environmental conditions such as temperature, humidity, acidity, moisture, fertility, contamination, and storage conditions. For example, recall how the sweet taste of fruits changes after a period of storage.

We ingest most of our carbohydrates from sugar and the starch in grains, vegetables, and fruits, though some carbohydrates are also available in milk and dairy products. Whether it comes from a plant or the milk of a dairy animal that has eaten green plants, a carbohydrate is always made up of carbon, hydrogen, and oxygen in the ratio of 1:2:1. The chemical formula for glucose is $C_6H_{12}O_6$. Because there are two molecules of hydrogen to one of oxygen, as in water (H_2O), the term *carbohydrate* literally means "hydrated carbon" (that is, water attached to carbon).

Types of Carbohydrates

Chemically, there are many different kinds of carbohydrates. The major categories are monosaccharides, oligosaccharides, polysaccharides, and organic acids. Monosaccharides are considered to be the simplest carbohydrate molecules, for they cannot be hydrolyzed or "split" into simpler forms.

Sometimes reactive hypoglycemia merely means that a person has waited too long between meals.

When a carbohydrate contains many units and each unit is made up of 2–10 monosaccharides chemically joined, it is called an oligosaccharide or disaccharide. In polysaccharides, the repeating units contain hundreds to thousands of monosaccharides. Either in the laboratory or in the intestine, the individual units of oligosaccharides can be hydrolyzed so that all the monosaccharides are released and exit in their free forms.

Organic acids are also carbohydrates, since their carbon, hydrogen, and oxygen units exist in the ratio of 1:2:1. However, most consumers are not aware of this form of carbohydrate. For example, citric acid, tartaric acid, and others are common organic acids occurring in many foods we eat.

The Simple Sugars—Monosaccharides

One of the principal roles of carbohydrates in the diet is to supply energy in the form of glucose. Six common sugars are found in foods—glucose, fructose, galactose, sucrose, lactose, and maltose. A number of other sugars are familiar to the users of special dietary products, notably the sugar alcohols—maltitol, mannitol, sorbitol, and xylitol.

Glucose.—Glucose, also known as blood sugar, is found free in fruits, vegetables, and honey. However, these foods provide only about 18 grams of glucose per day, which is only a small fraction of the glucose used daily by the body. Glucose is the main source of energy for the central nervous system (CNS), which includes the brain and nerve fibers. The CNS uses about 140 grams (9 tablespoons) of glucose per day. Red blood cells need about 40 grams (3 tablespoons). This extra glucose comes from the breakdown of more complex carbohydrates or from some amino acids.

Glucose is the only form in which carbohydrates can be transported in the blood to all the tissues such as muscles, heart, and lungs. These tissues also rely on glucose to serve as a major source of energy. Usually the body tries to keep at least 100 milligrams of glucose per 100 ml of blood by converting carbohydrate stores or some amino acids into glucose. This minimal supply of glucose is sometimes referred to as the fasting glucose level. After a meal, however, when the carbohydrate in the diet is digested and the monosaccharides are absorbed, the amount of glucose in the blood will rise and then gradually fall as the glucose is removed from the blood by the tissues to meet their immediate energy needs or to be stored for future use.

Whenever the amount of glucose in the blood increases above 160 mg/100 ml, a person is described as having hyperglycemia, or too much sugar in the blood. Hyperglycemia occurs most often in people suffering from diabetes when the hormone insulin is not produced fast enough by the pancreas to help cells remove glucose from the blood. Under these circumstances the blood glucose levels get so high that the kidneys, which usually reabsorb glucose so that it will not be lost, cannot keep up. The result is that sugar spills over into the urine. When this loss of glucose occurs, more urine must be produced to dilute the glucose being excreted; and urination is more frequent. A person who urinates more frequently feels thirsty because of the need to replace the fluids being lost. As a result, the symptoms of diabetes are high blood glucose levels, glucose in the urine, thirst, and frequent urination.

When blood glucose levels fall below 60 mg/100 ml, the condition is known as hypoglycemia. In addition to feeling hungry, people with low blood glucose levels can also experience weakness, sweating, and light-headedness. Hypoglycemia is not a disease but rather a symptom (like fever) by which other diseases can be diagnosed.

A mild form of hypoglycemia sometimes called *reactive hypoglycemia* occurs from time to time in almost everyone. Sometimes reactive hypoglycemia merely means that a person has waited too long between meals. Reactive hypoglycemia results when the cells have taken up the blood glucose faster than it can be replaced from the liver, where reserves of carbohydrates are stored. It tends to occur several hours after eating and lasts only a short time.

Reactive hypoglycemia may also occur after eating a diet high in carbohydrates, especially simple sugars that are absorbed rapidly. This causes a sudden increase in blood glucose, which in turn signals the pancreas to produce more insulin and release it into the blood. The insulin travels to the cells and stimulates them to take up more glucose from the blood quickly. Sometimes the pancreas overreacts and continues to produce insulin longer than necessary. This overreaction causes the cells to take up too much glucose, which causes the blood glucose levels to fall to a low level. Symptoms usually include a lack of neuromotor coordination. Because this form of hypoglycemia occurs after eating, it is sometimes known as *postprandial* (*post,* meaning "after," and *prandium,* meaning "meal") *hypoglycemia.*

In spontaneous hypoglycemia the pancreas constantly puts out too much insulin which causes low blood glucose levels. This occurs whether or not there has been a surge of glucose into the blood to stimulate the pancreas. The symptoms are the same and indicate that the brain and nerves, which can use only glucose as a source of energy, are literally starved and are reacting by sending out distress messages.

Because symptoms such as anxiety, weakness, and dizziness are common to both reactive and spontaneous hypoglycemia, many people are misdiagnosed as having true hypoglycemia when they do not.

Sorbitol is a reduced form of glucose. It has had one hydrogen atom added. Sorbitol is found in fruits such as apples, pears, and peaches and in several vegetables. Because it is absorbed from the intestine into the blood at about one third the rate of glucose, sorbitol permits blood glucose levels to remain above fasting levels for a longer time following a meal, thus delaying the onset of hunger sensations. It may be included as an ingredient in weight-reducing aids. However, in some people sorbitol causes flatulence (gas produced in the colon) and diarrhea, which greatly reduces its acceptance. Sorbitol is also used extensively in chewing gum because it is less likely to lead to dental cavities.

Fructose.—Fructose is also known as fruit sugar or levulose. It occurs naturally in many fruits and berries and makes up over one third of the sugar in honey. Recently, scientists have been able to use enzymes to produce crystalline fructose and a high fructose corn syrup (HFCS) from cornstarch or from sucrose. Crystalline fructose and HFCS are sweeter per calorie than sugar and were first used commercially in the early 1970s. They are now being used in a large number of processed foods, especially beverages.

Fructose does not cause a rise in blood sugar in the diabetic because insulin is not required for it to be taken up by the cell. However, we have not had enough experience with diets high in fructose to be sure that it is entirely safe as a sugar replacement for diabetics. We do know that it is less likely to be cariogenic (tending to cause tooth decay) than other sweeteners. Dental caries are produced when bacteria in the mouth act on carbohydrate to produce acid. Acid production depends on the type of carbohydrate available.

Galactose.—Galactose, the third monosaccharide, occurs only as a result of the digestion of the disaccharide lactose, which is the sugar in milk. Galactose is the only monosaccharide obtained primarily from animal foods. Galactose does not occur free in nature; it is always bonded to something else, but it is freed during digestion. Glucose, fructose, and galactose are the three monosaccharides (simple sugars) common in foods.

The Double Sugars—Disaccharides

The three disaccharides found in food are sucrose, lactose, and maltose. They are formed when one unit of the monosaccharide glucose is combined with one unit of either fructose, galactose, or glucose. For example, (1) sucrose = glucose + fructose; (2) lactose = glucose + galactose; (3) maltose = glucose + glucose.

After we eat these sugars, they are broken down to monosaccharides so they can be small enough to be absorbed through the intestinal wall. This can occur when the disaccharide comes into contact with acid or when an enzyme facilitates the split.

The average amount of added sucrose consumed in the U.S. per person per day is 81 grams (about 3 ounces or 6 tablespoons).

Sucrose.—Sucrose, or table sugar, is the most familiar of the three disaccharides. Sugar cane (70%) and sugar beets (30%) are two sources from which it is purified and granulated to various extents to provide the brown, white, and powdered sugars available in the supermarket. Brown sugar is 97 percent sucrose and is made by adding some molasses to white sugar.

The average amount of added sucrose consumed in the U.S. per person per day is 81 grams (about 3 ounces or 6 tablespoons). There is some concern that the increase in total sweetener (sucrose plus HFCS) to 125 grams per person may have adverse health consequences.

Lactose.—Lactose is the principal carbohydrate of milk, making up about 5 percent of its weight. Lactose serves to enhance the absorption of calcium. A human baby is born with the digestive enzymes necessary to hydrolyze lactose into its two monosaccharide parts, glucose and galactose, so that they can be absorbed. Babies can digest lactose at birth, but they don't develop the ability to digest starch until they are several months old. This is one of the many reasons breast milk and formula are such good foods for babies; they provide simple, easily digested carbohydrates which supply the right amount of energy.

Many adults, especially those of Asian or African ancestry, suffer from a deficiency of the enzyme *lactase*, which is produced normally in the wall of the intestine and is essential for the conversion of dietary lactose to glucose and galactose. This lactase insufficiency results in lactose intolerance. If the lactose in the intestine is not rapidly hydrolyzed and absorbed, then numerous small sugar molecules remain in the intestine undigested, attract water, and cause fullness, discomfort, cramping, nausea, and diarrhea. The lactose also becomes food for intestinal bacteria, which multiplies and produces irritating acid and gas, making a person more sick.

People who can't or won't drink milk urgently need to find another food source of the calcium and riboflavin it provides in abundance. The availability of enzymes produced by yeasts and molds makes it possible for lactose-intolerant people to drink milk. When those enzymes, which are available in tablet form, are mixed with milk, they split lactose into glucose and galactose before the milk is ever consumed. Thus, the lactose never reaches the colon.

Maltose.—The third disaccharide is found at only one stage in the life of a plant. When the seed is formed, it is packed with starch-glucose units strung together in long arrays to be used as fuel for the germination process. When the seed begins to sprout, an enzyme cleaves the bonds between pairs of glucose units, making maltose. Another enzyme then splits the maltose units into two glucose units, which are then absorbed into the blood. Thus maltose, like other disaccharides, contributes glucose to the body.

The Complex Carbohydrates—Polysaccharides

While the sugars contain three monosaccharides in different combinations, the polysaccharides are composed almost entirely of only one—glucose. The difference between them has to do with the ways glucose is condensed into the large molecules of starch, glycogen, and cellulose.

> Nutritionally the body does not discriminate among starches.

Starch.—As a chemist sees it, starch is a long or branched chain of hundreds of glucose units connected together. A starch molecule may contain as many as 2,000 glucose units (one with 26,000 units has been identified). These giant molecules are packed side by side in the rice grain or potato tuber, as many as a million in a cubic inch of food. In addition, each of these starches has unique characteristics of solubility, thickening power, and flavor. Nutritionally the body does not discriminate among starches. The body is able to break down all cooked starches into their component glucose units for absorption and use by the body cells.

All starchy foods are, in fact, plant foods. Grains (rice, corn, oats, wheat, barley, rye) are the richest source. A second important source of starch is the legume (beans and peas) family, including peanuts and dried beans such as butter beans, kidney beans, baked beans, black-eyed peas, and soybeans. These legumes are not only rich in starch but also contain a significant amount of protein. A third major source of starch is the tubers, such as the potato, yam, and cassava. Usually, one to four hours after a meal, all the starch has been digested and circulated to the cells as glucose.

Glycogen.—Animals store a limited amount of carbohydrate as the polysaccharide glycogen, primarily in the liver and in the muscle. These are the two animal tissues besides milk and blood that contain carbohydrates. The adult human stores only about 340 grams of glycogen, which is enough to last about one half of a day. One third of the glycogen is stored in the liver, and two thirds is stored as muscle glycogen.

Glycogen is more complex and more highly branched than starch. Its structure permits rapid breakdown. Enzymes can attack all the branches of glycogen simultaneously, producing a surge of energy for emergency action.

Cellulose.—The third polysaccharide of importance in nutrition is cellulose. Cellulose, like starch, is found abundantly in plants and is composed of glucose units connected in long, branching chains. However, the bonds holding its glucose units together are not digestible by human enzymes; only bacteria enzymes can digest them. Cellulose is not, therefore, of much significance as an energy source for humans but is of great importance as one of the food fibers, which we will discuss in detail.

The Fibers

Two types of fiber are found in food—crude fiber and dietary fiber. Cellulose is the major component of crude fiber. It provides the structural framework for all plant material; that is, it gives the shape to a carrot, a bean, or a squash. Cellulose is the most abundant organic compound in the world, being found in fruits, vegetables, and whole-grain cereals as well as wood and leaves. Like starch, it is composed of many glucose units. Unlike starch, however, these units are linked together in such a way that human digestive enzymes are unable to break them apart to form separate glucose units; nor can the chemist digest them with acid in the laboratory.

In addition to cellulose or crude fiber, several other complex carbohydrates and related compounds, pectins, and hemicelluloses resist digestion. Together these are known as dietary fiber. In summary, crude fiber is the portion of a plant that resists chemical breakdown, whereas dietary fiber is any material that remains undigested in the intestine. When nutrition scientists talk about fiber, they are referring to dietary fiber. *Crude fiber* is an outmoded term. Other outmoded terms for dietary fiber include *roughage* and *bulk.*

Dietary fiber can be further classified as soluble and insoluble fiber. Soluble fiber found in fruits, some legumes, and

In countries whose populations ingest low-calorie, high-fiber diets, there is evidence of growth retardation primarily due to negative zinc-balance.

grains, such as oats, rye, and barley, dissolves in water to form a gel. This gel slows the rate at which digested food passes through the large intestine and thus increases the rate of absorption. Soluble fiber also binds cholesterol from the bile and prevents its reabsorption and recirculation in the blood, accounting for its effectiveness in controlling or lowering blood cholesterol levels. Also soluble fiber may act by binding the bile acids that normally promote the absorption of dietary cholesterol, thus causing less to be absorbed. Oat fiber appears to be more effective than fibers from other cereals in reducing cholesterol absorption.

In contrast, the insoluble fiber found in vegetables and wheat bran that consists of cellulose, hemicellulose, and legnins does not dissolve in water. Instead, it tends to absorb water and increase bulk, contributing to the volume of the stools. This helps keep the food moving through the gastrointestinal tract, especially the colon, and prevents constipation and diverticulosis.

Why do we need fiber in our diet?—Dietary fiber supplies mass to the feces, making elimination easier. When enough fiber is consumed, the stool will be large and soft because many types of plant fibers attract water. The large size stimulates the intestinal muscles, which aids peristalsis. Consequently, less pressure is necessary to expel the larger stool. The stool may also have a tendency to float in water.

When eating too little dietary fiber, the opposite can occur: The stool may be small and hard. Constipation may result, which may force one to exert high pressures in the large intestine during defecation. These high pressures can force parts of the large intestine wall to pop out from between the surrounding bands of muscle, forming small pouches. A person can have many of these pouches, called diverticula. About 50 percent of elderly people have diverticula. Hemorrhoids (dilated veins in the anus) may also result from excessive straining during defecation. If the diverticula become filled with food particles, such as hulls or seeds, bacteria can metabolize these food particles into acids and gases. The acids and gases irritate the diverticula and may eventually cause them to become inflamed. This condition is known as diverticulitis. Antibiotics may be needed to counter the bacterial action, and dietary fiber intake will be reduced to limit further bacterial activity. Once the inflammation subsides, a high dietary fiber intake (but free of seeds) is begun to ease stool elimination and reduce the risk of a future attack. In the past low fiber diets were recommended after an attack, but research has shown that high-fiber diets work much better.

Can we eat too much fiber?—In countries whose populations ingest low-calorie, high-fiber diets, there is evidence of growth retardation primarily due to negative zinc-balance. All fibers bind positive ions, such as zinc, calcium, and magnesium. There is always the danger that a diet too high in fiber will lead to a mineral imbalance. It is easy to overshoot fiber in the diets of certain groups such as elderly people, whose energy intake is normally low. In addition, some people can tolerate more fiber than others. In any case, if you want to increase fiber consumption, do so gradually because your body needs time to learn to deal with the added bulk and to let you know when enough's enough. If the change is made too fast, your body will complain by producing gas and bloating.

How much dietary fiber do we need?—Expert panels convened in Canada and the United States arrived independently at similar suggestions for fiber intake. They proposed that it be geared to energy intake and recommended 10–13 grams of fiber per 1,000 calories. This amount would provide 20–35 grams of dietary fiber for a healthy American adult. The ratio of insoluble to soluble fiber should be about 3:1, as it is in nature. The same panels suggested that the fiber we eat come from the grocery and not the pharmacy.

How can we increase our dietary fiber?—Before increasing your dietary fiber intake, first calculate the amount of fiber you are already eating. If it is less than 20–35 grams per day, find some higher-fiber foods to substitute for foods you already eat, or add some new ones (see table 11.1). Eating a high-fiber cereal for breakfast is one possibility. It's better to eat whole food sources over bran supplement sources because foods can provide a broader variety of nutrients. This is especially true for many natural high-fiber foods such as whole-grain breads and cereals. The way you check for whole grains is to read the label. Manufacturers are now listing enriched white flour as wheat flour on food labels. Most people think that if "wheat bread" is on the label they are getting a whole-wheat product. This is not so; the label must say whole-wheat flour in the ingredient list (stone-ground whole wheat is best). If it does not say whole-wheat flour, it is not whole-wheat bread and so probably will not contain as much dietary fiber as it could. See table 11.2 for tips on increasing dietary fiber.

Table 11.1
Dietary Fiber Value for Fiber-Containing Foods

Food Group	Serving	Calories	Dietary Fiber(g)
Fruits			
Apple	1 medium	80	3.5
Apricot, fresh	3 medium	50	1.8
Apricot, dried	5 halves	40	1.4
Banana	1 medium	105	2.4
Blueberries	½ cup	40	2.0
Cantaloupe	¼ melon	50	1.0
Cherries	10	50	1.2
Dates, dried	3	70	1.9
Grapefruit	½ cup	40	1.6
Orange	1 medium	60	2.6
Peach	1 medium	35	1.9
Pineapple	½ cup	40	1.1
Prunes, dried	3	60	3.0
Raisins	¼ cup	110	3.1
Strawberries	1 cup	45	3.0
Breads and Cereals			
100% bran	½ cup	75	8.4
Air-popped popcorn	1 cup	25	2.5
All Bran	⅓ cup	70	8.5
Brand Buds	⅓ cup	75	7.9
Bran Chex	⅔ cup	90	4.6
Corn bran	⅔ cup	100	5.4
Cracklin' Oat Bran	⅔ cup	110	4.3
Bran flakes	¾ cup	90	4.0
Grapenuts	¼ cup	100	1.4
Oatmeal (cooked)	1 cup	144	2.2
Whole-wheat bread	1 slice	60	1.4
Legumes, Cooked			
Kidney beans	½ cup	110	7.3
Lima beans	½ cup	130	4.5

Food Group	Serving	Calories	Dietary Fiber(g)
Vegetables, Cooked			
Beans, green	½ cup	15	1.6
Broccoli	½ cup	20	2.2
Brussels sprouts	½ cup	30	2.3
Cabbage	½ cup	15	1.4
Carrots	½ cup	25	2.3
Cauliflower	½ cup	15	1.1
Corn	½ cup	70	2.9
Green pepper	½ cup	12	0.8
Green peas	½ cup	55	3.6
Kale	½ cup	20	1.4
Lettuce	1 cup	7	0.8
Parsnip	½ cup	50	2.7
Potato, with skin	1 medium	95	2.5
Tomato, chopped	½ cup	17	1.5

Table 11.2
Tips on Increasing Fiber in Diet

Try This	Instead of This
Whole-wheat bread	White bread
Brown rice	White rice
Baked potato in the skin	Mashed potatoes
Unpeeled apple (or applesauce made with unpeeled apples	Regular applesauce
Orange segments	Orange juice
Whole-grain cereals (hot or ready to eat)	Sweetened cereals
Popcorn (lightly seasoned with butter or salt, if at all)	Potato chips
Bean dip	Sour cream dip
Kidney beans on salad	Bacon bits on salad

How the Body Uses Carbohydrates

All carbohydrates are converted into glucose which each cell of the body uses. Cells can't use lactose, sucrose, or starch; they require glucose. The task of the digestive system, then, is to disassemble the disaccharides and polysaccharides to monosaccharides, to absorb these into the blood, to convert the glucose not already in the form of glucose, and to transport the glucose to the cells. The cells then have three options: They may store this glucose as glycogen, split the glucose for energy, or convert it to fat. Let's see how the body does all three.

Storing Glucose as Glycogen

Glycogen is the body's form of stored glucose. If the blood delivers more glucose than the cells need, the liver and muscles take up the surplus. The muscles hoard two thirds of the body's total store of glycogen and use it themselves during intensive exercise. The liver stores the other one third, making it available when the brain or other organs need to draw on the supply. God wondrously designed glycogen for its task. Instead of having long straight (amylose) or branched (amylopectin) chains like starch, which are cleaved one unit after the other during digestion, it is highly branched, so that hundreds of ends stick out at the surface. On the tip of each chain is a glucose whose attachment to the next glucose is easily accessible to the glycogen-splitting enzymes. When quick energy (glucose) is needed by the cells, a hormone (epinephrine) floods the bloodstream. Thousands of enzymes within the liver cells respond by attacking a multitude of ends simultaneously and releasing an abundance of glucose into the blood for use by all the body's cells. This response is part of the body's defense mechanism in time of danger.

Splitting Glucose for Energy

The main function of the simple sugar, glucose, is to supply energy for the body. Certain tissues in the body derive energy only from glucose, such as the red blood cells and most parts of the brain. Some people refer to glucose as the "brain's food."

Body fat can never regenerate glucose to feed the brain. This is one reason fasting can be dangerous and low-carbohydrate diets are also dangerous.

Inside the cell, glucose breaks in half, releasing some energy. These halves have two pathways open to them. They can be put back together to make glucose, or they can be further broken apart into smaller fragments. If they are broken into smaller fragments, they can never again be used to form glucose. They can yield still more energy and in the process break down completely to carbon dioxide and water, or they can be hitched together into units of body fat.

Body fat can never regenerate glucose to feed the brain. This is one reason fasting can be dangerous and low-carbohydrate diets are also dangerous. When there is a severe carbohydrate deficit, the body has two problems.

First, having no glucose, the body has to turn to protein to make some. This action diverts protein from vitally important functions such as producing antibodies, muscle tissue, and cellular structures. Protein's importance to the body is so great that carbohydrates should be kept available precisely to prevent this use of protein for energy. This is called the protein-sparing action of carbohydrate. Therefore, if you do not eat enough carbohydrates to yield that glucose, your body is forced to make it from other nutrients, such as proteins. This process is termed gluconeogenesis, which means "production of new glucose." Proteins (amino acids) usually provide carbon atoms for these new glucose molecules.

Second, without a sufficient amount of carbohydrate, the body can't use its fat in the normal way. This is because carbohydrates are needed to combine with the fat fragments so they can be used for energy. Amino acids from the proteins in muscles, heart, liver, kidneys, and other vital organs supply the carbon atoms needed to make the glucose. If the process occurs over weeks, the body has to go into ketosis, which means using fat without the help of carbohydrate. Without sufficient carbohydrates, carbon dioxide (CO) and water (H_2O) molecules are not formed during fat metabolism. Instead, fats are turned into ketones. Ketosis during pregnancy can cause brain damage and irreversible mental retardation in the infant, but even in adults it is a condition to avoid.

The amount of carbohydrate needed to ensure complete sparing of body protein and avoidance of ketosis is around 100 grams a day in an average-size person. This has to be digestible carbohydrate (not fiber), and considerably more than this minimum is recommended. In fact, the dietary goals state that an intake of available carbohydrate (starch and sugar), which might be ideal to support long-term health, should be 55 to 60 percent of total calories. A person consuming 1,500 calories a day should therefore have 825–900 calories of carbohydrate, or about 200 to 225 grams. A person consuming 3,000 calories a day should have twice that, or 400–450 grams. Most of this would be starch, with its accompanying fiber; some would be the naturally occurring sugars of fruits, vegetables, and milk; only 10 percent or less would be concentrated sugar. The recommended intakes of 200–500 grams of carbohydrate a day are generous in comparison with the minimum amount of carbohydrate necessary to spare protein. They are even more generous in comparison with the "less than 60 grams" recommended by most low-carbohydrate diets.

Regulating This Energy Source in the Bloodstream

Before we discuss the third way the body uses glucose (converting glucose to fat), let's look at how glucose is regulated in the bloodstream. The maintenance of a normal blood glucose level depends on two types of safeguards. First, when the level gets too high, it can be corrected by siphoning off the excess into liver and muscle glycogen. Second, when the level gets too low, it can be raised by the hormone *glucagon.*

The correction of a too-low level has already been mentioned. The hormone epinephrine is involved in bringing about the release of glucose from liver glycogen. Other hormones also act in this manner, including some that promote the

The simple sugars have a number of different names and are hidden in many products that don't necessarily taste sweet.

conversion of protein into glucose. However, the liver can store only half a day's worth of glycogen; then the available supply is depleted. As for protein, none can be spared without cost. When body protein is used, it has to be taken from muscle, organ, or blood proteins. No surplus of protein is stored for emergencies. As for fat, you have already seen that it can't regenerate glucose.

Under normal circumstances, blood glucose usually varies between 70 and 120 milligrams per 100 milliliters of blood. If blood glucose rises above 160 milligrams, it begins to spill over into the urine. If blood glucose falls below 40–60 milligrams, a person begins to feel nervous, irritable, and hungry and may develop a headache. Having high levels of blood glucose is called hyperglycemia. Having low levels of blood glucose is called hypoglycemia.

If you eat a meal high in concentrated sugar, your blood glucose concentration may rise too high, so that the pancreas oversecretes insulin and drives glucose into the cells too fast. Then the blood glucose level may fall too low or too fast. This effect is called the glycemic effect of foods. Certain carbohydrate foods are absorbed more quickly than others, producing a sudden rise in blood glucose.

Most people have had the impression that simple sugars produce a major surge in blood glucose while complex carbohydrates produce a flatter response curve, but now we know that the case is not so simple. The effects of different foods on blood glucose apparently depend on many factors:

- The digestibility of the starch in the food.
- Interactions of the starch with the protein in the food.
- The amount and kinds of fat, sugar, and fiber in the food.
- The presence of other constituents, such as molecules that bind starch.
- The form of food (dry or liquid, coarsely or finely ground, etc.).

All these factors working together produce the food's glycemic effect, and it is not always what a person might expect. Ice cream, for example, produces less of a response than potatoes.

The glycemic effect of a food is important to people with abnormalities of blood glucose regulation, notably diabetes and hypoglycemia. Such people are wise to avoid foods that have been studied; the ones with the lowest glycemic indexes appear to be legumes, especially lentils. In fact, lentils taken for breakfast have a moderating effect on blood glucose that extends even through lunch.

The way you eat can help your body keep a happy medium between the glycemic extremes. Two guidelines apply. First, when you are hungry, you should eat and not wait until you are famished. Second, when you do eat, you should eat a balanced meal, including some protein and fat as well as complex carbohydrate. The fat slows down the digestion and absorption of carbohydrate, so that it trickles gradually into the blood, providing a steady, ongoing supply. The protein elicits the secretion of glucagon, whose effects are generally opposite to those of insulin; and this reduces insulin's effect.

Converting Glucose to Fat

After the glycogen stores are full and the cell's immediate energy needs are met, the body takes a third path for using carbohydrate. Let's say you are eating potato chips and drinking soda pop while watching a baseball game (Chicago Cubs) on television. If your digestive tract is delivering glucose from the potato chips and soda to the liver, the liver will break the extra energy compounds into smaller fragments and put them together into the more permanent energy-storage compound—fat. The fat is then released, carried to the fatty tissues of the body, and deposited there. Unlike the liver cells, which can only store about half a day's worth of glycogen, the fat cells can store unlimited quantities of fat. Moral: You had better play the game if you are going to eat the food.

Sources of Carbohydrate

Many foods contain carbohydrate; it is present in all parts of the food pyramid. Carbohydrate can also be found in groups known as "limited extras," in which various sweeteners are placed. The sources are divided into groups for discussion: simple carbohydrate and complex carbohydrate.

Simple Carbohydrate

Derived from sugar beets and sugarcane, affordable table sugar has been available for about one hundred years. As the technique for refining sugar improved, table sugar was produced in large quantities. The refining process shreds, strains, boils, centrifuges, dissolves, clarifies, filters, crystallizes, and dries sugarcane and sugar beets into a concentrated end product known as raw sugar. Raw sugar is not commonly used due to contaminants in the

Table 11.3
Some Hidden Sources of Sugar

Food	Size Portion	No. Teaspoons Granulated Sugar
Cakes and Cookies		
Angel food	1 (4 oz. piece)	7
Cheesecake	1 (4 oz. piece)	2
Chocolate cake	1 (4 oz. piece)	10
Poundcake	1 (4 oz. piece)	5
Strawberry shortcake	1 (4 oz. piece)	4
Brownie	1 (¾ oz.)	3
Chocolate cookies	1	1½
Fig Newtons	1	5
Oatmeal cookies	1	2
Chocolate eclair	1	7
Doughnut (glazed)	1	6
Candies		
Hershey chocolate bar	1 (1½ oz.)	2½
Chewing gum	1 stick	1/2
Chocolate mints	1 piece	2
Gumdrop	1	2
Hard candy	4 oz.	20
Lifesavers	1	½
Peanut brittle	1	3½
Canned Fruits and Juices		
Canned fruit juices	½ cup	2
Canned peaches	2 halves	3½
Fruit salad	½ cup	3½
Dairy Products		
Ice cream	⅓ pt. (3½ oz.)	3½
Ice cream bar	1	5
Ice cream cone	1	3½
Ice cream soda	1	5
Ice cream sundae	1	7
Malted milk shake	1 (10 oz.)	5

Food	Size Portion	No. Teaspoons Granulated Sugar
Jellies and Jams		
Apple butter	1 T	1
Jelly (grape, strawberry, etc.)	1 T	5
Orange marmalade	1 T	5
Strawberry jam	1 T	4
Desserts		
Apple cobbler	½ cup	3
Blueberry cobbler	½ cup	3
Custard	½ cup	2
Jello	½ cup	4½
Apple pie	1 slice	7
Cherry pie	1 slice	10
Cream pie	1 slice	4
Lemon pie	1 slice	7
Pumpkin pie	1 slice	5
Banana pudding	½ cup	2
Chocolate pudding	½ cup	4
Rice pudding	½ cup	5
Tapioca pudding	½ cup	3
Sherbet	½ cup	9
Soft Drinks		
Cola drinks	1 12oz.	9
Ginger ale	1 12oz.	10
Root beer	1 12oz.	7
Seven-up	1 12oz.	10
Soda pop	1 12oz.	10
Sweet cider	1 12oz.	12
Syrups and Icings		
Brown sugar	1 T	3
Chocolate icing	1 oz.	5
Corn syrup	1 T	3
Granulated sugar	1 T	3
Honey	1 T	3
Karo syrup	1 T	3
Maple syrup	1 T	5
Molasses	1 T	3½
White icing	1 T	3

The average per capita consumption of sugar is about 25 teaspoons per day. Children eat even more sugar, with much of their intake originating from soft drinks, fruit drinks, and sugared cereals.

product, and it must be sanitized.

In the U.S. consumption of sugar averages 18 percent of each person's calories, or about 154 pounds per person each year. Most people don't believe that they eat that shocking amount. However, the simple sugars have a number of different names and are hidden in many products that don't necessarily taste sweet. When you are in the supermarket someday, check labels for the following terms, which equate with simple sugars: honey, brown sugar, dextrose, sucrose, maltose, molasses, fructose, levulose, corn syrup, and high fructose corn syrup.

Some products contain more sugar than one might expect. For example, table 11.3 shows the number of teaspoons of sugar that can be found in some commonly eaten foods. A 12-ounce can of soft drink contains 9–12 teaspoons, and a banana-split ice-cream sundae has a whooping 25 teaspoons. The average per capita consumption of sugar is about 25 teaspoons per day. Children eat even more sugar, with much of their intake originating from soft drinks, fruit drinks, and sugared cereals. Soft drinks are now the number-one beverage used in the U.S. The annual per capita consumption in 1997 was 51 gallons—2.5 times the consumption in 1962. It is alarming to note that soft drinks, pastries, and sugar contribute almost 20 percent of the total carbohydrate intake in America.

Complex Carbohydrate

Complex carbohydrate is rich in starch, fiber, or both. Starch and fiber are usually found together in unprocessed foods, and the food is referred to as "whole." Whole starches have not been concentrated or separated from the plant food. Legumes (dried beans and peas), fruits, vegetables, and whole grains can be found in this category.

Dietary Guidelines for Carbohydrate

The dietary guidelines for carbohydrate suggest the following changes in food selection and preparation:

1. Increase the consumption of whole fruits and vegetables and whole grains. Decrease consumption of juices, which usually have the fiber removed. The recommended servings from high-fiber, complex carbohydrate food groups are: Whole-grain products (4–6 servings per day); fresh fruits (2–3 servings per day); vegetables (2–5 servings per day); and legumes (3 servings per week).

2. Don't remove edible peels from fruits or vegetables unless absolutely necessary. Wash fruits and vegetables well.

3. When choosing breads, cereals, pasta, crackers, and other grain products, look for the term *whole* before the listing of the grain. The term *enriched* before the grain indicates that the product is refined and probably contains little fiber.

4. Read ingredient labels and screen for sugars and refined carbohydrate. Remember that the ingredients are listed by amount on the label, with the larger amounts in the product listed first.

5. Drink more water. Soft drinks are high in sugar, so substitute juices and beverages in which you can control the amount of sugar that is added (e.g., lemonade).

6. Choose cereals, drinks, fruits, and desserts that allow the individual to add sugar. Add sugar sparingly.

7. Include legumes in your diet.

God's story of carbohydrate turns out to be a cycle. Carbon dioxide, water, and energy are combined in plants to form glucose. The glucose may be stored in the polysaccharide starch. Then, in the body, the starch becomes glucose again, and this may be stored as the polysaccharide glycogen. Ultimately, the glucose delivers the sun's energy to fuel the body's activities; the waste products, carbon dioxide and water, are excreted to be used again by a plant, which completes the cycle. "And the earth brought forth vegetation, plants yielding seed after their kind, and trees bearing fruit, with seed in them, after their kind; and God saw that it was good" (Gen. 1:12).

[CHAPTER 12]

Understanding the Lipids

Have you ever thought about eating a hamburger without mayonnaise, mashed potatoes without the gravy, or perhaps a salad with just vinegar and herbs? The usual toppings on these foods consist of a large proportion of lipid (fats).

Lipids (from Greek *lipos* meaning fat) are an integral part of our diet, adding flavor and nutrients to the foods we eat. However, they have recently received a bad reputation for being the related cause of several chronic diseases as well as providing hidden calories to our foods. Nonetheless, God made lipids essential to our diet.

Lipids are fatty substances that usually do not dissolve in water but do dissolve in ether. Fats (solid lipids) and oils (liquid lipids) are general terms that apply to many members of the lipid group. Traditionally fat has held a prominent place in the American diet. We have maintained a relatively rich fare in our basic food patterns with approximately 45 percent of our total caloric intake coming from fat, more than any other country in the world.

Although recommendations remain somewhat controversial, dietary guidelines encourage Americans to reduce the amount of fat consumed. After water and carbohydrate, the most plentiful nutrient in the American supply is lipid. Some sources of lipid are easily recognized as visible fats and oils such as the fat surrounding meat, butter, margarine, and salad oils. These sources, however, account for less than half of the lipid in the diet; the rest is invisible fat. Invisible fat includes fat that is marbled throughout meat fibers, dispersed in finely divided form in egg yolk or homogenized whole milk, and found in whole-grain cereals and nuts.

Your Body Needs Fat

We need fat in our food and in our bodies to keep us healthy. This need is indicated by the number of functions fat performs in nutrition, both in our diets and in our overall body metabolism. Lipids have seven important functions.

Supply fuel source.—Fats supply a basic continuing source of fuel for the body to store and burn as needed for energy. Food fat yields 9 cal/g when oxidized in the body, whereas carbohydrates and protein yield 4 cal/g. Body fat, which is called adipose tissue, is energy stored in compact form.

Provide essential nutrients.—An essential nutrient in lipids is a compound called *linoleic acid.* If children do not get enough of this essential fatty acid, their growth will be impaired. If your diet is deficient in linoleic acid for many months, your skin will become scaly and rough. Fortunately, linoleic acid is widespread in the food supply, so most people who eat a varied diet are likely to fulfill their own needs.

Carry fat-soluble vitamins into the body.—Vitamins A, D, E, and K are absorbed into the body much more easily if they are dissolved in fat.

Provide components for body structures.—Lipids are necessary components of cell membranes, some hormones, nerve coverings, vitamins, and some digestive secretions. In fact, cholesterol is lipid that performs a variety of these functions. It is important to keep in mind that cholesterol, which has had so much negative publicity, is a necessary substance. It is so important that God made our bodies in such a way that they actually produce it, usually in a larger amount than we consume in our diets. Fat serves a vital constituent of the cell membrane structure, helping transport nutrient materials across the cell membranes. Fat also surrounds nerve fibers which help provide electrical insulation and transmit nerve impulses.

Insulate the body thermally.—If you are of average weight, roughly half of the adipose tissue in your body is just under the skin and is called subcutaneous fat. Located there, it constitutes an internal blanket that helps hold in your body heat. Whether you consider this an advantage or a disadvantage depends on how much subcutaneous fat you have and the usual temperature of your environment.

> Fats in the diet supply flavor to food, which contributes to a feeling of satisfaction that lasts longer after eating than do the feelings of satisfaction after eating carbohydrates.

Protect vital organs.—A weblike padding of adipose tissue surrounds vital organs such as the kidneys, protecting them from mechanical shock and providing a supporting structure.

Produce food satiety.—Fats in the diet supply flavor to food, which contributes to a feeling of satisfaction that lasts longer after eating than do the feelings of satisfaction after eating carbohydrates. This satiety (a feeling of fullness) is enhanced by the fuller texture and body that fat contributes to food mixtures and the slower gastric emptying time it brings.

What Are the Types of Lipids?

Lipids are categorized according to their structural similarities. We will examine glycerides, phospholipids, and sterols. They are of major importance because of their prevalence in the diet and body and their implications for health.

Glycerides

Glycerides are the most common forms of lipids. By definition, glycerides consist of a molecule of the three-carbon compound glycerol to which one, two, or three fatty acids are attached. They are called monoglyceride, diglyceride, and triglyceride. Triglycerides account for about 95 percent of the weight of lipids in foods; fats and oils are largely triglycerides. Mono- and diglycerides also occur in nature, as do some unattached or "free" fatty acids.

Even though the name of these compounds draws attention to the glycerol portion of the lipid molecule, the attached fatty acids are the components responsible for giving different glycerides their characteristics. Fatty acids differ from one another most significantly in their chain length and in their degree of saturation.

Chain length refers to the number of linked carbon atoms in the fatty acid skeleton. Chain length is significant because the shorter the fatty acid chains, the more likely a glyceride is to be liquid at room temperature. For example, milk fat has many short-chain fatty acids. Triglycerides with long fatty acids, such as those found in red meats, are solid at room temperature. Fatty acids may have anywhere from 4 to 22 carbons. Oleic acid, the most common fatty acid, has 18 carbons in its chain.

A characteristic with even more far-reaching significance than chain length is the degree of saturation. Saturation refers to the number of hydrogen atoms attached to the carbons in the fatty acid skeletons. If the fatty acid chain can accommodate more hydrogen than it currently does, the fatty acid is said to be unsaturated, and the unsaturated carbons will be connected by double bonds.

Triglycerides containing mostly SFAs (saturated fatty acids) are usually solid at room temperature and are generally found in animal products such as beef fat and butter. Triglycerides containing mostly PUFAs (polyunsaturated fatty acids) are usually liquid at room temperature and are generally found in plant products such as cottonseed oil and corn oil. Notable exceptions to this generalization are that coconut and palm oils, which are plant oils commonly used in processed foods, contain a high proportion of SFAs. Another exception is fish oils, which might be expected to contain primarily SFAs but, in fact, contain many PUFAs.

Phospholipids

Phospholipids are compounds that resemble triglycerides except that a phosphorous-containing unit is substituted for one of the fatty acids. Lecithin, a common and important group of phospholipids found in cell membranes, have the biologically useful characteristic of mixing well with both watery and oily substances, which is an unusual trait that few types of lipids have. This property classifies them as emulsifiers (substances which break up fats).

Sterols

Sterols are unlike other lipids in the organization of their carbon, hydrogen, and oxygen components. Nonetheless, they qualify as lipids because of their physical insolubility in water and solubility in ether.

Undoubtedly the most well-known sterol is cholesterol, a

compound produced by animals, including humans. Cholesterol is found particularly in eggs and organ meats such as liver. Although cholesterol and saturated fats are lipids typically found in animal products, they are distinctly different from each other. Cholesterol will be discussed in detail later in the chapter.

Digestion, Absorption, and Transport of Lipids

In this section we will focus on only two of the many varieties of lipids transported into the body. Triglycerides are discussed because they are the most common lipid in foods (95%), and dietary cholesterol is included because of the current concern about heart disease.

The Small Intestine

Bile is the first of these substances. It is made in the liver, stored in the gallbladder, and released into the small intestine upon the entrance of triglycerides. Bile is composed of cholesterol, lecithin, and bile salts (sterols). Large droplets of triglycerides are emulsified, or broken down into smaller droplets, by bile. This increases the surface area that can be exposed to digestive enzymes.

Lipase is a digestive enzyme produced in the pancreas and small intestine. They break down the triglycerides into glycerol, fatty acids, and monoglycerides. These products are then incorporated with bile salts in a package called a micelle. Micelles deliver their contents of the intestinal cell membrane for transport into the body.

Dietary cholesterol is usually attached to a fatty acid in foods. This is first removed in the small intestine by lipase; then cholesterol can be incorporated into the micelles. Again the micelles deliver the cholesterol to the intestinal cell for transport into the body.

The absorption of triglycerides depends on the availability of bile salts. If sufficient quantities are present, 97 percent of all fat will be absorbed. In contrast, only 50 percent of cholesterol is commonly absorbed. Its absorption depends on the presence of micelles to move it into the intestinal cells.

Transport from the Intestine

There are two mechanisms for the transport of the products of lipid digestion into the bloodstream, based on the solubility of these products in water. The blood is a water medium and can therefore transport only water-soluble forms of lipid material.

Glycerol and fatty acids with short- and medium-length chains are water soluble. They may be transported from the cells of the small intestine directly to the liver, moving through bloodstream via the portal vein.

Long-chain fatty acids, cholesterol, and phospholipids are insoluble in water. If they were to enter the bloodstream, they could potentially clump together and clog blood vessels. A water-soluble packaging must therefore be constructed for transport. The long-chain fatty acids are reformed into triglycerides and packaged along with cholesterol, phospholipids, and protein. The result is a soluble aggregate known as a lipoprotein. This particular type of lipoprotein is approximately 85 percent triglyceride and is called a chylomicron. Chylomicrons are the principal lipoprotein made in the intestinal wall. They are released into the lymphatic system and soon link with the bloodstream. The fate of the triglycerides in the chylomicrons is that they will be used for energy production or for storage as fat in muscle, adipose, or liver tissue.

Transport Between Body Tissues

The level of lipids in the bloodstream is not only determined by those absorbed by the intestine but also by those released from the liver. The liver can take fatty acids directly from the bloodstream or synthesize them from other nutrients, such as glucose, amino acids, or alcohol. These fatty acids are combined with glycerol to form triglycerides. The triglycerides are packaged with cholesterol, phospholipids, and protein before being released to the bloodstream. These protein packets are known as lipoproteins and are necessary to allow lipids to move through the water medium of the blood.

LDL is often referred to as "bad cholesterol" because it may be taken up by muscle cells in arteries, and it has been implicated in the development of atherosclerosis.

There are three major lipoproteins in addition to the chylomicrons.

Very low density lipoprotein (VLDL).—These consist mainly of triglycerides that are being transported to provide fatty acids and glycerol to tissues.

Low density lipoprotein (LDL).—They contain a high proportion of cholesterol. LDL transport cholesterol from the liver to other body cells. LDL is often referred to as "bad cholesterol" because it may be taken up by muscle cells in arteries, and it has been implicated in the development of atherosclerosis, a hardening of the arteries that leads to coronary heart disease, strokes, and other diseases.

High density lipoprotein (HDL).—HDL is dense because it is made up of a large proportion of protein. It also contains a high proportion of cholesterol; however HDL transports cholesterol in an opposite direction from LDL. HDL removes cholesterol from peripheral tissues and returns it to the liver for possible degradation. This function is beneficial to the prevention of atherosclerosis and coronary heart disease; therefore, HDL is often referred to as "good cholesterol." We will discuss cholesterol and heart disease later in the chapter.

Recommendations for Fat Intake

There are no RDAs for fat. A good goal is to consume about 4 percent of energy from plant oils in order to get the essential fatty acids (linoleic acid and alpha-linoleic acid). The RDA suggests that people need to consume 1–2 percent of their total calories from linoleic acid. Currently Americans consume about 7 percent. Up to 10 percent of calories from polyunsaturated fatty acids is generally recommended as a safe upper level. Since plant oils (corn, soybean, cottonseed, sunflower, and safflower oils) all contain over 50 percent of fatty acids as linoleic acid, they should supply about 4 percent of our total calorie intake. On a 2,500-calorie diet this corresponds to 1 tablespoon of plant oil per day.

The RDA also suggests that in the future an allowance for omega-3 fatty acids should be considered. Leading researchers support this suggestion. They think that diet planning should include a regular supply of alpha-linoleic acid or its related omega-3 form eicosapentenoic acid (EPA). This would essentially require weekly consumption of fatty fish, such as salmon, tuna, and sardines, or canola or soybean oil. All are good sources

Table 12.1
Dietary Cholesterol and Saturated Fat in Foods

Food	Amount	Percent Calories from Total Fat	Percent Calories from Saturated Fat	Cholesterol (mgs.)
Fruits		Low	Low	0
Vegetables		Low	Low	0
Grains		Low	Low	0
Nuts		High	Moderate	0
Avocado		88	17	0
Coconut, dried		88	76	0
Milk, nonfat	1 cup	—	—	5
Milk, low fat	1 cup	30	17	22
Cottage cheese (4%)	½ cup	35	20	24
Cheese pasteurized	1 oz	73	40	25
Cream (half & half)	¼ cup	79	58	26
Ice cream, regular	½ cup	49	27	27
Cheese, cheddar	1 oz.	72	40	28
Milk, whole	1 cup	48	27	34
Butter	1 tbsp	100	55	35
Margarine	3 tbsp	100	18	0
Tuna, canned	3 oz.	38	10	55
Chicken, cooked	3 oz.	19	6	74
Pork, cooked	3 oz.	73	26	76
Beef, cooked	3 oz.	77	37	80
Lamb, cooked	3 oz.	61	34	83
Egg, yolk	one	71	43	210
Liver, fried	2 oz.	43	13	273

Source: U.S. Department of Agriculture, Food Handbook

of omega-3 fatty acids.

The U.S. diet contains about 40–45 percent of total calories as fat. Vegetable sources supply about half this fat, and animal sources supply the other half. Major sources of fat in the U.S. diet include animal flesh, whole milk, and pastries.

The ratio of saturated to monounsaturated to polyunsaturated fatty acids in the U.S. diet is about 42:40:18, respectively. Sometimes the ratio of polyunsaturated fatty acids to saturated fatty acids (P:S ratio) is calculated for a diet. The P:S ratio for the U.S. diet is 18:42, or about 0.43. A ratio of 1 is generally recommended to reduce the risk of heart disease.

The American Heart Association (AHA) recommends a fat intake of 30 percent of total calories, with a ratio of about 10:10:10 for saturated to monounsaturated to polyunsaturated fatty acids (ratio of 1). The AHA further recommends lowering fat intake to 20 percent of total calories in cases where elevated serum cholesterol level does not respond to this moderate recommendation. The National Cholesterol Education Program, established in 1985, recommends reducing saturated fatty acids to 7 percent of total calories if a high serum cholesterol level does not respond to reducing it to 10 percent. By encouraging a reduction in total fat and saturated fat intake, all these suggestions are in line with the Dietary Guidelines for Americans.

What Are Some Sources of Fats in the Diet?

The first step in improving lipid consumption is to know which foods are high or low in triglycerides, the main source of lipid. The top five foods eaten in the U.S. that contribute the most fat to an average adult's diet are burgers, hot dogs, whole milk, doughnuts, and beef steaks. Three out of the five are meats. On a typical day, almost 30 percent of adults eat a hot dog, ham, or lunch meat; 26 percent consume burgers; and 23 percent have at least one serving of steak or roast beef.

Table 12.1 reveals the percentage of calories from fat in various food choices. In general, whole fruits and vegetables have little or no fat, with avocados and olives being notable exceptions (about 80 percent of their calories is fat). Red meats, whole-milk dairy products, and eggs contain considerable amounts of fat. Other sources of dietary fat are more obvious, such as gravies, butter or margarine, salad dressings, mayonnaise, sour cream, creamed soups, and sauces.

Saturated Fat

The AHA recommends a 30–50 percent reduction in the amount of saturated-fat calories that Americans currently eat. This will take considerable effort. A person who now eats 2,200 calories per day would have to consume no more than 220 calories, or 25 grams, as saturated fat. Table 12.2 shows the number of grams of saturated fat in some commonly eaten foods.

Most foods that contain fat have a combination of saturated and unsaturated fats. Some general rules apply for pinpointing foods that are made up of more saturated than unsaturated fats. Saturated fats are usually solid at room temperature. For example, think about the fat surrounding a piece of steak; it doesn't melt at room temperature. Some saturated fats are surrounded by watery mediums, and this particular property is not obvious—whole milk, for instance.

Most foods that contain fat have a combination of saturated and unsaturated fats.

Saturated fat tends to raise blood cholesterol levels. Foods high in saturated fats include red meats, whole milk products and butter, many solid and hydrogenated (saturated) vegetable shortenings, and coconut and palm oils (which are often used in commercial baked goods).

Polyunsaturated Fat

Although polyunsaturated fats are associated with lower blood cholesterol levels, AHA guidelines recommend a maximum consumption of 10 percent of the total calories. This caution is necessary because overconsumption of polyunsaturates may be related to other diseases, like cancer.

Like most of the plant oils, polyunsaturated fats are usually liquid at room temperature. Both coconut and palm oils are highly saturated and are exceptions to the rule. They are often used in food processing because of their flavor and low cost. Safflower oil and canola oil are good substitutes for coconut and palm oil.

One group of polyunsaturated fats has been experiencing considerable publicity recently. The omega-3 fatty acids, which are commonly found in fish oils, are apparently beneficial in reducing blood pressure and blood cholesterol. The omega-3 fatty acids promote the production of one type of prostaglandin, a hormone-like substance that seems to play a regulatory role for blood pressure and blood cholesterol levels in the body. As mentioned before, cold-water fatty fish (herring, mackerel, salmon, tuna, and rainbow trout) are the best natural sources of the omega-3 fatty acids.

Consumers should not purchase supplements containing

Table 12.2
Amounts of Total Fat, Saturated Fat, and Dietary Cholesterol in Foods

	Total Fat (milligrams)	Saturated Fat (grams)	Cholesterol (grams)
Dairy Products			
Milk, whole, 1 cup	8.1	5.1	33
Milk, 2% fat, 1 cup	4.7	2.9	18
Milk, 1% fat, 1 cup	2.4	1.5	10
Skim milk, 1 cup	0.6	0.4	5
Cottage cheese, ½ cup	5.2	3.3	17
Cheddar Cheese, 1 oz.	9.4	6.0	30
Mozzarella cheese, 1 oz.	4.5	2.9	16
Sour Cream, 1 Tbsp.	2.5	1.6	5
Cream, half & half, 1 Tbsp.	1.0	1.1	6
Vanilla ice cream ½ cup	0.2	4.4	30
Vanilla ice milk, ½ cup	2.8	1.8	9
Frozen yogurt ½ cup	1.5	1.0	6
Orange sherbet ½ cup	1.9	1.2	7
Meats, Poultry, Fish, Beans, Eggs			
Beef rib roast, choice, roasted,			
2 oz. lean and fat	18.4	7.8	48
2 oz. lean only	8.1	3.5	46
Beef rump, choice, roasted,			
2 oz. lean and fat	8.9	3.5	47
2 oz. lean only	4.4	1.6	46
Ground-beef patty, cooked,			
2 oz. regular	11.7	4.6	51
2 oz. lean	10.5	4.1	49
2 oz. extra lean	9.3	3.6	48
Pork loin, lean, roasted,			
2 oz. lean and fat	13.8	5.0	51
2 oz. lean only	7.9	2.7	51
Liver, beef, cooked with fat, 2 oz.	4.5	1.6	273
Chicken, roasted, 2 oz.			
Light meat with skin	6.2	1.7	48
Light meat without skin	2.6	0.7	48
Dark meat with skin	9.0	2.5	52
Dark meat without skin	5.6	1.5	53
Turkey, roasted, without skin			
2 oz. light meat	1.8	0.6	39
2 oz. dark meat	4.1	1.4	48
Halibut fillets, broiled, 2 oz.	0.8	0.1	35
Tuna, canned, oil pack, 2 oz.	4.6	1.2	37
Great Northern (navy beans) (½ cup)	0.4	0.1	0
Canned beans without pork (½ cup)	0.6	0.2	0
Egg, large, 1			
Whole	5.6	1.7	210
Yolk	5.6	1.7	210
White	Trace	0	0

	Total Fat (milligrams)	Saturated Fat (grams)	Cholesterol (grams)
Fats and Oils			
Animal fats, 1 tbsp.			
Butter	11.5	7.2	31
Vegetable oils, 1 tbsp.			
Corn	13.6	1.7	0
Peanut	13.5	2.3	0
Safflower	13.6	1.2	0
Soybean	13.5	2.0	0
Olive	13.5	1.8	0
Coconut	13.6	11.8	0
Palm	13.6	6.7	0
Margarine			
Hard (stick)	11.4	2.1	0
Soft (tub)	11.4	1.8	0
Vegetable shortening, hydrogenated	12.8	3.9	0
Salad dressings, 1 tbsp.			
Mayonnaise	11.0	1.6	8
Italian	7.1	1.0	0
Blue cheese	8.0	1.5	3
French	6.4	1.5	0
Thousand Island	5.6	0.9	4
Selected Snacks			
Potato chips, 10	8.0	2.0	0
French fries, 10 long strips, salted	10.3	2.6	0
Corn chips, ½ cup	6.1	1.3	0
Popcorn, plain, 1 cup	0.3	Trace	0
Popcorn, salted and buttered, 1 cup	2.0	0.9	4
Saltine crackers, 4	1.4	0.3	0
Whole-wheat crackers, 4	2.2	0.5	0
Pretzels, salted, 10 thin	0.1	Trace	0
Nuts and Seeds			
Peanuts, roasted, salted, ¼ cup	17.9	3.9	0
Peanuts, dry roasted, salted, ¼ cup	17.6	3.1	0
Peanut butter, 2 tbsp.	15.3	2.8	0
Sunflower seeds, roasted, salted, ¼ cup	16.8	3.2	0
Desserts			
Chocolate chip cookies, 2	4.4	1.3	8
Frosted brownie, 1	6.6	2.2	12
Gingersnaps, 2	1.2	0.3	5
Oreo cookies, 2	4.5	1.2	8
Chocolate cupcake, 1	4.5	1.8	17
Doughnut, 1	11.2	2.8	10

Source: U.S. Department of Agriculture, Food Handbook, 1982

Margarine is made up of both hydrogenated and polyunsaturated fat. To make the best choice in margarine, choose the one that is in liquid form at room temperature.

fish oils or omega-3 fatty acids. Such extracts are expensive, have not been proven beneficial, and have not been tested for safety. Incorporating fish meals into weekly menus is a better strategy for increasing omega-3 fatty acids in the diet.

Hydrogenated Fat

Polyunsaturated liquid oil is often changed into a saturated fat (also referred to as trans-fat) by a process known as hydrogenation. The double bonds that characterize a polyunsaturated fat are broken by adding hydrogen atoms, thus creating a saturated fat. The body is not able to tell the difference between a hydrogenated fat and a saturated fat. Hydrogenated fats have the same detrimental effects on blood cholesterol as do saturated fats. Margarine, vegetable shortening, and processed foods are the major source of hydrogenated fats in the diet.

One reason the food industry changes an unsaturated fat to saturated fat is, for example, to make margarine spreadable (it would otherwise be liquid). The hydrogenated fat allows margarine to be more solid at room temperature. This property may at times be beneficial for the texture of baked or cooked products.

Why use margarine instead of butter if the hydrogenated fat in the margarine is really saturated? Margarine is made up of both hydrogenated and polyunsaturated fat. To make the best choice in margarine, choose the one that is in liquid form at room temperature. Also, check the ingredient list on the product for the term *hydrogenated* or *partially hydrogenated* corn, soybean, or another oil. If the liquid oil is listed before the hydrogenated oil, the food probably has a P:S ratio that is greater than one, which is beneficial.

Monounsaturated Fat

The AHA recommendations do not limit the percentage of calories that are derived from monounsaturated fatty acids (MUFA) above the 30 percent total fat limitation. This is based on recent research that has shown that MUFA lower total and LDL cholesterol but not HDL. This research is consistent with evidence that MUFA are safe and effective in lowering heart disease risk in Mediterranean countries. Though MUFA may be beneficial in reducing heart disease, they are still a concentrated form of calories.

Cholesterol

Cholesterol is not an essential nutrient that has to be consumed. Your liver is manufacturing it now at the rate of perhaps 50,000,000,000,000,000 molecules per second. The raw materials the liver uses to make cholesterol can all be taken from glucose (carbohydrate), amino acids (proteins), or fatty acids (fats).

After manufacture, cholesterol either leaves the liver or is transformed into related compounds like the hormones previously mentioned. The cholesterol that leaves the liver has four possible destinations:

1. It may be made into bile and move through the gallbladder into the intestine, then be recycled back to the liver.
2. It may be made into bile, move into the intestine, and then be excreted in the feces.
3. It may be incorporated into the body's cell membranes.
4. It may wind up accumulating in arteries and causing artery disease.

The first possibility is that some of the cholesterol the liver makes becomes part of the bile salts, and these are released into the intestine to emulsify fat. After doing their job, most are reabsorbed from the intestine. The cholesterol is thus recycled.

The second possibility is that, once out in the intestine, some of the bile salts can be trapped by certain kinds of soluble dietary fibers (notably pectin and gums), which carry them out of the body with feces. The excretion of bile salts reduces the total amount of cholesterol remaining in the body.

The third possibility is that cholesterol, packaged with other lipids, leaves the liver by way of the bloodstream, for transport to the body tissues. These packages are the lipoproteins. The blood carries them through all the arteries, and any tissue can extract lipids from them; some cells take them up whole. More than nine tenths of all the body's cholesterol is located in the cells, where it forms part of the multitude of external and internal membranes that make up the cell's structure and perform their work.

The fourth possibility is that, on its way into the cells from the bloodstream, cholesterol will be deposited in the artery walls. Cholesterol deposits in arteries create disease conditions leading to heart attacks and strokes.

Artificial Fats

The development of two new additional fats may help some individuals reduce their total fat consumption. Olestra™ is a calorie-free fat replacement that was formerly known as sucrose polyester. Although Olestra is a synthetic combination of sucrose and fatty acids, it is not digestible. Olestra passes through the digestive tract unabsorbed but will interfere with the absorption of dietary cholesterol and cholesterol that is being recycled from bile. This results in a reduction in blood cholesterol.

Olestra looks, feels, and tastes like dietary fat and has some similar cooking properties. It can be used in oils, margarines, snacks, and desserts. Current research suggests that Olestra is safe. Its only undesirable effect is that it interferes with the absorption of Vitamin E. For some individuals it causes gastrointestional problems. Vitamin E may be fortified in products that contain Olestra.

The second fat substitute, Simplesse,™ has been approved by the FDA. This product is manufactured from protein of egg white and milk. In a manufacturing process the protein is altered into tiny round particles that feel creamy on the tongue. Simplesse provides one and one-third calories per gram, a substantial reduction from the 9 calories per gram offered by fat. Simplesse is available only to manufacturers and is used in products such as ice cream, yogurt, sour cream, and oil-based products. Since Simplesse gels when heated, it is unsuitable for products that are heated or baked.

How Can You Cut the Fat in Your Diet?

Each person must devise his or her own plan for reducing dietary fat. Foods that contain visible fats, the ones you can see, are often the easiest to change first. These include gravies, sour cream, sauces, salad dressings, margarine, and the fat around meat.

Surprisingly though, as much as 60 percent of the fat Americans eat is invisible and can go unnoticed. The fat inside the meat (known as marbling), ice cream, cheese, baked goods, and casseroles are in this category. Both visible and invisible sources of fat need to be examined when developing a plan to reduce intake.

The following are practical suggestions for cutting down on visible and invisible fats and dietary cholesterol. Use these suggestions to develop your own plan.

Foods to Eat More Often

- **Fish and poultry** (without the skin). These are low in saturated fat, so try substituting them more often for beef, lamb, or pork.
- **Lean cuts of meat.** When you do eat red meat, choose lean cuts and trim visible fat.
- **Fruits, nuts, and raw vegetables** (except coconut and avocado). Try them as snacks.
- **Skim milk or low-fat dairy products.** Skim milk or low-fat milk and low-fat cheese offer a triple treat—less saturated fats, dietary cholesterol, and calories.

Each person must devise his or her own plan for reducing dietary fat. Foods that contain visible fats, the ones you can see, are often the easiest to change first.

- **Grains and starchy foods.** These will give you important vitamins, minerals, and fiber.
- **Liquid vegetable oils and margarine high in polyunsaturated or monounsaturated fats.** Go easy on all fats, but when you do use them, substitute these fats because they help to lower blood cholesterol.

Foods to Eat Less Often

- **Fatty luncheon and variety meats and organ meats.** Sausage, bacon, salami, bologna, liver, and kidney are high in fat and cholesterol.
- **Egg yolks.** People who are concerned about cholesterol should eat fewer egg yolks, which are particularly high in cholesterol.
- **Butter.** When you have to use fat, try a margarine that is high in polyunsaturated and/or monounsaturated fat instead.

Foods to Eat Cautiously

- **Processed and convenience foods.** Read the labels on foods, and don't assume that *cholesterol free* means "good for you." Remember that coconut and palm oils are saturated fats used in many processed foods. The terms *light, lean,* or *lower fat* may also be misleading. Interpret the label for fat content.
- **Fast foods.** Avoid deep-fried foods. Instead broil, boil, roast, or stew your food. These cooking methods help remove fat from food.

Some Health Problems Associated with Lipids

Insufficient Lipid Consumption

Insufficient lipid consumption (less than 3% of the total calorie intake) most often occurs in infants who are fed low-fat or nonfat milk or formulas made from these. Overzealous parents may also try to restrict the lipid consumption of an infant or toddler under the age of three for health benefits. Parents need to be cautioned that limitations in lipids are not meant for individuals under three years of age. Essential fatty acids are needed in the diet. This is particularly important for growth stages. If a child does not get enough of the essential fatty acids, his or her growth will be impaired. Older children and adults may only experience rough, scaly skin.

Excess Lipid Consumption

Four major threats to the health of Americans are associated with excess lipid consumption.

Obesity.—Much of the obesity today is in part due to calorie-rich foods that are high in fat. Both animal and human research studies provide evidence to support this theory.

Calories from any source can create obesity, but many researchers suggest that a high-carbohydrate, low-fat diet will help individuals remain lean or lose excess fat.

The most commonly used means of inducing obesity in laboratory rats is feeding them a high-fat diet. Lean human subjects had difficulty gaining weight on a mixed diet but gained weight easily on a high-fat diet. Research also shows that it costs the body less energy to store dietary fat as body fat (3% of ingested calories) than to store carbohydrate as body fat (23% of ingested calories).

Calories from any source can create obesity, but many researchers suggest that a high-carbohydrate, low-fat diet will help individuals remain lean or lose excess fat. See chapter 16 for a discussion on obesity and how to achieve and maintain reasonable weight.

Diabetes.—Individuals with diabetes have twice the risk of developing cardiovascular disease than those without diabetes. Therefore, a diet low in total fat, saturated fat, and cholesterol that is consistent with the American Heart Association (AHA) guidelines is recommended for individuals with diabetes. In addition, by restricting fatty foods, individuals are better able to decrease their body weight. When most individuals with diabetes lose weight, their metabolic disorder returns to normal.

Cancer.—Dietary fat is also associated with the second leading cause of death in the U.S.—cancer. A diet high in total fat may be a factor in the development of breast, colon, rectal, uterine, and prostate cancer.

Cardiovascular disease.—Cardiovascular disease is a group of heart and blood-vessel diseases that include heart attack, stroke, high blood pressure, and atherosclerosis. They are responsible for one of every two deaths in the U.S. Let's examine in detail how lipids affect cardiovascular disease.

Cardiovascular Disease

Heart disease is the major killer of North Americans. About 600,000 people die of heart disease each year in the U.S. This figure rises to almost 1 million if we include strokes and other circulatory diseases. Heart disease is a chronic disease. It takes years to develop symptoms. There is no single cause of heart disease, but many factors increase the risk for its development. What are its causes? How can it be prevented? Can it be reversed?

Atherosclerosis

The single biggest cause of heart and blood-vessel disease is atherosclerosis, or "hardening of the arteries." Atherosclerosis is characterized by plaque formation on the inner walls of the arteries (figure 12.1). One commonly accepted theory of plaque formation suggests that there is a minor injury to the lining of a blood vessel. Lipid material is deposited at the injured spot and covered by platelets, the clotting mechanism of the blood. The blood vessels in turn produce more cells to cover over this area. As the process continues, hardening (or calcification) occurs. This newly formed material is called plaque. Arteries undergoing plaque formation soon lose their ability to expand and contract, and their diameter also narrows, making blood flow more difficult.

Normally, blood surges through the arteries with each beat of the heart, and the arteries expand with each pulse to accommodate the flow. Arteries hardened and narrowed by plaque cannot expand, and so the blood pressure rises. This increased pressure puts a strain on the heart and damages the artery walls further.

There are two possible consequences to the continued plaque formation. The first is a narrowing of the artery to the point that a total blockage occurs. Any tissue beyond that point would lose its oxygen and nutrient supply. The tissue would quickly die, and if it were a large organ or one important enough to the functioning of the body, the person might die. Otherwise, varying degrees of functioning might be impaired.

Another consequence is that a blood clot could form on top of the plaque. This itself may occlude or block an artery and is known as a thrombus. A thrombus may break loose into the bloodstream, then referred to as an embolus, and can lodge in a smaller artery. This results in a sudden loss of blood to the area the artery previously supplied.

Any area of the body could be affected by atherosclerosis, but two of particular concern are the heart and brain. Interruption of blood flow to the brain results in a cerebrovascular accident, or stroke. In the heart, myocardial infarction, or a heart attack, occurs if blood flow through the coronary arteries that supply the heart muscle is blocked (figure 12.1).

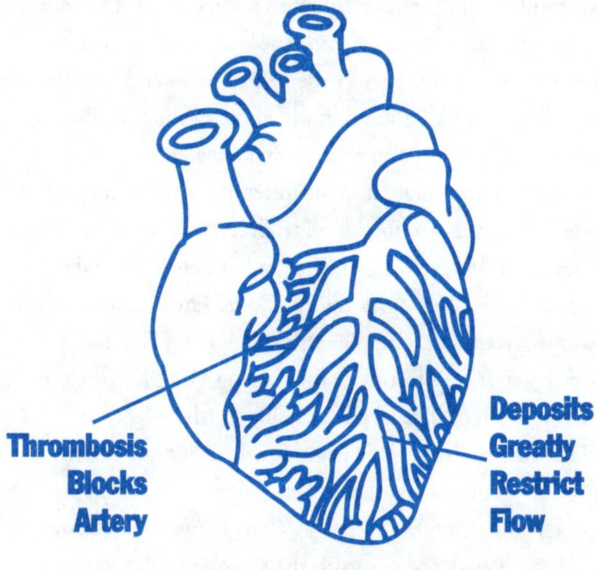

Atherosclerosis begins early. Fatty streaks have been observed in the aortas of infants less than a year old, and plaques are well developed in most individuals by the time they are 30. No one is free of the condition. The question is not whether you have it but how far advanced it is and what you can do to retard or reverse it.

Atherosclerosis takes a heavy toll among people in the productive periods of their lives, long before retirement. Many health agencies have devoted millions of hours to the battle against atherosclerosis, but so far all that can be said for sure about its cause is that it is multifactorial in origin. There are many risk factors—perhaps 30 or so in all. Extensive clinical and statistical studies have identified several risk factors for cardiovascular disease. Some of the risk factors cannot be changed, such as heredity, sex, race, and age. The three primary risk factors for heart disease are changeable—cigarette smoking, high blood pressure, and high blood-cholesterol levels. Let's examine all three.

Any area of the body could be affected by atherosclerosis, but two of particular concern are the heart and the brain.

Cigarette smoking.—The recent Surgeon General's report on the cardiovascular disease consequences of smoking has stated: "Cigarette smoking should be considered the most important of the known modifiable risk factors for coronary heart disease in the U.S." This report estimates that smokers who average one pack per day have a 70 percent greater coronary heart disease (CHD) death rate than nonsmokers. Heavy smokers who consume more than two packs per day experience death rates from CHD more than two hundred times those of nonsmokers.

Carbon monoxide, tar, and nicotine (substances found in cigarettes) are judged as the most likely contributors to the health hazards of smoking. Carbon monoxide, tar, and nicotine might cause irregular rhythms to occur in the heart rate, increase the clumping of platelets, and decrease blood-vessel-wall oxygen supply, thus increasing the coronary arteries' permeability to cholesterol. Cigarette smoking also lowers HDL cholesterol in the blood.

A person who stops smoking reduces his or her CHD death risk to that of nonsmokers within approximately 15 years. Yet every two minutes a day, 5 teenagers begin smoking.

High blood pressure.—There are several ways to reduce high blood pressure:

1. Weight reduction provides a powerful means of reducing high blood pressure. This occurs even if ideal weight is not achieved. For every pound of adipose tissue gained in weight, it takes approximately 200 miles of new capillaries to supply that extra tissue. Gaining 20 pounds requires 4,000 miles of new capillaries. Blood pressure will be affected.

2. Salt restriction may be another way of decreasing high blood pressure. Approximately 30 percent of Americans are salt (NaCl) sensitive. That is, their bodies retain sodium. Sodium (Na) causes their bodies to retain fluids in the blood vessels. This extra fluid retention in the vessels sometimes causes the blood pressure to elevate in order to circulate this extra fluid.

A major study recently demonstrated that a combination of weight loss and salt restriction allowed 39 percent of hypertensive individuals to be reclassified as normal. Several other lifestyle factors have been associated with a decrease in high blood pressure, including calcium and magnesium intake, high potassium, high dietary fiber, high polyunsaturated/saturated fat ratio, and aerobic exercise.

Regular eating habits (three balanced meals per day), an energy intake matched to energy output, and a lower total fat intake often help by lowering blood triglyceride levels.

High blood cholesterol levels.—Recently, a 12-year study concluded that a 49 percent drop in coronary heart disease incidence can be predicted for individuals who reduce their blood-cholesterol levels by 25 percent. Blood-cholesterol level is determined by analyzing a small sample of blood. A typical blood test will usually include a measurement of blood cholesterol. The average blood-cholesterol level for middle-aged adults is 215 mg/dl. This means that there are 215 mg of cholesterol in every one-tenth liter of blood. An optimal level of total blood cholesterol is 160 mg/dl, with 190 mg/dl being an attainable level for most Americans. One in every five Americans has a high blood-cholesterol level.

A more sophisticated report will include measurements of LDL and HDL cholesterol. The ratio of LDL cholesterol to HDL cholesterol (LDL-C/HDL-C) has been found to be highly predictive of heart disease risk, more so than total blood cholesterol alone. When LDL is not available, the total blood cholesterol to HDL cholesterol ratio can be used. Individuals with LDL-C/HDL-C of 2.0 or a total blood-cholesterol/HDL-C of 3.4 have about one half the heart disease risk of the average American.

If you do not currently know your blood-cholesterol level but have had a blood test recently, call your doctor to find out. You may want to request a blood test at your next visit; or take advantage of a local health fair that may be doing blood tests, provided the fair is sponsored by a hospital and trained personnel are performing the tests.

How Can You Lower Your Total Blood Cholesterol/LDL Cholesterol?

Listed below are some factors that help to lower LDL cholesterol:

1. Decrease calories from fat.
2. Decrease saturated fat.
3. Decrease dietary cholesterol.
4. Increase polyunsaturated/saturated fat ratio.
5. Increase monounsaturated fat.
6. Increase water-soluble fibers in the diet (mainly found in fruit, vegetables, grains, and legumes).
7. Lose weight.
8. Do aerobic exercise.

How Do You Raise HDLs?

An important first step in lowering a total blood-cholesterol level is not to lower the blood HDL cholesterol level. Only the LDL cholesterol level should fall. If the HDL cholesterol level does fall, an emphasis on monounsaturated fat, rather than polyunsaturated fat, is a good idea. Exercising at least 30–45 minutes 4 times a week will also protect the HDL cholesterol level and usually will even raise it. In addition, regular eating habits (three balanced meals per day), an energy intake matched to energy output, and a lower total fat intake often help by lowering blood triglyceride levels. Lowering blood triglyceride levels often results in increased HDL levels. The goal is to have fasting blood triglyceride levels below 150 mg/dL. Certain medications also act to lower triglyceride levels. When this happens, HDL levels also often increase. It is unfortunate that raising HDL levels is usually difficult. Lowering LDL levels is usually much easier.

The factors affecting the health of the heart and arteries are all tangled together. The exact relationships among them are not completely understood. Though we don't know which factors cause what, all evidence points in the same general direction. For good health and to avoid CVD, you should stop smoking; reduce blood pressure and weight, if necessary; eat a balanced, adequate, and varied diet; reduce fat intake, especially saturated fat; and do aerobic exercise. And now that you have it all under control, you can serve God longer and better.

[CHAPTER 13]

Understanding the Proteins

When you think of protein, do you picture a person who has strength, muscle mass, leanness, and can kick sand in anybody's face? Everybody knows that protein is the material of muscles and that it is important in the diet. It is associated with strength and power, and every cereal box boasts of its presence. In fact, protein has been so overemphasized that many people eat more than enough, sometimes at the expense of other nutrients that are equally important. An understanding of the quantity and quality of protein is needed to help put it in its proper place as only one of the nutrients needed in correct proportions to achieve a balanced diet.

Structure of an Amino Acid

To understand the structure of a protein, you must first examine the structure of an amino acid. An amino acid contains carbon, hydrogen, and oxygen, which makes it an organic substance. (It contains carbon.) Unlike other organic nutrients (carbohydrate and fat), amino acids also contain nitrogen as a necessary part of their structure. Sometimes they may contain sulfur as well. Every amino acid consists of an amino group which contains the nitrogen, an acid group, and a side group of one or several connected atoms, which gives the amino acid its identity.

Approximately 22 amino acids are commonly found in nature. Two amino acids are found to be rare in nature, so most physiologists classify the body with 20. Every living cell can produce some but not all of the 20, as long as it has the elemental ingredients—carbon, hydrogen, oxygen, and nitrogen. Since carbon, hydrogen, and oxygen are liberally available from other dietary sources, the cell has no trouble coming up with those elements, but it has a critical need to obtain nitrogen in order to synthesize (make) amino acids.

Once amino acids have been produced, they can then be linked together by peptide bonds. If two amino acids have been joined, the resulting substance is a dipeptide; three amino acids create a tripeptide. A larger number of connected amino acids constitute a polypeptide. A protein may be made of one or more polypeptides.

Structure of a Protein

The structure of a protein is infinitely more complicated. There are sometimes hundreds of amino acids in a single protein molecule. Furthermore, a molecule of a particular protein is bent, folded, or coiled into a specific three-dimensional shape that is hard to depict in a drawing. However, structures of the smaller and simpler proteins can be "flattened out" for artistic convenience (see figure 13.1). Each three-letter abbreviation represents an amino acid.

Notice that the same kind of amino acid appears many times in a single molecule of a protein. Also notice that the amino acids are in a specific order. If one is in the wrong place or if one amino acid substitutes for another, a different protein may result. Severe illness can result. Sickle-cell disease is an example of a hemoglobin protein mistake in the amino acid sequence. Normal hemoglobin contains two kinds of chains. One of the chains in sickle-cell hemoglobin is an exact copy of that in normal hemoglobin. But in the other chain, the sixth amino acid, which should be glutamine, is replaced by valine (see table 13.1). The character and shape of the protein are so much affected by this difference that the protein is unable to carry and release oxygen. The red blood cells collapse into crescent shapes instead of remaining disc-shaped as they normally are. If too many abnormal hemoglobins appear in the blood, the result is illness and death.

The great variety of proteins in the world is due to the infinite number of sequences of amino acids. If you consider the size of the dictionary, in which every word is constructed from just 26 letters, you can visualize the variety of proteins that are designed from 20 or so amino acids. The letters in a word must alternate between consonant and vowel sounds, but the amino acids in a protein need follow no such rules. Also, there is no restriction on the length of the chain of amino acids. Thus, there are many more possible proteins than words possible in the English language. There may be as many as 10,000 different proteins in a single human cell. Amazing! We are "fearfully and wonderfully made" by God.

Figure 13.1
The Structure of a Protein: Insulin

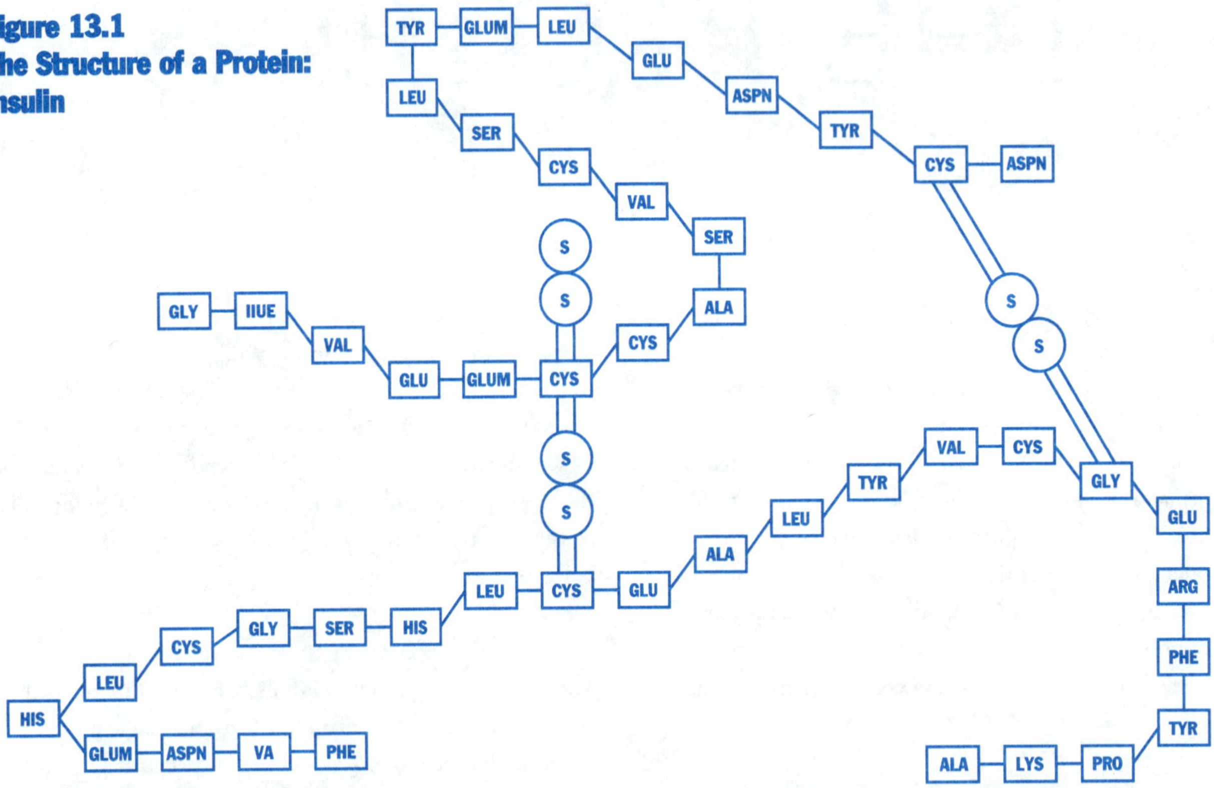

Each abbreviation represents an amino acid.

The amino acid cysteine can form crossing links between parts of the amiono acid chain, giving shape to the module.

Table 13.1
The First Eight Amino Acids in One of the Chains of Human Hemoglobin

Normal		Sickle-Cell Disease
Valine	1	Valine
Histidine	2	Histidine
Leucine	3	Leucine
Threonine	4	Threonine
Proline	5	Proline
Glutamine	6	Valine
Glutamine	7	Glutamine
Lysine	8	Lysine

How does the body know how to assemble its different proteins? The answer is found in the nucleus of every body cell, where material called deoxyribonucleic acid (DNA) and ribonucleic acid (RNA) contain the information that governs the synthesis of each protein. DNA and RNA direct the "spelling" of proteins in the body's dictionary.

When a cell needs to make a particular protein, it draws from the assortment of amino acids available to it at that time. The foods we take in contain proteins but not the same ones from which our own bodies are made. The fact that food proteins are not identical to human proteins is not a problem. Digestion dismantles food proteins so we use the components for reassembling our own body proteins. Now let's look at exactly what humans need from dietary protein.

Need for Nitrogen and Essential Amino Acids

We first and foremost need sufficient nitrogen from food proteins, and we need enough of certain amino acids that are necessary for human protein synthesis but cannot be produced within the body. These are called essential amino acids. Sufficient nitrogen and the essential amino acids are often referred to as issues of protein quantity and quality.

Quantity of Protein—Adequate Nitrogen

Remember that cells can synthesize some amino acids if they have a nitrogen source. Once they have the amino acids, they can synthesize their own unique proteins. Therefore, the most important protein intake issue is quantity, getting enough protein in the diet to provide the necessary nitrogen for amino acid production.

Protein is in almost all of the foods in the basic food groups of the food pyramid. Dairy products, meats and alternates, and foods made from these offer the greatest amount of protein per serving. When protein in your diet is low in calories, it is also likely to be low in protein and therefore nitrogen. On the other hand, if you eat enough of the basic foods to satisfy your energy needs, you will usually get enough protein at the same time. If, however, a large proportion of your calories comes from the foods in the very-low-protein limited extra group, your protein intake may be inadequate.

Quality of Protein—Adequate Amounts of Essential Amino Acids

The second protein intake issue is one of quality. To be judged of good quality, a food protein must contain adequate amounts of essential amino acids the body needs for protein synthesis but cannot produce by itself.

Nine amino acids are essential in the diet. Table 13.2 lists them, as well as the 11 nonessential amino acids (the ones the body can produce). Not only have scientists learned that these amino acids are indispensable, but they have also estimated what amounts of most of them are needed by the human body. To be judged of good quality, a food protein should contain them in those approximate proportions.

Table 13.2
Essential and Nonessential Amino Acids

Amino Acids Essential in the Diet	Amino Acids not Essential in the Diet
Histidine	Alanine
Isoleucine	Arginine
Leucine	Asparagine
Lysine	Aspartic Acid
Methionine	Cysteine
Phenylalanine	Glutamic Acid
Threonine	Glutamine
Tryptophan	Glycine
Valine	Proline
	Serine
	Tyrosine

The amino acids cysteine and tyrosine are not essential but can substitute in part for methionine and phenylalanine, respectively.

In general, higher quality food proteins come from animal sources, whereas lower quality proteins generally come from plant sources. More specifically, the best food proteins are those that match human needs best and are found in eggs, milk, and fish. The proteins in eggs and milk are of such high quality that scientists sometimes refer to them as "reference proteins" and compare the quality of others to them. Good quality proteins are also found in meats, poultry, cheese, and soybeans (a good plant source).

The proteins in other legumes, nuts and seeds, grains, and vegetables get a fair rating; that is, some may have relatively low levels of one or two essential amino acids and high levels of others, whereas different proteins may be low (or high) in different amino acids. At any rate, the proportion of amino acids in a fair quality does not match our essential amino acid needs particularly well. A protein of blatantly poor quality is gelatin.

Protein quality is not a widespread concern because the assortment of amino acids present in one individual food is not as important as the whole assortment available from everything that is eaten at the same time. People eat different foods together, with some foods having greater or lesser amounts of particular amino acids in them than others. Several foods eaten together often contain in combination about the right proportions of amino acids.

This phenomenon of one food supplementing low levels of amino acids in another is called mutual supplementation. Examples of foods whose amino acids complement each other are shown in table 13.3. Note that many of these combinations have been commonly used in various world cultures.

If you consume your RDA for proteins, you'll probably get as much as you need of the essential amino acids. Many North Americans take in almost double the protein they need, which gives them an abundant supply of both essential and nonessential amino acids.

Some groups of people limit or completely eliminate animal protein from their diet. Vegetarians who abstain from all animal products could probably achieve better overall dietary protein quality by using protein supplementation rather than by leaving their food combinations to chance. This is particularly true for growing children and pregnant and lactating women, whose protein needs are higher.

There are many different kinds of vegetarians. Not all need to be concerned about mutual supplementation. To make the distinction, let's first describe the better known types of vegetarians.

1. Semivegetarian—avoids only selected kinds of meat, fish, or poultry (flesh)
2. Lacto-vegetarian—avoids eating flesh and eggs but uses dairy products
3. Vegan—avoids all food of animal origin
4. Lacto-ovo-vegetarian—includes dairy products and eggs but no animal flesh

The types of vegetarians who can easily meet their protein quantity and quality needs by following basic dietary guidelines are semi-, lacto-, and lacto-ovo vegetarians. Vegans, especially those who are growing, may profit from complementing protein sources as just described. We will discuss vegetarians later in this chapter.

Table 13.3

Complementary Protein Combinations	
Lentils	+ Wheat, rice
Legumes	+ Cereals (enriched or whole grain)
Sesame or sunflower seeds	+ Leafy vegetables, whole grains
Brewer's yeast	+ Peanuts, legumes, seeds, nuts, whole grains, corn, leafy vegetables
Leafy vegetables	+ Seeds, whole grains, yeast
Traditional Protein Combinations	
Soybeans	+ Rice (Indochina)
Peas	+ Wheat (Fertile Crescent)
Beans	+ Corn (Central and South America)

The Role of Protein

Protein has three general functions in the body. Protein provides structure, regulates body processes, and supplies energy. Within these three categories, a wide variety of different proteins have various roles, depending on the particular function they are asked to perform.

Provides Structure

Protein provides the structure or framework on which the body is built. Bone, teeth, the muscles, skin, hair, tendons, and ligaments are all constructed of proteins. Proteins also ensure that amino acids are available to build proteins of new tissue. The new tissue may be in a growing child, in the scar tissue that helps heal wounds, or in new hair and nails. Each cell in the body contains protein—in the cell membrane that surrounds the cell and holds it together, in the organelles in the cytoplasm, and in the nucleus itself, where DNA is housed. For this new growth, amino acids must be supplied constantly from food.

Regulates Body Processes

Enzymes and hormones.—Enzymes are among the most important of the proteins formed in cells. Enzymes are catalysts; they help chemical reactions take place. Life continues from minute to minute due to thousands of these biochemical reactions. Enzymes are responsible for allowing these reactions to take place at a fast enough pace to support life. Enzymes take part in digestion, blood clotting, muscle contraction, nerve transmission, the production of energy, growth, and many other life-sustaining activities.

Similar to the enzymes in the profoundness of their effects are the hormones. However, these molecules differ from the enzymes in that not all of them are made of protein and they don't catalyze chemical reactions directly. Instead, they signal the appropriate enzymes to start working on what the body needs. Hormones regulate overall body conditions such as the blood glucose level (insulin) and the metabolic rate (thyroxin), and they do it through the work of enzymes.

Antibodies.—Of all the great variety of proteins in the living body, the antibodies best demonstrate that proteins are specific for one organism. Antibodies are formed in response to the presence of foreign particles (bacteria, virus, toxin, food allergy) that invade the body. The body, after recognizing that it has been invaded, manufactures antibodies, and they attack and inactivate the foreign protein. In many cases, once the body has encountered a particular foreign protein, it doesn't forget it and can quickly recall the recipe for the antibody. This is referred to as immunity.

Fluid balance.—Proteins help regulate the quantity of fluids in the compartments of the body to maintain the fluid balance. To remain alive, a cell must contain a constant amount of fluid. Too much might cause it to rupture, and too little would make it unable to function. Although water can diffuse freely in and out of the cell, proteins cannot; and proteins attract water. By maintaining a store of internal proteins, the cell retains the fluid it needs. Similarly, the cells secrete proteins into the spaces between them to keep the fluid volume constant in those spaces. The proteins secreted into the blood can't cross the vessel walls, and thus they maintain the blood volume in the same way. This process is called osmosis. Individuals with protein-deficiency disease often suffer from edema, an accumulation of fluid due to the shift of water into inappropriate areas because protein is not present to exert its influence.

Bone, teeth, muscles, skin, hair, tendons, and ligaments are all constructed of proteins.

Salt balance.—Transport proteins in the membranes of all the cells respond sensitively to small changes in the circulating fluids and work to maintain equilibrium by pumping substances into and out of cells. Thus, for example, sodium (Na) is concentrated outside the cells, and potassium (K) is concentrated inside. A disturbance of the salt balance can impair the action of the indispensable heart, lungs, and brain, triggering a red-hot medical emergency.

Acid-base balance.—Normal processes of the body continually produce acids and their opposite, bases, which must be carried by the blood to the organs of excretion. The blood must do this without allowing its own acid-base balance to be affected. This magical feat is another trick of the proteins in the blood, which act as buffers. They pick up hydrogen (acid) when there is too much and release hydrogen again when there is too little.

Excess acid can disrupt normal body functioning and in severe cases result in coma or death. Protein will buffer this acid until it can be removed from the body by the kidneys or lungs. A buffer is any agent that will bring the pH toward neutral, not acidic or alkaline. The normal pH of the blood ranges between 7.3 and 7.4, or slightly alkaline.

Carrier proteins.—Some proteins help to carry other important substances through the bloodstream to their destination. Two examples are lipoproteins (which carry triglycerides and cholesterol in the blood because they are not soluble), and hemoglobin, which transports oxygen from the lungs to all the cells of the body.

Energy

Only protein can perform all the functions described above, but protein will be sacrificed to provide needed calories if insufficient fat and carbohydrate foods are eaten. The body's top-priority need is for energy. All other needs have a lower priority.

When amino acids are degraded for energy, their amine groups are usually incorporated by the liver into urea and sent to the kidneys for excretion in the urine. The fragments that remain are composed of carbon, hydrogen, and oxygen, as are carbohydrates and fats, and can be used to build those substances or be metabolized like them.

Not only can amino acids supply energy, but most of them can also supply energy as glucose, as fat can never do. Thus, if need be, protein can help maintain a steady blood glucose level and so serve the brain.

Carbohydrates offer energy; fat offers concentrated energy; and protein, if needed, can offer energy plus nitrogen.

Let's review the three energy nutrients and look at their similarities and differences. Carbohydrates offer energy; fat offers concentrated energy; and protein, if needed, can offer energy plus nitrogen.

Only if the protein-sparing calories from carbohydrate and fat are sufficient to power the cells will the amino acids be used for their most important function—making proteins. Thus energy deficiency (starvation) is always accompanied by the symptoms of protein deficiency.

If amino acids are oversupplied, the body has no place to store them. It will remove and excrete their amine group and then convert the residues to glucose and glycogen or to fat for energy storage. In case there is a great shortage of amino acids, tissues like blood, muscle, and skin have to be degraded so that their amino acids can be used to maintain the brain, heart, and lungs.

In summary, when insufficient carbohydrate and fat are provided to meet the body's energy need, food protein and body protein are sacrificed to supply energy. The nitrogen part is removed from each amino acid and excreted in the urine. The resulting fragment is oxidized for energy.

How Does the Body Handle Protein?

When a person eats food proteins, whether from cereals, vegetables, beef, or cheese, the body must break them down into amino acids in order to rearrange them into its own unique sequence.

Digestion in the Stomach

Other than being crushed and mixed with saliva, nothing happens to protein until it reaches the strong acid of the stomach. There the acid helps to uncoil (denature) the protein's tangled strands so that stomach enzymes can attack the bonds. You might expect that the stomach enzymes themselves, being protein, would be attacked; but these (especially pepsin) are the only proteins in the body that God designed to resist strong acid and to become most active in it. After the protein is denatured, pepsin breaks the long strands into polypeptides (small chains of amino acids), which are moved along to the small intestine where they will be further broken apart.

Digestion in the Small Intestine

By the time proteins enter into the small intestine, they are already broken into different-sized pieces. A barrage of proteases (protein-digesting enzymes) awaits the polypeptides in the small intestine. These enzymes have been released from the pancreas and will break the polypeptide strands into tripeptides, dipeptides, and single amino acids. The raising of the pH (to about 7) enables the next enzyme team to accomplish the final breakdown of the strands. Digestion continues until almost all pieces of protein are broken down into smaller fragments and more free amino acids.

Absorption Across Intestinal Cells into Blood

The end products of digestion are absorbed by the small intestine and travel through the portal vein to the liver, where they can enter the general circulation. Surprisingly, dipeptides and tripeptides are absorbed more rapidly than single amino acids.

The cells of the small intestine possess different sites for the absorption of different classes of amino acids. A specific protein carrier helps the neutral amino acids across the cell membranes; another helps the acidic ones; and another, the basic ones. Within each class, amino acids compete for the carriers.

The presence of specific sites for the absorption of amino acids explains why supplementing the diet with specific amino acids might be dangerous. For example, lysine supplements have

The nitrogen of egg protein tends to be retained in the body, indicating that it is used with little waste.

been proclaimed to cure fever blisters. But if one amino acid floods the absorptive carriers, another similar one may travel by the site without having a chance to be absorbed. Competition for transport will cause loss by excretion of that amino acid, creating an imbalance. The best guarantee of having a good balance of amino acids is to supply the dietary protein from foods.

If a nonessential amino acid is unavailable for a growing protein strand, the cell will synthesize it and continue attaching amino acids to the strand. If an essential amino acid is missing, the building of the protein will be halted. Partially completed proteins are not held for later completion (for example, the next day). Rather, the partial structures are dismantled, and the surplus amino acids are returned to circulation to be made available to other cells. If they are not soon inserted into protein, their amine groups will be removed and excreted, and the residues will be used for other purposes. The need that prompted the calling for that particular protein will not be met.

It is imperative that all the essential amino acids be eaten within the same time period, probably about four hours. This presents no problem to people who eat complete proteins, such as those of eggs, fish, poultry, cheese, or milk. The proteins of these foods contain ample amounts of all the essential amino acids. An equally sound choice is to eat two incomplete protein foods from plants, each of which supplies the amino acids missing in the other. This strategy is a must to supply a sufficient amount of dietary protein to the vegetarian's protein needs.

In summary, amino acids in the cell can be used to:

- Synthesize protein.
- Provide glucose (most of them can).
- Provide nitrogen in the form of amine groups to build nonessential amino acids.
- Provide energy if there is a scarcity of energy nutrients.
- Increase the stored energy in glycogen and fat.

Amino acids are wasted (not used to build protein) whenever there is:

- Not enough energy from carbohydrate and fat.
- An imbalance, with not enough essential amino acids (low-quality protein).
- Too much protein so that not all is needed.

Factors that must be supplied in the diet for the body to be able to synthesize protein include:

- All essential amino acids simultaneously and in the proper amounts.
- An adequate total amount of protein (to supply amine group to synthesize the nonessential amino acids).
- Adequate carbohydrate and calories (to supply energy).

The Quality and Use of Proteins

A diet that contains an imbalance of amino acid so severe as to limit body protein synthesis is said to be a diet containing protein of poor quality. A person in good health can be expected to use dietary protein efficiently. However, malnutrition or infection can seriously impair digestion (by reducing enzyme secretion). Malnutrition or infection can also impair absorption (by causing degeneration of the absorptive surface of the small intestine or causing losses from diarrhea), and malnutrition or infection can impair the cell's use of protein by forcing amino acids to meet other needs.

Amino acids from animal proteins have the best percentage of absorption (over 90%). Those from legumes follow (about 80%), and those from grains and other plant foods vary (from 60% to 90%). Cooking with moist heat generally improves protein digestibility, whereas dry heat methods may impair it. Protein will be used most efficiently if accompanied by carbohydrate, fat, and the full array of vitamins and minerals.

A protein that supplies all the essential amino acids in exactly the right ratio will be the most completely used. If an essential amino acid is in short supply, it limits the use of all the others for building protein. Remember, a protein that almost entirely lacks an essential amino acid can't be used for protein synthesis at all unless that amino acid is supplied from some other source.

When amino acids are wasted, their amine groups (which contain their nitrogen) can't be stored. Therefore, the efficiency of a protein can be assessed experimentally by measuring the amount of nitrogen lost from the body. The higher the amount of nitrogen retained, the higher the quality of the protein. This is the basis for determination of the biological valve (BV) of proteins.

The most perfect protein by this standard is egg protein. The nitrogen of egg protein tends to be retained in the body, indicating that it is used with little waste. Egg protein has been designated the reference protein for purposes of measuring protein quality and has been assigned a biological value of 100 by the Food and Agriculture Organization (FAO), which sets world standards. Eggs are a highly valued protein source in

Complete protein foods include all meat, fish, poultry, milk, milk products, and eggs. Small daily amounts of any of these easily meet human needs.

less-developed nations where protein-rich foods are scarce. They offer high-quality protein; they are relatively inexpensive, and they store well. Rice protein has a high biological value, but other plant proteins are of poorer quality (see table 13.4).

Table 13.4
Biological Value of Some Common Protein Foods

Protein	Chemical Score	Net Protein Utilization
Eggs	100	100
Milk	93	75
Rice	86	67
Beef	75	80
Fish	75	83
Corn	72	56

The protein efficiency ratio (PER) is yet another method used to measure protein quality. This is done by determining the efficiency by which protein supports growth. For example, a laboratory experiment will measure how well a growing rat will gain weight if given a fixed amount of dietary protein.

All of these measurements are used to determine recommendations for protein intake. For instance, the higher the PER or net protein utilization (NPU) (which measures both the amino acid pattern and the digestibility of food) of a particular food, the less the individual would need to consume. If a person's diet contains mainly low-quality (low PER) protein source, more protein needs to be consumed.

Certainly these standards have their limitations. For those who choose not to tangle with the BV or PER, a convenient way to distinguish among proteins is to use the following guidelines:

1. Complete protein foods include all meat, fish, poultry, milk, milk products, and eggs. Small daily amounts of any of these easily meet human needs.

2. Other protein-rich foods such as grains, nuts, and legumes have to be used in strategic combinations.

3. Not much protein is found in other vegetables or fruits, but each makes a supportive contribution to the total.

Recommended Protein Intake

Recommendations for protein intakes can be stated in three ways:

- As a percentage of total energy.
- As grams per kilogram of body weight per day.
- As an absolute number (grams per day).

Dietary guidelines generally recommend that people's protein intakes contribute about 12 percent of the total energy consumed. (This allows almost 60% of energy or more to come from carbohydrate.) Most people in this country already eat this much protein and more.

The recommended daily allowances for protein are guidelines that vary with both weight and age (see table 13.5). An adult needs .8 grams of protein per kilogram of weight. Infants, because of their tremendous rate of growth, need more than double that, or 2.2 grams per kilogram of body weight. The need gradually decreases with age until adulthood is reached. Of course, this is not really a change with age but with growth requirements. In addition, the RDA allots extra allowances for protein during pregnancy (plus 30 grams) and while lactating (plus 20 grams).

Table 13.5
RDA for Protein

Age (years)	RDA (g/kg)
0–½	2.2
½–1	2.0
1–3	1.8
4–10	1.1
11–14	1.0
15–18	.9
19 and up	.8

The RDA increases by 30 grams during pregnancy and by 20 grams during lactation.

The table of RDA actually recommends 56 grams of protein for a male and 44 grams for a female. This calculation is based on the reference male weighing 154 pounds (70 kilograms) and reference female weighing 121 pounds (55 kilograms). Protein

Plant foods can provide more than enough of all the essential amino acids and can sustain people in good health as long as there are not too many empty-calorie foods in the diet.

needs vary from individual to individual, but the RDA is generous. The RDA recommends a protein intake that is more than that needed by 96 percent of healthy Americans.

Sometimes guidelines for protein consumption are given as 10–12 percent of a person's caloric intake. Most Americans eat far more than this. Studies estimate that from 16 to 20 percent of all calories come from protein in the American diet. For example, for a 70-kilogram (154 lb) person, the RDA for protein would be 56 grams of protein per day.

The two guidelines for protein intake, based on weight and calories, will not necessarily produce the same recommendation. For example, physically active persons may require larger quantities of calories. This would increase the protein guideline based on calories but not change the recommendation based only on weight. Recall that an RDA is an allowance, not a requirement. Some people require less than this amount. Even so, the average man and woman in the U.S. consume about 70 and 90 grams of protein, respectively, per day, a level in excess of the RDA. This excess protein cannot be stored as such. As noted before, the amine group is removed and the carbon skeleton is turned into glucose or fat and then either stored or burned for energy needs.

Mental stress, physical labor, and sports activity do not require an increase in the RDA for protein. Elderly people might need 1 gram of protein per kilogram of body weight. In addition, to support either substantial gains in muscle tissue from sports activities or a large muscle mass formerly acquired, increasing the allowance up to twice the RDA might be considered. But keep in mind that many Americans eat that much protein already. Extra protein intakes above usual adult intakes for athletes are generally not needed. In addition, there is usually no reason for athletes to take either protein or individual amino acid supplements. All of us, athletes included, can meet our protein needs using basic foods.

Food Sources of Protein

There are two categories of protein sources—animal and plant. Animal sources of protein contain all the essential amino acids. Examples of this group are beef, tuna, salmon, eggs, cheese, yogurt, milk, lamb, and pork. Animal sources are somewhat of a mixed blessing. While containing high-quality protein, some also contain high amounts of fats. Since many Americans eat more than double the RDA for protein, unfortunately they receive the extra fat, too.

Plant protein, however, is not necessarily of high quality, legumes being the exception. This group includes the seeds of plants such as lima beans, pinto beans, garden peas, soybeans, and lentils. Legumes provide protein with almost as high a quality as meat; and they are also an excellent source of B-vitamins, iron, fiber, and other nutrients (see table 13.6)

Protein for the Vegetarian

The vegetarian has the same nutritional tasks as any other person and so must plan a diet that will deliver a variety of foods providing all the 45 known nutrients within an energy allowance that won't cause weight gain or loss. The added challenge comes from doing so with at least one less food group.

The lacto-ovo vegetarian who each day consumes two cups of milk, or the equivalent in milk products, and two cups of legumes is guaranteed an adequate intake of complete protein. The vegan, who cannot rely on milk and milk products should learn the method of mutual supplementation and use it wisely to achieve a balance of all the needed amino acids. Some recent studies indicate that adequate consumption of the essential amino acids is possible without practicing mutual supplementation. Plant foods can provide more than enough of all the essential amino acids and can sustain people in good health as long as there are not too many empty-calorie foods in the diet.

Assuming the vegan consumes enough energy, the possibility of a protein deficiency is remote. Only when fruits and certain poorly chosen vegetables define the core of the diet might protein deficiency result. Fruits provide adequate energy, but most are low in protein. A wise vegan can improve the quality of protein consumed by practicing mutual supplementation, even though he should probably not be overly concerned about it. A wiser use of time and energy should be to obtain, prepare, and eat a wide variety of foods from the vegetarian food groups (table 13.7) to obtain adequate energy, protein, and other nutrients.

An advantage of vegetarian protein foods is that they are generally lower in fat than meats and are often higher in fiber and richer in certain vitamins and minerals. Vegetarians can

Table 13.6 Protein Sources			
Food	**Amount**	**Protein (g)**	**Energy (cal)**
Animal Protein			
Meat, cooked:			
Ground Beef	3 oz.	20–23	185–235
Liver	3 oz.	23–28	160–215
Pork	3 oz.	23–28	310
Poultry (w/out skin)	3 oz.	25	145–175
Fish, light and dark, cooked	3 oz.	20–25	125–175
Cheese			
Cheddar	1 oz.	7	115
Cottage	½ cup	12–15	85–130
Egg	1 large	7	80
Milk			
Nonfat	1 cup	9	90
Whole	1 cup	9	160
Good Sources of Plant Protein			
Vegetables, cooked:			
Broccoli	1 med. stalk	6	45
Brussels Sprouts	1 cup	7	55
Cauliflower	1 cup	3	30
Greens	1 cup	3–7	30–65
Legumes:			
Dried, cooked	½ cup	7–8	90–115
Mung Sprouts, raw	½ cup	2	20
Tofu (soybean curd)	4 oz.	9	85
Significant Quantities of Protein from These Foods (If You Can Afford the Calories)			
Cereal, whole grain, cooked			
Barley, whole grain, cooked	½ cup	4	135
Bran, unprocessed	½ cup	4	55
Bran cereal (100% bran)	½ cup	5	90
Breads	1 slice	2–3	60–80
Cornmeal, unrefined	½ cup	5	215
Oatmeal, cooked	1 cup	5	130
Pasta, enriched	1 cup	5–7	15–200
Rice, cooked	1 cup	4–5	225–230
Wheat, bulgur	½ cup	7	225
Wheat, cracked	½ cup	4	110
Wheat berries	½ cup	5	110

Food	Amount	Protein (g)	Energy (cal)
Starchy Vegetables			
Corn	½ cup	3	70
Peas	1 cup	9	115
Potato, baked	1 large	4	145
Squash	1 cup	4	130
Miscellaneous			
Nut butter	1 tbsp.	4	95
Nuts	2 tbsp.	2–5	80–115
Seeds	2 tbsp.	3–5	95–100
Yeast, brewers	2 tbsp.	6	40–45

These items are high in fat and should be used in moderation.

Table 13.7
Vegetarian Food Group Plan

Milk and milk products—2 servings
Protein-rich foods—2 servings
Legumes—2 servings
Fruits and vegetables—4 servings
Breads and cereals (whole grain only)—4 servings

If not using milk or milk products, use soy milk fortified with calcium and vitamin B_{12}.

Examples of protein-rich foods are cheese and tofu.

Women should eat legumes (2 cups daily) in addition to protein-rich foods to help meet iron requirements; count 4 tbsp. peanut butter as one serving.

Women should include 1 cup dark greens daily to help meet iron requirements.

therefore enjoy a nutritious diet that is low in fat, provided they also limit other high-fat foods like butter, cream cheese, sour cream, cheese, nuts, and avocados.

Health Effects of Protein

Imagine what havoc can occur to the body if there is a deficiency of dietary protein! An excess of dietary protein has its own consequences as well. Let's briefly examine the health effects of inadequate and excessive protein intake.

Protein Shortage

Unlike Americans, people in other parts of the world do not consume enough protein. Let's look at the health results that can occur if the body doesn't receive its appropriate protein.

Marasmus.—Marasmus is a disease that occurs when a child receives insufficient protein, calories, and other nutrients. The condition is also generally referred to as protein energy malnutrition. The word *marasmus* means "to waste away." Children do just that. They have the "skin and bones" appearance seen on posters from relief agencies. The body appears wasted because most of the muscle tissue is used to supply energy just for staying alive. Marasmus deprives the body of nutrients at the time when growth of the infant is critical.

Even if a child with marasmus is helped in time and fed, he may never fully recover from the disease. Most brain growth takes place between conception and the first birthday. In fact, the brain is growing at its most rapid rate at birth. If the diet does not support brain growth during the first months of life, the brain may not grow to its full size. This reduced growth can lead to a decrease in intelligence.

Animal foods are excellent sources of both protein and phosphorus.

Kwashiorkor.—Kwashiorkor, a word from Ghana, means "the disease that the first child gets when the new child comes." From birth the child is probably breast-fed. By the time the child reaches 1–1.5 years, the mother is probably pregnant or has already given birth again, and breast feeding is no longer possible for the first child. The child abruptly switches from nutritious breast milk to native starchy roots and gruels. These foods have such low protein densities compared with total calories that they cannot meet the child's protein needs.

The major symptoms of kwashiorkor are apathy, listlessness, failure to grow and gain weight, withdrawal from the environment, and most important, an increased susceptibility to infections. This can make conditions such as measles, a disease that normally makes a healthy child ill for only a week or so, a severely debilitating and fatal disease.

If a child with kwashiorkor is helped in time and fed a diet ample in protein, calories, and other essential nutrients, the disease symptoms reverse. The child begins to grow again and may even show no signs of the previous condition, aside perhaps from shortness of stature. However, by the time many of these children reach a hospital or care center, they already have severe infections. In spite of the best care, they still die. Or, if they survive, they return home and repeat the cycle. Can Christians make a difference for these starving children?

An Excess of Protein

While protein shortages are of world concern, perhaps protein excess is of personal concern. This section points out some of the problems associated with a high protein intake.

High cholesterol.—Several studies show that diets containing animal protein induce higher cholesterol levels in most subjects than do diets containing vegetable protein, probably because the high-saturated fat intake that usually accompanies the animal protein is the responsible culprit. Some research studies have now found that the protein itself may have an effect on cholesterol. Animal protein seems to raise blood-cholesterol levels, and plant proteins have the opposite effect. Current data reveals that the protein in the diet does not change synthesis or absorption but does change the turnover time of cholesterol in the blood. Plant protein decreases the time cholesterol remains in the blood. The accelerated excretion of cholesterol may account for its lack of accumulation in the blood.

Dehydration.—There is some concern that high protein intakes may unduly burden the kidneys to excrete the resulting excess nitrogen (mostly as urea) into the urine. In the process of excretion, large amounts of water are needed to dilute the urea as it leaves the body. For every 100 calories of protein metabolized, the body loses 350 grams of water, whereas carbohydrate or fat uses only 50 grams when metabolized. High-protein diets are particularly hazardous to the athlete, who already has difficulty remaining hydrated. Perspiration and metabolic losses can leave the athlete with too little water to function safely. The solution is simple: Consume lots of water and reduce protein intake to reasonable levels, closer to the RDA.

Preserving kidney function is especially important for people with diabetes mellitus and for people who have only one functioning kidney. Presently many U.S. medical centers are studying whether a conservative protein intake preserves kidney function better in people with diabetes mellitus than does the typical North American high-protein intake. For people without diabetes the risk of suffering kidney failure is low; therefore the risk of a high-protein diet contributing to kidney disease in later life is probably also low.

Calcium loss.—Research in the 1970s suggested that a high-protein diet might cause greater calcium loss in the urine. This worried researchers because they thought protein caused calcium to leak out of the bones. In the long run this depletion can demineralize bones and lead to osteoporosis, a severe bone disease. However, follow-up studies show that if extra phosphorus is also consumed urine calcium does not increase so much. Animal foods are excellent sources of both protein and phosphorus. So typical North American intakes probably don't threaten calcium balance as long as the RDA for calcium is met.

[CHAPTER 14]

UNDERSTANDING THE VITAMINS

The term *vitamin* comes from *vita*, meaning "life," and *amine*, because vitamins were believed to contain the chemical structure called an amine. Before vitamins were discovered, whole groups of people were only half alive (or were going blind or had an "incurable" sickness). Then an alert scientist stumbled onto the substance missing in their diets. According to the plot, the scientist usually confirmed the discovery by feeding the vitamin-deficient food to laboratory animals. The animals responded to the diet just as the humans did, by becoming unable to walk (or going blind or bleeding profusely). Then, miraculously, they recovered when one missing ingredient was restored to their diet. They walked in "newness of life."

Having read of dramatic events like these happening in real life, people continue to believe that a vitamin supplement will cure a wide variety of ailments. But the truth is that the only disease a vitamin will cure is the one caused by a deficiency of that vitamin. Vitamins, in general, are not cure-alls for such vague symptoms as tiredness. But if there is a deficiency of one of the vitamins essential to the release of energy from glucose, tiredness may be one of the symptoms. Only the restoration of that vitamin to the diet will alleviate the symptom.

Definition and Classification of Vitamins

Vitamins are organic (carbon-containing) compounds needed for important metabolic reactions in the body. Most plants can synthesize all the vitamins they need. But human bodies cannot make them, and so we rely on our diets. However, we need vitamins in only small quantities, about 28 grams (1 ounce) for every 70 kg (150 pounds) of food we eat.

Vitamins yield no energy for the body. Instead, they facilitate energy-yielding chemical reactions and promote body growth and development. Vitamins A, D, E, and K dissolve in fat, while the B vitamins and vitamin C dissolve in water. In addition, the B vitamins and vitamin K function as part of coenzymes—molecules that directly help enzymes function.

Most people adhere to the belief that "if a little is good, more must be better." Approximately 40 percent of the U.S. adult population takes vitamin supplements. This totals out to be a 3-billion-dollar-a-year industry. Many Americans take extremely large doses in belief that this will provide extra energy, health, and protection from disease. Each year more than 4,000 cases of vitamin poisoning are reported in the U.S. alone. A recent survey of the U.S. adults showed that 8 percent take potentially toxic doses of vitamin A, 11 percent take potentially harmful doses of vitamin C, and 16 percent take excessive doses of vitamin E.

High intakes of vitamins and minerals beyond body needs are not beneficial, for they can upset the law of homeostasis or balance within the body cell. Too much or too little of any one of the nutrients can lead to various health problems. Moderation is the key to health, and this moderation is best achieved by eating a variety of wholesome foods. In other words, there is no need to use vitamin supplement pills.

Classification of Vitamins

Vitamins are usually grouped and distinguished according to their solubility in either fat or water. The fat-soluble vitamins are A, D, E, and K. They are closely associated with lipids in the body. They can be stored, and their functions are generally

Vitamins in foods should be consumed daily, but an occasional lapse in the intake of one of more water-soluble vitamins should cause no harm.

related to structural activities. The water-soluble vitamins are the B-complex ones and C. These have fewer problems in absorption and transport. They cannot be stored except in the general "tissue saturation" sense. The B vitamins function mainly as coenzyme factors in cell metabolism. Vitamin C is a vital structural agent.

Vitamins in foods should be consumed daily, but an occasional lapse in the intake of one of more water-soluble vitamins should cause no harm. It takes an average person 10 days to develop the first symptoms of a thiamin deficiency and 20 to 40 days for vitamin C deficiency to develop when these vitamins are completely lacking in the diet. This shows that all vitamins are stored to some extent in the body.

Because fat-soluble vitamins are not readily excreted, some can build up in the body and cause toxic reactions. Vitamins A and D are especially likely to do so, from heavy and regular consumption of supplements of foods such as liver. Regular use of "one-a-day" types of multivitamin and mineral supplements will not cause toxicity problems if this yields less than two times the RDA, except perhaps during pregnancy.

Isolated reports in scientific literature show that vitamin E and the water-soluble vitamin B_6 and niacin can be toxic, but only when consumed in very high amounts (50 to 100 times the RDA). So except for vitamin pill use these three vitamins are unlikely to cause toxic symptoms. In comparison, vitamins A and D can cause toxicity with long-term use at just 5 to 10 times the RDA.

The people who actually need extra vitamins are those who experience fat malabsorption. For example, those with cystic fibrosis, celiac disease, or Crohn's disease usually experience fat-soluble vitamin malabsorption also. Unabsorbed fat carries fat-soluble vitamins to the colon and into the feces. Such persons are especially susceptible to a vitamin K deficiency because it is not as readily stored as are the other fat-soluble vitamins. People who use mineral oil as a laxative at mealtime are also susceptible to fat-soluble vitamin deficiencies. Some B vitamins (such as folacin) and minerals (such as calcium and magnesium) are also susceptible to malabsorption during intestinal disease.

Water-soluble vitamins can be lost in cooking due to heat, alkalinity, and leaking into the cooking water. Steaming, stir-frying, microwaving, or simmering vegetables in minimal moisture allows them to retain most of the B vitamins and vitamin C. Although baking soda is sometimes added to vegetables during cooking to make them greener or to beans to make them softer, it is not a good nutritional practice, because the alkalinity destroys much of the thiamin and vitamin C found in the vegetables. You may wonder if there are still more vitamins lurking in foods, waiting to be discovered. After all, the structure and chemical formula of the first known vitamin (thiamin) was not determined until 1937, and the last known vitamin (B_{12}) was characterized in 1948. Though some optimistic researchers hope to discover one more vitamin, most scientists are confident that all vitamin needs by humans have been discovered. Let's review first the fat-soluble vitamins and then the water soluble.

The Fat-Soluble Vitamins (A, D, E, K)

Fat-soluble vitamins are absorbed along with dietary fat. These vitamins then travel in chylomicrons with other dietary fats through the lymphatic system and reach the bloodstream. They are then carried by the chylomicrons and other lipoproteins (VLDL and LDL) to body cells. Other carriers in the bloodstream also help distribute vitamins A and K.

When fat absorption is efficient, that is, the actions of bile salts and lipase promote adequate digestion and there is adequate absorptive capacity from a healthy intestinal wall, about 40–90 percent of the fat-soluble vitamins are absorbed. As the blood lipoprotein is metabolized by cells lining the bloodstream, the lipoprotein remains are picked up by the liver. In this way the fat-soluble vitamins contained in the remains also enter the liver, which is a major storage site, especially for vitamin A. In disease states in which fat digestion is poor or lipoprotein synthesis is hampered, fat-soluble vitamins status may be deficient, especially for vitamins K and E. Supplements may then be appropriate, with a physician's guidance.

Vitamin A

Vitamin A has the distinction of being the first fat-soluble vitamin to be discovered. There are three different forms of vitamin A: retinol (an alcohol), retinal (an aldehyde), and retinoic acid (an acid). These forms are found in the diet and to some extent can be converted into one another. Together, all three are referred to as retinoids. Vitamin A activity in the diet is also present in the form of the common plant pigments, called provitamin A. The most potent form is beta-carotene. Combining the retinoids

Vitamin A is undeniably an important nutrient, if for no other reason than that it plays a vital role in vision.

with the provitamin A carotenoids yields what is generically referred to as Vitamin A.

Most vitamin A is stored in the liver. To leave the liver, retinol must bind to a retinol-binding protein, which requires zinc for its synthesis. Thus a zinc deficiency will result in a secondary vitamin A deficiency.

Roles vitamin A plays in the body.—Vitamin A may be the most versatile of the fat-soluble vitamins because of its roles in several important body processes. Its roles in promoting good night vision, the health of mucous membranes and skin, and growth of the body's tissues are well documented by research. The following are some other roles vitamin A plays in the body:

1. It maintains the stability of cell membranes.
2. It helps the adrenal glands to synthesize cortisol (a hormone).
3. It helps the normal output of thyroxin (a hormone) from the thyroid gland.
4. It helps with immune reactions.
5. It helps maintain the nerve cell sheaths.
6. It helps in manufacturing red blood cells.
7. Beta-carotene may inhibit certain types of cancers.

Vitamin A is undeniably an important nutrient, if for no other reason than that it plays a vital role in vision. Only God could have designed such a system as vision. Light itself cannot be conducted through the solid material of the brain, so it is changed into signals transmitted by nerves. But light comes in different colors (wavelengths), which convey needed information. To keep the colors sorted out, the eye uses different light-sensitive cells (cones) to receive them. Blue light is absorbed by one set of cells, green by another, and yellow-red by a third. By day, combinations of these give the full range of color vision. By night, the light entering the eye is of low intensity, and the set of cells (rods) that can receive this light are of one kind only; so by night, a person can normally see only the presence of light, not its color.

After receiving light and sending a message about it, the molecule of retinal is converted back to its original form and rejoined to opsin to regenerate the pigment rhodopsin. Many molecules of retinal are involved in this process. There are about 6 to 7 million cone cells and 100 million rod cells in the retina of the eye, and each contains about 30 million molecules of visual pigment. Repeated small losses incurred by visual activity necessitate the constant replenishment of retinal from the blood, which brings a new supply from the body stores. Ultimately, vitamin A is the source of all the retinal in the pigments of the eye. But only one thousandth of the vitamin A in the body is in the retina. Much more is in the body's skin and linings. All surfaces, both inside and outside, are maintained with the help of vitamin A.

It is important that each of these mucosa (linings) surfaces be smooth. The linings of the mouth, stomach, intestines, trachea, lungs, urinary tract, and eyelids are examples of mucosa linings. Vitamin A helps to maintain the integrity of these mucous membranes.

Vitamin A plays an important role in fighting infection. Children with even mild vitamin A deficiency develop respiratory diseases and diarrhea at two to three times the rate of children with normal vitamin A status. By maintaining strong epithelial tissue (linings), vitamin A prevents the invasion of bacteria and viruses. In addition, vitamin A is required for the growth of many of the body's tissues, including the lymph glands where antibodies are produced.

Vitamin A also supports growth. Some of the cells involved in bone formation contain sacs of degradative enzymes that can take apart the structure of bone. With the help of vitamin A in a sensitively regulated process, these cells release their enzymes, which eat away at selected sites in the bone, removing the parts that are not needed as the bone grows longer.

Sources of vitamin A.—Vitamin A in foods exists in two forms, animal and plant. Animal vitamin A is found in liver, fish, oils, fortified milk, and eggs. Butter and margarine are also fortified with vitamin A, but we don't eat enough of either to make them significant sources. Plant vitamin A is mainly found in dark green and orange vegetables and some fruits. Carrots, spinach, squash, broccoli, papayas, and apricots are examples of sources. About 50 percent of the vitamin A in the American diet comes from animal sources.

The major contributors of vitamin A to the U.S. diet are liver, carrots, eggs, tomatoes, vegetable soups, whole milk, and greens. Foods with the highest nutrient density (per calorie) for vitamin A are carrots, liver, spinach, broccoli, tomatoes, and romaine lettuce. Beta-carotene accounts for the yellow-orange color of carrots. The yellow-orange color is often hidden, however, by dark-green chlorophyll pigments in vegetables such as broccoli. Consuming a varied diet rich in green vegetables and carrots ensures efficient sources for meeting vitamin A needs.

RDA for vitamin A.—The current RDA for vitamin A for adults is 1,000 RE for men and 800 RE for women. RE stands for retinol equivalents. Previously, vitamin A content foods were expressed in international units (I.U.). Both measurements are widely found in charts, graphs, and food labels. To convert, one retinol equivalent is 3.33 I.U. of retinol or 10 I.U. of carotene. Data from national surveys indicate that the average college male is consuming 5,629 I.U. (approximately 1,705 RE), and the average college female 3,951 (approximately 1,197 R.E) per day, which is more than adequate. Children require less, whereas pregnant and lactating women should strive for 1,000 and 1,200 R.E., respectively.

Vitamin A deficiency.—Vitamin A deficiency commonly occurs together with protein and zinc deficiency. Both zinc and protein deficiency impair protein synthesis, including that of the retinol-binding protein that transports vitamin A around the body. A specific connection between zinc and vitamin A is evident in the retina of the eye, where zinc assists the enzyme that regenerates retinal from retinol.

Up to a year's supply of vitamin A may be stored in the body, 90 percent of it in the liver.

Vitamin A deficiency depends on the adequacy of vitamin A stores and protein (to provide its carrier). Up to a year's supply of vitamin A may be stored in the body, 90 percent of it in the liver. If a healthy adult were to stop eating good food sources of the vitamin, deficiency symptoms would not begin to appear until after stores were depleted, which would take one to two years. Then, however, the consequences would be profound and severe.

Night blindness.—This is one of the first detectable signs of vitamin A deficiency and aids in diagnosis of the condition. Night blindness occurs if there is insufficient vitamin A available to resupply the visual pigment, rhodopsin. As light strikes the eyes, the rhodopsin bleaches, triggering nerve impulses to the brain and allowing interpretation of the scenery. Then, amazingly enough, clear sight does not resume until the rhodopsin is regenerated with vitamin A. If vitamin A stores are low, there will be a delay. In dimly lit settings, such as movie theaters, or night driving, this delayed sight recovery is called night blindness. Thus, because vitamin A stores are slowly used up in this process, daily dietary replenishment is necessary.

Xerophthalmia (zer-off-thal-mee-uh).—Vitamin A is important for the maintenance of mucus-forming cells. Without vitamin A, mucus-forming cells deteriorate and no longer synthesize mucus, a lubricant needed throughout the body. The cells then make a hard protein, called keratin, which is typically found in hair and nails. The eyes are first affected by this loss of mucus-synthesizing capacity, especially the cornea. Mucus in the eye is critical for lubricating its surface and washing away dirt and other particles that land on the eye.

Xerophthalmia (which means "dry eye") is a disease of the eye. With severe vitamin A deficiency, xerosis, or drying of the conjunctiva, occurs. The conjunctiva is the mucus membrane lining the eyelids. Xerosis of the cornea may follow. In this serious development, the cornea becomes opaque and distorted. Proper treatment, including vitamin A supplementation, is urgently needed to prevent the advanced state of keratomalacia (softening of the cornea) and subsequent blindness.

Vitamin A deficiency is the second-leading cause of blindness in the world, the first being accidents. American children are at little risk because of generally good diets. Children in less-developed nations, however, are especially susceptible to vitamin A deficiency because their poor intakes and stores of the vitamin fail to meet their high needs due to rapid childhood growth. More than half a million children in poorer nations of the world become blind each year because of vitamin A deficiency.

Immune function.—During vitamin A deficiency, mucus production in the intestines and lung cells and poor health of epithelial cells in general increase the risk of infection. A vitamin A deficiency also reduces the activity of some immune cells, such as T-lymphocytes. Together these effects leave a person more vulnerable to infections.

Growth and development.—Vitamin A is necessary for the growth and development of cells. Vitamin A can travel into a cell and interact with the DNA in the cell nucleus. By doing so, vitamin A causes the DNA to increase the synthesis of some cell proteins that in turn stimulate proper growth and development.

Cancer prevention.—The ability of retinoids (three forms of vitamin A) to influence epithelial cell development, coupled with its ability to increase immune system activity, could make vitamin A valuable in the fight or prevention of cancer, especially skin, lung, bladder, and breast cancer. Researchers have been encouraged by work using animals and also by the fact that most forms of cancer arise from epithelial cells.

Carotenoid precursors of vitamin A, especially beta-carotene, may also help prevent cancer because they are excellent antioxidants. The many double bonds present in some carotenoid molecules make them effective traps for free oxygen atoms and peroxides. Some evidence shows that regular consumption of vegetables high in carotenes decreases risk of lung cancer in smokers. However, much investigation is needed in this area before specific recommendations regarding carotenes and cancer prevention can be made—other than eating fruits and vegetables. Cancer and the diet are discussed later in this chapter.

An excess of vitamin A.—Toxicity symptoms from excessive vitamin A can appear with long-term supplement use at just 10 times the RDA. High vitamin A intakes are especially dangerous during pregnancy because they can cause fetal malformation. Loss of appetite, dry skin, hair loss, bone pain, cessation of menstruation, nausea, enlarged liver and spleen, abnormal skin pigmentation, headaches, and hyperirritability are among the symptoms of vitamin A toxicity.

Vitamin A toxicity is the result of supplementation with vitamin A pills. Food alone, with the exception of liver, cannot induce vitamin A poisoning. Early accounts of arctic explorers consuming large amounts of polar bear or dog livers in their attempts to survive indicate symptoms of vitamin A toxicity.

If someone consumes a large amount of carrots, or beta-carotene supplements, in the form of carrot juice, for example, the high carotene levels in the bloodstream that result can turn skin yellow-orange. The result is hypercarotenemia. The person appears to have jaundice; but unlike a case of jaundice, the sclera (whites of the eyes) are white (instead of yellow); and the liver is enlarged. Moderation is the answer.

Vitamin D

Vitamin D is not just a vitamin. It is also considered a hormone because skin cells can make it in the presence of sunlight. Therefore, in a sense, vitamin D is not an essential nutrient. The amount of sun time to produce vitamin D depends on the darkness of the skin. Young, light-skinned people need approximately 15 minutes a day in the sun, while dark-skinned people need more sun exposure. This process is also more efficient in younger people than in the elderly. Anyone who does not receive enough sunshine to make vitamin D must consume vitamin D instead. For these people, vitamin D is a vitamin and an essential nutrient.

Vitamin D occurs in two major forms, vitamin D_2 (made from plant foods) and vitamin D_3 (made from animal foods). Vitamin D_2 is formed when ergosterol, found in plants, is exposed to ultraviolet light on the skin. Vitamin D_3 is a natural substance occurring in animal cells and formed by the action of sunlight on a cholesterol derivative in the skin.

The main function of vitamin D is to help regulate calcium and bone metabolism. To do this, it performs three functions.

1. Vitamin D helps regulate absorption of calcium and phosphorus from the intestine.
2. It reduces kidney excretion of calcium.
3. It helps regulate the deposition of calcium in the bones.

Vitamin D is not just a vitamin. It is also considered a hormone because skin cells can make it in the presence of sunlight.

Vitamin D deficiency.—The net result of vitamin D is to increase calcium and phosphorus deposition in bones. Without adequate calcium and phosphorus deposition, bones weaken and bow under pressure. When these symptoms occur in a child, the disease is called rickets. Symptoms of rickets include enlarged head, joints, rib cage, deformed pelvis, and bowed legs. The diets of infants, especially, and of others as well, should contain a food or supplement source of vitamin D if sufficient exposure to sunlight is not possible. This is especially important for breast-fed infants in their first six months of life. Today, rickets is most commonly associated with fat malabsorption, as is seen in children with cystic fibrosis.

Adult rickets, or osteomalacia (meaning "soft bones"), occurs most often in women who have low calcium intakes and little exposure to sun and who go through repeated pregnancies and periods of lactation. The bones of the legs may soften to such an extent that a young woman who is tall and straight at 20 may be condemned by repeated pregnancies to become bent, bowlegged, and stooped before she is 30. Combinations of sun exposure and/or treatment with vitamin D can be used in women with osteomalacia.

Vitamin D toxicity.—Of the 13 vitamins, vitamin D is the most toxic. An excess of vitamin D increases calcium absorption, causing abnormally high concentrations of the mineral in the blood (hypercalcemia). It promotes return of the bone calcium into the blood as well. The excess calcium in the blood will cause formation of stones. This is especially likely to happen in the kidneys, which concentrate calcium in the effort to excrete it. Calcification and hardening of the blood vessels (arteriosclerosis) may also occur and is especially dangerous in the major arteries of the heart and lungs, where it can cause death.

The range of safe intakes of vitamin D is narrower than that of vitamin A. Half the recommended intake is too little, but over a few times the recommended intake may be too much. Intakes of 100 micrograms per day causes high blood-calcium levels in infants, and some infants are sensitive to lower doses than this. Intakes of 250 micrograms per day for four months or 5,000 micrograms per day for two weeks cause toxicity in children and, if further prolonged, in adults. The amounts of vitamin D found in foods in America are well within these limits, but pills containing the vitamin in concentrated form should definitely be kept out of the reach of children and used cautiously by adults.

High levels of vitamin E are found in the lungs, which is good because oxygen is concentrated there. The lungs need protection from the oxygen.

Sources of vitamin D.—The way to meet your vitamin D needs is to synthesize it yourself with the help of sunlight. Some foods contain the performed vitamin (chiefly animal foods, such as milk, fish, eggs, and liver); but unless they are fortified, they are not likely to meet the RDA. The recommendations for vitamin D in rapidly growing children is twice as high as that for mature adults. Neither cow's milk nor human breast milk supplies enough vitamin D to meet human needs reliably; hence cow's milk is fortified, and infants are given either fortified formula or supplements. The fortification of milk is the best guarantee that children will meet their vitamin D needs and underscores the importance of milk in children's diets. The milk-drinking vegetarian is protected, but there is no practical source of vitamin D in plant foods. Without fortification or supplementation, diet alone cannot meet the body's vitamin D needs. The vegan needs exposure to sunlight for at least 20 minutes a day.

RDA for vitamin D.—Recently the accepted unit for measuring vitamin D became the microgram (mg). International units (I.U.) were previously used and are still found on food labels. For conversion to micrograms, one I.U. is equal to 0.025 mg (or 2.5 mg are equal to 100 I.U.). The RDA is 10 mg (400 I.U.) for infants, children, and adolescents to ensure proper skeletal growth. Young adults (ages 19–22) have an RDA of 7.5 mg (300 I.U.). Individuals older than 22 have an RDA of 5 mg (200 I.U.). During pregnancy and lactation, the RDA is increased to 10 mg (400 I.U.).

Because vitamin D is fat soluble, the fatty tissues of the human body can build up large amounts of this vitamin. Intakes above the RDA are thus potentially dangerous and strongly discouraged.

Vitamin E

What we call vitamin E is actually a family of compounds called tocopherols and tocotrienols. Vitamin E is one of the body's fat-soluble antioxidants. An antioxidant has the ability to step between a compound seeking electrons and the compound's target molecule, such as a fatty acid in a cell membrane. The antioxidant donates electrons and/or hydrogens to the electron-seeking compound, thus neutralizing it. This then protects other molecules or parts of the cell from an attack by the electron-seeking compound.

If vitamin E does not step in, the electron-seeking compound can pull electrons from cell membranes, DNA, and other electron-dense cell parts. That either alters the cell DNA, which may increase the risk for cancer, or destroys the cell membrane, causing cell death and possibly speeding the aging process.

The best known electron-seeking compounds likely to be found in cells are free radicals. These short-lived forms of compounds exist in a state in which an oxygen or carbon atom in the molecule contains only one electron, rather than two, in its outer shell. Consequently it seeks an electron to fill that outer shell. The special chemical-structure natures of oxygen and carbon atoms readily allow them to form a free-radical structure.

Free radicals are a necessary part of cell metabolism. But because free radicals cause chain reactions, it is important for vitamin E to buffer their assault on cell membranes to prevent significant cell destruction. Within minutes, one free radical can generate thousands of others. A small amount of cell destruction can lead to great destruction. After vitamin E donates two electrons, it is broken down itself and can no longer function.

High levels of vitamin E are found in the lungs, which is good because oxygen is concentrated there. The lungs need protection from the oxygen. People who smoke need even more vitamin E because of the oxidant stress smoking puts on the lung. A recent study, however, showed that even when consuming 240 times the adult RDA, smokers still had lower vitamin E concentrations in their lung fluids. The safest way to protect the lungs against illness (cancer, etc.) is not to smoke!

Another function of vitamin E is that it protects red blood cell membranes. A deficiency of vitamin E causes breakdown (hemolysis) of red blood cells, especially in infancy. The polyunsaturated fatty acids in the red blood cell membrane are

Vitamin E can help improve vitamin A absorption if the dietary intake of vitamin A is low. In this case vitamin E acts to protect the double bonds in vitamin A from damage.

sensitive to attack by free radicals. Since vitamin E can neutralize these agents, it can protect the red blood cell membrane from damage. Red blood cell hemolysis is common in premature infants because they did not receive sufficient vitamin E from their mothers.

Vitamin E can help improve vitamin A absorption if the dietary intake of vitamin A is low. In this case vitamin E acts to protect the double bonds in vitamin A from damage. Vitamin E is also needed for iron metabolism in the cell and the maintenance of nervous tissues and immune function.

Vitamin E deficiency.—Unlike the other vitamins, a deficiency of vitamin E does not produce its own unique disease. It is actually difficult for humans to develop a deficiency state. Most of the few cases on record coincide with fat malabsorption in adults and inadequate intake in premature infants. These individuals experience hemolysis (red blood cell destruction). Some adults have increased excretion of creatinine, which is a sign of muscle breakdown, and pigmentation in small intestinal muscles. Far more is known about vitamin E deficiency in animals, but these results do not seem to parallel human metabolism.

Vitamin E toxicity.—Vitamin E is relatively nontoxic. Some studies show that amounts in excess of approximately 500 milligrams (800 I.U.) per day of vitamin E can cause nausea, weakness, headache, diarrhea, and fatigue, as well as antagonize vitamin K metabolism. However, other studies show that intakes up to 2,100 milligrams (3,200 I.U.) may be safe for months. People with diseases such as phlebitis, in which blood clots form easily, sometimes benefit from large supplements of vitamin E but should follow such a regimen under the careful eye of a physician. Otherwise, hemorrhages may result.

RDA for vitamin E.—The RDA, as expressed in alpha-tocophenol equivalents (åTE), is 10 mg åTE for boys and men (15 I.U.) and 8 mg åTE for girls and women (12 I.U.). During pregnancy and lactation, the RDA increases to 10 mg and 11 mg åTE, respectively. People whose diets are higher in polyunsaturated fatty acids (plant oils) or omega-3 fatty acids (fish oils) need more vitamin E to inhibit oxidation. In some animal studies, when fish oil capsules are included in the diet, vitamin E deficiency develops.

Sources of vitamin E.—The most nutrient-dense food sources of vitamin E are plant oils, some fruits and vegetables, such as peaches and asparagus, and margarine. Animal fats have practically no vitamin E. Careful processing of plant oils to remove pesticide residues does not reduce much of vitamin E present. Other sources include wheat germ oil, whole grains, dark-green leafy vegetables, nuts, seeds, and legumes.

Vitamin K

Vitamin K was the last of the four fat-soluble vitamins to be discovered. It comes from a family of compounds known as quinones. The K stands for *koagulation,* as it is spelled in Denmark, because a Danish researcher first noted the relationship between vitamin K and blood clotting. It is stored primarily in the liver. However, these stores of vitamin K are relatively small and are rapidly used up. Vitamin K is stable to heat and oxidation but is destroyed by light, acid, alkali, and alcohol.

Functions of vitamin K.—Vitamin K contributes especially to the synthesis of several blood-clotting factors, including prothrombin. Vitamin K is needed for adding carbon dioxide molecules to these compounds. Prothrombin levels in the blood determine the rate at which the blood will clot.

A deficiency of vitamin K most likely occurs when a person takes antibiotics or has severe fat malabsorption. Antibiotics destroy many bacteria in the intestine that normally account for half the vitamin K absorbed.

An anticoagulant called Dicumarol, which is chemically similar to vitamin K, stimulates the formation of vitamin K oxide in the liver. Dicumarol can antagonize the action of vitamin K and so act as a potent anticoagulant. People who tend toward increased blood clotting greatly benefit from this drug. Heart attack victims are usually given dicumarol to prevent future blood clots. However, people taking drugs must be warned against consuming supplements of vitamin K and foods especially rich in vitamin K, since that would reduce the action of the drugs.

Sources of vitamin K.—Small amounts of vitamin K are found in a wide variety of foods. The most nutrient-dense food sources of vitamin K are peas, green beans, broccoli, cabbage, spinach, and turnip greens. Significant amounts are also present in milk and dairy products, cereals, fruits, and liver.

Most vitamin K consumed in a day is gone by the next.

Vitamin ads would have you believe that B vitamins give you energy. They don't.

However, vitamin K is so abundant in the diet that there is low risk of suffering a deficiency.

Not much vitamin K is found in human milk. In addition, an unborn child is not well adapted to store or synthesize vitamin K. So at birth, infants run the risk of poor blood clotting and eventual hemorrhage. To prevent this possible vitamin K deficiency condition, physicians routinely treat infants at birth with a form of vitamin K. This protection is intended to last until the infant's intestinal bacteria begin to synthesize vitamin K.

RDA for vitamin K.—Not only is vitamin K found in different foods, but it is also synthesized in the intestinal tract, especially in the jejunum and ileum. Approximately 50 percent of the daily requirement for vitamin K is supplied by intestinal bacteria. The RDA for adults is 60–80 micrograms per day. The U.S. diet contains 300 to 500 micrograms per adult per day of vitamin K, so a deficiency is unlikely.

Toxicity from vitamin K is likewise highly unlikely because, although it is fat-soluble, it is poorly stored in the body. One form of vitamin K, menadione, can be toxic; but it is available only by prescription. Symptoms include jaundice and a type of anemia.

The Fat-Soluble Vitamins—in Summary

To summarize, the four fat-soluble vitamins play many specific roles in the growth and maintenance of the body. Their presence affects the health and function of the skin, bones, teeth, eyes, blood, and nervous system.

Consuming excesses of the fat-soluble vitamins can cause toxicity, especially when people use supplements. The body cannot excrete excesses as it does with water-soluble vitamins; but rather, it stores them. The roles the fat-soluble vitamins play differ from those of the water-soluble vitamins, and they appear in different foods. Yet they are just as essential to life, and the need for them underlines the need to eat a wide variety of nourishing foods daily. Eating the right foods will help you "walk in newness of life" for your Lord.

The Water-Soluble Vitamins

As mentioned, the water-soluble vitamins include vitamin C and the eight B vitamins. The B vitamins, and possibly vitamin C, act as part of coenzymes. A coenzyme is a small molecule that can combine with an inactive protein to make it an active enzyme.

Unlike fat-soluble vitamins, water-soluble vitamins are generally absorbed directly from the intestine into the blood and need no carriers to travel around in the body fluids. Because they are water soluble, they are easily excreted in the urine, should more than the needed amount be present. Under ordinary circumstances you need not be concerned about taking small excesses; however, there have been reports of toxicity occurring after mega-dosing for long periods of time.

The B Vitamins

Vitamin ads would have you believe that B vitamins give you energy. They don't. The energy-yielding nutrients (carbohydrate, fat, and protein) can be used as energy, and the B vitamins help to burn that energy, but the vitamins do not serve as energy themselves.

It is true, though, that without B vitamins you would lack energy. Some of the B vitamins serve as helpers to the enzymes that release energy from carbohydrate, fat, and protein.

B vitamins also help cells to multiply, and this is especially important in population of cells with short life spans that must replace themselves rapidly. Such are the red blood cells and the cells lining the GI tract. Both of these cells are key members of the team of cells that deliver energy to all the body's tissues.

Each B vitamin plays several roles in metabolism. The roles they play as parts of coenzymes are the best understood. Remember, coenzymes are small nonprotein molecules that associate closely with some enzymes. There are differences in the details of the relationships between coenzymes and enzymes, but one thing is true of all: Without its coenzyme, an enzyme cannot function.

Thiamin (B_1)

The discovery of thiamin occurred in 1937 because of the high incidence of the disease beriberi. Fifty years earlier, one researcher, concerned with the high incidence of beriberi among Japanese sailors, noted that the addition of meat and milk to the diet seemed to prevent the disease. Shortly thereafter, another researcher observed that chickens fed polished rice developed symptoms similar to patients with beriberi. He experimented and found that feeding the chickens brown rice or rice bran

Riboflavin is light sensitive. It can be destroyed by the ultraviolet rays of the sun or by fluorescent light. For this reason milk should not be sold or stored in transparent glass containers.

eliminated the disease symptoms. In both cases, the original diets were deficient in thiamin, and the addition of thiamin-rich foods alleviated the problem.

Functions of thiamin.—The principal function of thiamin is to act as a coenzyme in the reactions that release energy from carbohydrate and trap the energy in a compound that the cells can briefly keep on hand to use when they need to do work. A thiamin deficiency produces nausea, severe exhaustion, loss of appetite, tenderness in the calf muscles; and, if prolonged, beriberi occurs. Emaciation, loss of control of the limbs (polyneuritis), and abnormal heart action are symptoms of beriberi. Unless treatment is initiated, beriberi is fatal. The effects are felt in every body cell and especially in those that are most dependent on carbohydrate. It is as if thiamin is the signal that allows traffic to flow across an intersection. When the signal isn't there, a massive traffic jam results. When thiamin is returned to the diet, the metabolic traffic flows again; and recovery can occur in a matter of a few hours. If thiamin deficiency is prolonged enough and severe enough, however, and occurs during the period of critical brain development in children, full recovery is impossible. Permanent brain damage results.

Recommended intakes of thiamin.—Because thiamin cannot be stored and is used up in the metabolism of energy nutrients, sufficient whole foods that provide it should be eaten daily. The RDA for the average adult woman is 1 milligram a day; and for the average man, 1.4 milligrams. As a general rule, the more calories a person needs in a day, the more thiamin is also needed. The thiamin requirement can be expressed as a proportion of the calorie allowance, as 0.5 milligrams per 1,000 calories. Thus athletes, especially runners, swimmers, and other endurance athletes, need more thiamin. Because athletes tend to eat more than sedentary people, however, more than enough of the extra thiamin is ingested, with no supplementation being necessary. The average college male and female consume 1.84 mg and 1.06 mg thiamin per day, respectively.

Sources of thiamin.—Sunflower seeds, wheat germ, cereals, and lean pork stand out as the richest sources of thiamin. Refined flour and polished rice are among the poorest, for thiamin is lost in the refining of wheat and rice. Enriched procedures for bread and cereal products replace the thiamin content. Other good sources are legumes, nuts, and fresh green vegetables.

Riboflavin (B_2)

Like thiamin, riboflavin acts as a coenzyme in energy-releasing reactions. Riboflavin also helps prepare fatty acids and amino acids for breakdown. Because of riboflavin's important role in the energy schema, some athletes believe that supplementation of riboflavin will improve performance. However, there is no evidence to support this claim.

Deficiency of riboflavin.—Riboflavin deficiencies are rare but sometimes appear in alcohol abusers. One riboflavin deficiency is called ariboflavinosis. This deficiency is characterized by inflammation of the mouth and tongue, dermatitis, cracking of tissue around the corners of the mouth, various eye disorders, and confusion. These symptoms develop after approximately two months of consuming a riboflavin-poor diet. A riboflavin deficiency often occurs with deficiencies of niacin, thiamin, and vitamin B_6; for these nutrients are often found in the same foods.

Recommended intake of riboflavin.—The RDA for men is 1.6 mg; and for women, 1.2 mg. Young children's needs begin about 1 mg a day and rise rapidly during the growing years. Teenagers need more riboflavin than adults (approximately 2 mg).

Sources of riboflavin.—Unlike thiamin, riboflavin is unevenly distributed among the food groups. The major contributors of riboflavin are milk and meat. The need for riboflavin provides a major reason for including milk in some form in every day's meals. People who don't use milk products can substitute generous servings of dark-green leafy vegetables. Among the meats, liver is the richest source; but all lean meats, as well as eggs, provide some riboflavin.

Riboflavin is light sensitive. It can be destroyed by the ultraviolet rays of the sun or by fluorescent light. For this reason milk should not be sold or stored in transparent glass containers. Cardboard or plastic containers screen out light, protecting the riboflavin.

Niacin (B_3)

A confusing array of names is attached to the vitamin niacin. Any of these may be found on food or supplement labels: niacin, nicotinic acid, nicotinamide. Both nicotinic acid and nicotinamide compounds can function as niacin in the body, but only nicotinic acid lowers serum cholesterol levels when taken in high doses.

Functions of niacin.—Like thiamin and riboflavin, niacin is part of a coenzyme vital to obtaining energy. Without niacin to form this coenzyme, energy-yielding reactions come to a screeching halt. The disease that results is pellagra, with means "rough" or "painful skin." The symptoms of the disease are known as the four "Ds"—dementia, diarrhea, dermatitis, and death. Early symptoms include poor appetite, weight loss, and weakness.

The key nutrient that prevents the disease is protein. Tryptophan, an amino acid present in the protein of lean meats (but deficient in the protein of corn), is converted to niacin in the body. Thus a person eating adequate protein will not be deficient in niacin.

Recommended intakes of niacin.—The RDA of niacin for adults is 15–19 milligrams per day for men and 13–15 milligrams per day for women. The RDA is expressed as niacin equivalents to account for niacin received intact from the diet as well as that synthesized from tryptophan.

> Evidence exists that a vitamin B_6 deficiency lowers the body's ability to resist disease by impairing the immune response to invading organisms, toxins, or foreign proteins.

The U.S. food supply contains 1.4 times the RDA (26.8 milligrams of niacin) per person per day, without considering the contribution from tryptophan. As long as one follows the Daily Food Guide, developing a niacin deficiency is highly unlikely. People with alcoholism are generally the only group to show niacin deficiency.

Toxicity of niacin can occur if intakes of 100 milligrams or more of nicotinic acid are consumed. This excess can lead to an increase in blood flow to the skin, causing a general blood vessel dilation or "flushing" of the body. Headache and itching also may result. This excessive intake is sometimes used, under a physician's guidance, to lower elevated blood-cholesterol levels.

Sources of niacin.—The most nutrient-dense sources of niacin are mushrooms, wheat bran, tuna and other fish, chicken, and peanuts. Most niacin in the American diet comes from enriched white bread, rolls, crackers, breakfast cereals, beef, and turkey. Niacin has a high heat stability, and little is lost in cooking.

Vitamin B_6

Vitamin B_6 comes in three forms and three names: pyridoxine, pyridoxal, and pyridoxamine. It plays a vital role in many cellular reactions involving carbohydrate, fat, and protein. More than 60 enzyme systems depend on vitamin B_6. Its absence produces a myriad of symptoms but no specific disease.

Vitamin B_6 helps to change one amino acid of which the cell has an abundance to another amino acid the cell needs. This means it aids in the synthesis of nonessential amino acids. It also helps remove amine groups from amino acids that are fated to be used for energy. As a coenzyme, it acts in the conversion of the amino acid tryptophan to niacin. It also helps to convert the essential fatty acid, linoleic acid, to another important fatty acid. It plays a role in the synthesis of hemoglobin and the secretions of the adrenal glands. It is also part of the enzyme that releases glucose from stored glycogen and, therefore, is important for maintaining blood glucose levels.

Because the influence of vitamin B_6 is felt in so many areas, it is understandable that a deficiency should be expressed in generalized symptoms such as depression, nausea, and vomiting. Other symptoms include a greasy kind of skin disorder and some irritation of the nerves. Evidence also exists that a vitamin B_6 deficiency lowers the body's ability to resist disease by impairing the immune response to invading organisms, toxins, or foreign proteins.

Recommended intake of vitamin B_6.—The RDA of vitamin B_6 for adults is 2 milligrams per day for men and 1.6 milligrams per day for women. The RDA is set high in response to high protein intakes found in the U.S. The more protein eaten, the more vitamin B_6 needed. Athletes may need more vitamin B_6 because of their increased use of glycogen for fuel (glycogen metabolism requires vitamin B_6), their increased use of amino acids for fuel, and their high protein intakes. Dietary protein should easily supply any extra vitamin B_6 needed.

Average consumption of vitamin B_6 in the U.S. is 2.06 mg per person per day, or about the RDA. A national average intake that equals the RDA should be of concern because that means that about half the intakes are below the RDA. In such cases, some people are probably not meeting their needs.

Vitamin B_6 deficiency.—Studies reveal that about 35–40 percent of adolescents, adults, and elderly women have poor vitamin B_6 intakes. Poor vitamin B_6 status is often found in women who use oral contraceptives. While this relationship has been known for the past 15 years, there is still no consensus that would suggest women take vitamin B_6 supplements.

For adults, deficiency symptoms include muscular weakness, nervousness, insomnia, and a facial skin disorder. A type of anemia may also develop.

Vitamin B_6 toxicity.—Intakes of 2–6 grams of vitamin B_6 per day for 2 months or more can lead to irreversible nerve damage. These high doses have mostly been used by women with PMS. Symptoms include walking difficulties and hand and foot numbness. Some nerve damage in individual sensory neurons is probably reversible, but damage to the ganglions (where many nerve fibers converge) is probably permanent.

There is concern about toxicity from doses of vitamin B_6 as low as 25 milligrams per day. This concern deserves note, since 1,000 milligram tablets of vitamin B_6 are available in health food stores. Taking a toxic dose is easy to do.

Sources of vitamin B_6.—Small quantities of vitamin B_6 are found in a wide variety of foods. Legumes, dried fruit, seeds and nuts, bananas, rice, and many vegetables are good sources of vitamin B_6. Protein foods, especially meat, fish, and poultry (vitamin B_6 is stored in muscles), are also good sources; and the vitamin B_6 present in animal foods is often more absorbable than that in plant foods. This makes meat, fish, and poultry our best sources of vitamin B_6.

Folate

Folate is also known as folic acid and folacin. Folate is probably more often deficient in the diets of people around the world than any other vitamin. It is essential for the formation and maturation of both red and white blood cells and for the making of all new cells by cell division. Not only is folate deficiency the most common vitamin deficiency in people, but it is also the most likely to be caused by the taking of medication. Ten major groups of drugs have been shown to affect the body's use of folate, including aspirin, anticonvulsants, and oral contraceptives.

Folate deficiency.—Probably the most important role of folate is to contribute to the formation of purine and pyrimidine bases in RNA and DNA. One major change caused by a folate deficiency is that in the early phases of red blood synthesis, the precursor cells cannot divide because they cannot form new DNA. The cells grow larger and larger because they can still synthesize enough protein and other cell parts to make new cells. But when it is time for the cells to divide, there is insufficient DNA to form two nuclei. The cells then remain in a large immature form, known as a megaloblast. Since the bone marrow of a folate-deficient person produces mostly immature megaloblast cells, few mature red blood cells (erythrocytes) arrive in the bloodstream. Since fewer mature red blood cells are present, oxygen-carrying capacity decreases, causing anemia. In short, a folate deficiency anemic, as with any anemia, is tired, weak, and apathetic, and may have headaches, irregular heartbeats, and labored breathing. Megaloblastic anemia is also characterized by a sore tongue, intestinal injury and diarrhea, lack of appetite, and weight loss, and by behavioral symptoms such as irritability and forgetfulness. It is altogether a miserable condition.

Folate toxicity.—A high intake of folacin can mask the anemia caused by vitamin B_{12} deficiency. This tendency exposes the uninformed strict vegetarian to a special risk. Strict vegetarians are most apt to be deficient in vitamin B_{12} because it is obtainable only from animal products. In addition, they are more likely to be well supplied with folate because, as its name implies (foliage), it is abundant in vegetables and fruits. The amount of vitamin B_{12} that can be stored in the body is one thousand times the amount used each day, so it may take years to develop a deficiency in a new vegetarian; but when it does occur, it may be masked by a high folate intake. Sometimes the damage is first seen in the breast-fed infant of the vegan mother.

Legumes, dried fruit, seeds and nuts, bananas, rice, and many vegetables are good sources of vitamin B_6.

A deficiency of vitamin B_{12} must be detected early by the presence of large, immature red blood cells in order to prevent the severe nerve damage that otherwise will develop. The vegetarian's high intake of folate helps the red blood cells to develop (despite the lack of vitamin B_{12}) to normal size and maturity. This deceives the physician who examines a blood sample for signs of abnormality. However, the folate can do nothing toward repairing the nerve damage caused by vitamin B_{12} deficiency, so this damage proceeds unchecked. Because of the danger of masking a lack of vitamin B_{12}, the amount of folate supplements are regulated by the FDA, so that only low dosages are available without a prescription.

Recommended folate intake.—The RDA for adults is 180–200 micrograms per day. Because of new data showing that folate is better absorbed than once thought, the current RDA is about half the value given previously. These newer figures are much more in line with the current folate content of the foods in the U.S. diet, which is approximately 225 micrograms per person per day.

Sources of folate.—Good sources of folate are green leafy vegetables, organ meats, sprouts, other vegetables, and orange juice. In fact, one cup of orange juice contains about one hundred micrograms of folate, which is approximately one half of the RDA. The presence of vitamin C seems to protect folate from destruction. Although folate is present in many foods, only 25 percent is ready for immediate absorption. The other 75

Segments of the population have the mistaken view that vitamin B_{12} injections will provide extra vitality and energy.

percent must be converted by enzymes in the digestive tract. Food processing and preparation destroy 50–90 percent of the folate in food. Folate is susceptible to destruction by heat. This underscores the importance of regularly eating fresh fruit and lightly cooked vegetables. Vegetables are best cooked quickly in minimal water—steaming, stir-frying, or microwaving.

Vitamin B_{12}

An atom of cobalt is located in the middle of vitamin B_{12}, which explains why the term *cobalamins* is often used to describe vitamin B_{12}. The vitamin takes many different forms. Adults need about two micrograms of vitamin B_{12} a day. This is the tiniest amount imaginable (2 millionths of a gram). But what seems like such a tiny amount to the human eye contains billions of molecules of vitamin B_{12}, enough to provide coenzymes for all the enzymes that need its help.

Vitamin B_{12} is unique among the nutrients in being found almost exclusively in meats and animal products. Anyone who eats meat is guaranteed an adequate intake, and lacto-ovo vegetarians (who use milk, cheese, and eggs) are also protected from deficiency. But vegans must use vitamin B_{12} fortified soymilk, fermented foods, or other such products, or take vitamin B_{12} supplements.

A second special characteristic of vitamin B_{12} is that its absorption requires an intrinsic factor (a type of protein made by the stomach's acid-producing parietal cells). The design for this factor is carried in the genes. The intrinsic factor is synthesized in the stomach, where it attaches to the vitamin; the complex then passes to the small intestine and is absorbed into the bloodstream.

A few people have in their genetic makeup a gene for the intrinsic factor that becomes defective, usually in midlife. Without the intrinsic factor, they can't absorb the vitamin even though they are taking enough in their diets, and so they develop deficiency symptoms. In such a case vitamin B_{12} must be supplied by injection to bypass the defective digestive system.

Another vital function of vitamin B_{12} is maintaining the myelin sheaths that insulate nerve fibers from one another. People with vitamin B_{12} deficiencies show patchy destruction of the myelin sheaths. The destruction of the myelin sheaths eventually causes paralysis and perhaps death.

Deficiency of vitamin B_{12}.—Unlike the other B-vitamins, enough vitamin B_{12} can be stored in the body to last five to seven years. Since only a minute amount of vitamin B_{12} stores is lost daily, a deficiency from an inadequate dietary intake takes years to develop.

In the past, the inability to absorb vitamin B_{12} eventually led to death. Researchers noted a form of anemia that caused death within two to five years of initial illness. They called this pernicious anemia, which literally means "leading to death." Clinically, the anemia looks much like a folate deficiency anemia. Many macrocytes are seen in the bloodstream. Thus the vitamin B_{12} anemia is called a macrocytic anemia. A lack of vitamin B_{12} in the diet alone cannot cause pernicious anemia. Only a decreased ability to absorb vitamin B_{12} can cause it. Once pernicious anemia is noted, an injection of vitamin B_{12} reverses changes in red blood cell synthesis in one to two days.

Besides anemia, clinical signs and symptoms of pernicious anemia include weakness, sore tongue, back pain, apathy, and tingling in the extremities. It takes about three years for symptoms of nerve destruction to develop.

Toxicity of vitamin B_{12}.—Vitamin B_{12} toxicity has not been associated with daily doses as high as 100 mg. In a few rare cases, vitamin B_{12} injections have caused adverse reactions. Segments of the population have the mistaken view that vitamin B_{12} injections will provide extra vitality and energy. Some endurance athletes believe that vitamin B_{12} will enhance performance by building up their red blood cell supply. No evidence supports this. Vitamin B_{12} injections benefit only those rare individuals who already have a deficiency of the vitamin.

Recommended intake of vitamin B_{12}.—The RDA for vitamin B_{12} for adults is two micrograms per day. The average American diet yields approximately eight micrograms per day. This high intake provides the average meat-eating person two to three years' storage of vitamin B_{12} in the liver. Thus, if you eat animal foods regularly and can absorb vitamin B_{12}, a vitamin B_{12} deficiency is highly unlikely.

Sources of vitamin B_{12}.—The best sources of vitamin B_{12} are liver, oysters, beef, pork, eggs, milk, and hot dogs. Vitamin B_{12} is present only in animal foods; none is found in plant foods. Vitamin B_{12} is often added to breakfast cereal, soymilk, and meat-substitutes. When a vitamin is added to a food in which the vitamin is not normally present, the process is called fortification. Some cereals are fortified with vitamin B_{12}.

Pantothenic acid is present in all foods. Nutrient-dense sources include mushrooms, yeast, liver, peanuts, and eggs. Other good sources are meat, milk, and many vegetables.

Biotin

Biotin comes in two forms—the vitamin itself and biocytin, an inactive form that is simply biotin with the amino acid lysine attached. Biotin acts as a coenzyme in fat and carbohydrate metabolism. Specifically, biotin assists the addition of carbon dioxide molecules to other compounds. One problem in assessing biotin status is that there is no accurate measure for it. Symptoms of an overt biotin deficiency include a scaly inflammation of the skin, changes in the tongue and lips, decreased appetite, nausea, vomiting, anemia, depression, muscle pain, muscle weakness, and poor growth.

A substance present in egg whites, avidin, binds to biotin, preventing its absorption in the small intestine. Since one must consume at least two dozen raw egg whites daily to produce a deficiency, avidin binding of biotin is not a problem in the typical human diet. In cases of alcoholism, however, biotin deficiency symptoms resulting from raw eggs have been reported in people with a regular consumption of just three raw eggs a day. Be careful in consuming raw eggs for fear of salmonella bacteria food poisoning.

Recommended intake of biotin.—The estimated safe and adequate dietary intake for biotin is 30–100 micrograms per day for adults. The average American diet is thought to contain 100–300 micrograms per person per day. It is important to avoid a biotin supplement, for research knows little about this vitamin, especially its potential for toxicity.

Food sources for biotin.—Foods high in biotin are cauliflower, egg yolks, yeast, liver, peanuts, and cheese. These foods are also the most nutrient-dense sources of biotin. Fruits are generally poorer sources. Intestinal synthesis of biotin by bacteria probably supplies part of our needs, especially considering that a biotin deficiency is so unlikely. There are no known cases of toxicity from excessive biotin intake.

Pantothenic Acid

Pantothenic acid was named after the Greek word *pantos,* meaning "everywhere." This vitamin is found widely in all types of food. Therefore, there is no deficiency disease associated with pantothenic acid.

Pantothenic acid forms part of coenzyme A, which is necessary in the production of ATP (energy). It is also found throughout the body as part of an enzyme essential to fat, carbohydrate, and protein metabolism. As mentioned, pantothenic acid deficiency is virtually unknown, except in combination with other B-vitamin deficiencies. In animals with dark fur, pantothenic acid deficiency causes graying and loss of hair. This development does not occur in humans. Some entrepreneurs have promoted products containing pantothenic acid to help people prevent hair loss or graying. No evidence supports the claim that this will occur.

Research has not found any toxicity to occur when consuming large doses of pantothenic acid.

Recommended intakes of pantothenic acid.—The estimated safe and adequate daily intake for pantothenic acid is four to seven milligrams per day for adults. The current American diet intake is about six milligrams of pantothenic acid per person per day. Pantothenic acid is present in all foods. Nutrient-dense sources include mushrooms, yeast, liver, peanuts, and eggs. Other good sources are meat, milk, and many vegetables. Because pantothenic acid is not added to enriched grains, they are not especially good sources of this vitamin.

B-Vitamin Relatives

Three compounds called B-vitamins are inositol, choline, and lipoic acid. These are not essential nutrients for human beings, although deficiencies can be induced in laboratory animals in order to study the functions of these three compounds. Like the B-vitamins described above, they serve as coenzymes in metabolism. Even if they were essential for human beings, supplements would be unnecessary because they are abundant in foods.

Summary of the B Vitamins

In summary, the eight B vitamins play many specific roles in helping the enzymes perform thousands of different molecular conversions in the body. The B vitamins are active in carbohydrate, fat, protein metabolism, and in the making of DNA and thus new cells. They are found in every cell and must be present continuously for the cells to function as they should.

The meat and meat alternate group serves thiamin, niacin, vitamin B_6, and vitamin B_{12} well. The milk and milk products group stands out for riboflavin and vitamin B_{12}. The fruits and vegetables group excels for folate. The cereal and bread group delivers thiamin, riboflavin, and niacin. A diet that offers a variety of food from each of the food groups will provide an adequate intake of the vitamins. By emphasizing the low-fat items from each of the four food groups, a person will be able to achieve calorie control while still receiving adequate intakes of all the vitamins.

Vitamin C

The first nutrition experiment to be conducted on human beings was devised nearly 250 years ago to find a cure for scurvy. Scurvy is a vitamin C deficiency disease that was killing British sailors. Many sailors contracted the disease after traveling many months on the seas. A British physician found that giving citrus fruits to sailors with scurvy cured them within a short time. The British Navy used this information and required all navy vessels to provide lime juice to every sailor daily. The term *limey* was applied to the British sailors in mockery because of this requirement. The name later given the vitamin, *ascorbic acid*, literally means "no scurvy."

Function of vitamin C.—Vitamin C has four main functions in the body: (1) collagen synthesis, (2) antioxidant,

Because vitamin C is water soluble, the body rapidly excretes excesses.

(3) enhancing iron absorption, and (4) synthesis of vital cell compounds. Let's examine each.

Collagen synthesis.—Vitamin C helps to form the fibrous, structural protein collagen. Collagen is the most important protein of connective tissue. It serves as the matrix on which bones and teeth are formed. When your skin has been lacerated, collagen glues the separated tissues' faces together, forming scars. Cells are held together largely by collagen. This is especially important in the artery walls, which must expand and contract with each beat of the heart, and the walls of the capillaries, which are thin and fragile and must withstand a pulse of blood every second or so without rupturing.

The cross-bonding of collagen, which is increased by vitamin C, stabilizes collagen and so greatly strengthens the tissues it helps form. Widespread changes in tissue metabolism and structure occur when a person is deficient in vitamin C. One symptom of scurvy is a reduction in the rate of wound healing. The first symptoms of scurvy appear after about 20–40 days of no vitamin C intake and include weakness and tiny hemorrhages in the skin. In addition, gums bleed and joints become painful.

Antioxidant.—Remember, an antioxidant is any substance that can reduce (donate electrons to) another substance. When it reduces the other substance, it simultaneously becomes oxidized itself. Vitamin C is one of the cell's water-soluble antioxidants. Recall that vitamin E is a fat-soluble antioxidant in the cell membrane. Vitamin C is like a bodyguard for oxidizable substances; it stands ready to sacrifice its own life to save theirs.

Using its antioxidant capabilities, vitamin C can reduce the formation of carcinogenic nitrosamines in the stomach and also keep the folate coenzymes intact and so prevent their destruction. If vitamin C is found effective in preventing cancer, its effectiveness will probably be due to its antioxidant capabilities.

Enhancing iron absorption.—Vitamin C is important for iron absorption. For iron absorption to take place, about 50 milligrams of vitamin C (about 4 ounces of orange juice) must be consumed at the same meal with the iron. Increasing vitamin C intake is beneficial if one has poor iron stores. However, some people suffer from a disease called hemochromatosis, which is characterized by an overstorage of iron. These people are actually harmed if they increase their vitamin C intake; for likewise, their iron absorption would also increase. This is a perfect example in which recommending a vitamin intake above the RDA may have conflicting results. Some people may benefit, whereas others may be injured.

Synthesis of vital cell compounds.—Vitamin C is necessary for the synthesis of thyroxine (thyroid hormone), as well as epinephrine, carnitine, norepinephrine, serotonin, bile acids, steroid hormones, and purine bases used in DNA synthesis.

Vitamin C is vital for the function of the immune system, especially for the activity of certain cells in the immune system. In addition, vitamin C is used by chemical-detoxifying mechanisms in cells. Thus both disease states and drug use can increase the need for vitamin C, but it's unclear as to how much above the RDA to prescribe.

Deficiency of vitamin C.—Because vitamin C is water soluble, the body rapidly excretes excesses. With an adequate intake, the body maintains a fixed pool of vitamin C and rapidly excretes any excess in the urine. About 80–90 percent of vitamin C is absorbed when a person eats 30–180 milligrams of it per day. If someone ingests 6,000 milligrams per day, absorption efficiency drops to about 20 percent. With an inadequate intake, the pool becomes depleted at the rate of about 3 percent per day.

If the vitamin C pool is allowed to dwindle, latent scurvy appears. The gums around the teeth bleed easily, and capillaries under the skin break spontaneously, producing pinpoint hemorrhages. Atherosclerotic plaques grow rapidly in the arteries.

When the vitamin pool falls to about a fifth of its optimal size (this may take two months or more to occur), overt scurvy symptoms begin to appear. Failure to promote normal collagen synthesis causes further hemorrhaging. Muscles, including the heart muscle, degenerate. The skin becomes rough, brown, scaly, and dry. Wounds fail to heal because scar tissue will not form. Bones become softened, malformed, and painful; and fractures appear. Anemia and infections are common. Sudden death is likely, occasioned by severe atherosclerosis or massive bleeding into the joints and body cavities.

Once diagnosed, scurvy is readily reversed by vitamin C. Moderate doses in the neighborhood of 100 milligrams per day are sufficient, curing the scurvy within about five days.

Toxicity of vitamin C.—Vitamin C is the supplement which is most often added to the diet. Since the time Dr. Linus Pauling began advancing the concept that massive doses of vitamin C could prevent and cure the common cold and cancer, millions of people have dosed themselves with high quantities of vitamin C. Pauling advised people to consume 1,000–10,000 mg of vitamin C daily, 17–167 times the RDA. Other researchers have been unable to confirm Pauling's recommendation. Recent research by the Mayo Clinic, using a double-blind placebo design, has also not been able to show any benefit of massive vitamin C doses in curing cancer, contrary to Pauling's research findings.

Vitamin C is not highly toxic, but high doses can cause problems. Rebound scurvy can occur in individuals who suddenly stop their massive vitamin C doses. If a person suddenly reduces high intakes to normal, the accelerated disposal system may not be able to put on its brakes fast enough to avoid destroying too much of the vitamin. To avoid rebound scurvy, individuals who are using high amounts of vitamin C supplements should reduce their intake gradually.

Other complications from vitamin C megadosing include diarrhea, decreased copper absorption, and increased uric acid excretion leading to gout and kidney stones.

Recommended intake of vitamin C.—The RDA for men and women is 60 mg of vitamin C. Pregnant women need an additional 20 mg and lactating women an additional 40 mg. Care must be taken during food preparation to preserve vitamin C. Excess heat over a prolonged period, air exposure to cut surfaces, large amounts of cooking water, and exposure to baking soda reduce the level of vitamin C.

The amount needed to prevent overt scurvy is only 10 milligrams. However, 10 milligrams a day apparently does not saturate all the body tissues. Larger intakes increase the body's total vitamin C pool. At about 60 milligrams per day, the pool size in the average person stops responding to further increases in intake, and at 100 milligrams per day, 95 percent of the population probably reaches tissue saturation. After the tissues are saturated, all added vitamin C is excreted.

Sources of vitamin C.—The fruit and vegetable group supplies the highest concentration of vitamin C. Broccoli, brussels sprouts, greens, cabbage, cantaloupe, strawberries, and potatoes are rich sources of vitamin C. Foods from animal sources, such as milk, eggs, meat, poultry, and fish are largely devoid of vitamin C.

Nutrition scientists generally agree that most people can obtain the vitamins and minerals they need if they eat a healthy diet.

Do You Need Vitamin Supplements?

Americans spend nearly three billion dollars on vitamin pills each year. Forty-five percent of Americans use them. Yet nutrition scientists generally agree that most people can obtain the vitamins and minerals they need if they eat a healthy diet. The question that arises is, Why do people take vitamin and mineral supplements?

The answer may lie in the confusion and myths circulating throughout American society concerning vitamin consumption. Let's examine some of these myths and relate them to the facts.

Vitamin supplements prevent colds and other illnesses.—The fact is, if a vitamin is missing from the diet, taking that vitamin can prevent or cure the deficiency disease; however, taking extra doses of vitamins does not prevent or cure other diseases.

Vitamin supplements provide a hedge against an undesirable diet.—The truth is, consuming a poor diet high in fat, salt, and sugar, with little fiber, cannot be reversed with vitamins. Getting a good diet means more than just obtaining all the recommended amounts of vitamins. Many other nonvitamin aspects of the diet comprise good nutrition. To justify a poor diet by taking vitamin pills is a misguided practice.

Vitamin supplements are necessary because the soil is so depleted today.—The fact is, crops can't grow in depleted soil. If a nutrient is low, the yield will be low, but the vitamin content will be normal. Estimates of the nutrient content of our food supply by the U.S. Department of Agriculture indicate that the amounts of most nutrients available to the consumer have increased during this century.

A statement released from the American Medical Association emphasized that sound dietary practices should eliminate any need for supplemental vitamins after infancy in essentially all healthy children.

Vitamin supplements protect against harmful chemicals and pollutions.—The truth is, vitamins cannot ward off harmful chemicals or pollution. If a harmful chemical is consumed, no vitamin will negate its harmful effect.

Some people need high intakes of vitamins to be healthy.—The fact is, research studies have shown that it is extremely rare for anyone to need amounts higher than the RDA. People who may need higher amounts are discussed below.

Vitamin supplements give extra energy, especially during times of stress.—The truth is, only carbohydrates, fats, and proteins provide the body with energy (calories). Vitamins only assist in releasing this energy. The rate of this energy release is not affected by high vitamin intakes.

Vitamin pills from natural sources are always safe and are much better than synthetic ones.—The fact is, there is no difference between natural and synthetic vitamin pills except the price. Most vitamins labeled "natural" are actually synthetic, and both kinds can be toxic if taken in excess.

Vitamin supplements are harmless, so taking extra amounts will just give extra benefits and security.—Vitamin pills are not harmless extractions from food. When taken in high doses, vitamins are similar to drugs. Almost every vitamin is capable of producing toxic reactions in the body. The fat-soluble vitamins (A, D, E, and K) are especially dangerous. In addition to toxicity, vitamins also interfere with one another and with various minerals during intestinal absorption. For example, excessive vitamin C decreases copper absorption; high levels of folate decrease zinc absorption; and large amounts of niacin can counteract vitamin B_{12} absorption.

Recently a panel of nutrition scientists suggested a few cases in which vitamin and mineral supplementation might be considered:

1. Women with excessive menstrual bleeding may need extra iron.
2. Women who are pregnant or are breast-feeding may need extra calcium, iron, and folate.
3. People with low calorie intake need the range of vitamins and minerals.
4. Some vegetarians who are highly restrictive in their diets may need extra vitamin B_{12}, zinc, iron, and calcium.
5. Newborns may need vitamin K to prevent abnormal bleeding (only under the direction of a physician).
6. People with specific illness or diseases, such as a vitamin-resistance disease, may need supplements.
7. People who use certain medications may require supplementation of specific vitamins and minerals. For example, a physician might recommend extra calcium to treat osteoporosis.

A statement released by the American Medical Association emphasized that sound dietary practices should eliminate any need for supplemental vitamins after infancy in essentially all healthy children. Healthy adult men and women and healthy nonpregnant, nonlactating women consuming a usual, varied diet do not need vitamin supplements. All health practitioners should emphasize repeatedly that properly selected diets are the primary basis for good nutrition.

[CHAPTER 15]

Understanding the Minerals

Many of us have heard ministers quote at a funeral "ashes to ashes and dust to dust." Often, this familiar quotation is used to remind us of our mortality. But this familiar quotation used by ministers at funerals is inaccurate. For one thing, a person does not spring into being from the ashes. A living human being begins when the sperm penetrates the egg, and during the next nine months those two living cells multiply into a three-trillion, clay-colored, wrinkled package of screaming cells we call a baby. And when God takes our life force to be with Him, what is left behind is more than a small pile of ashes. Examination of these ashes reveals carbohydrates, proteins, fats, vitamins, minerals, and water, which soon disappear.

The carbon atoms in all the carbohydrates, fats, proteins, and vitamins combine with oxygen to produce carbon dioxide, which vanishes into the air; the hydrogens and oxygens of those compounds unite to form water; and this water, along with the water that was a large part of the body weight, evaporates. Then only the minerals are left behind as ashes. The small pile of ashes, about five pounds, is not impressive in size; but when you consider the tasks these minerals perform, you may realize their great importance in living tissue.

If you could separate calcium and phosphorus from the rest of the pile of ashes, you could take away about three fourths of the total. Crystals made of these two minerals, plus a few others, form the structure of the bones and so provide the architecture of the skeleton.

If a magnet were run through the one fourth of the pile that remains and picked up iron, it would not fill a teaspoon; yet it is billions and billions of iron atoms. As part of the protein hemoglobin, each iron atom has the special property of being able to attach to atmospheric oxygen and deliver it to all cells deep inside the body.

As you can see, minerals, like vitamins, are vital to our health. More than one third of the dietary nutrients you need to maintain life are minerals. These minerals play important roles in the human body and are also related to such diseases as cancer and high blood pressure. Minerals are categorized as major and trace minerals based on the amount humans need per day. Minerals of which we require 100 milligrams or more per day are considered major minerals; otherwise, they are considered trace minerals. In distinguishing between the major and the trace minerals, remember that one group is no more important than the other. A deficiency of the few micrograms of iodine needed daily by the body is just as serious as a deficiency of the several hundred milligrams of calcium. However, the major minerals, because of their larger total quantities, have a larger influence on the body fluids.

This chapter begins with a discussion of the characteristics of water, which is the most indispensable nutrient of all. The chapter then goes on to show how some of the major minerals affect it. Lastly, we will discuss the specialized role of each major mineral.

Water

Water is such an integral part of us that we seldom are conscious of its importance unless we are deprived of it. We can survive a deficiency of all the other nutrients for long periods of time, some of them even for months or years; but we can survive only a few days without water. You began life as a single cell bathed in

Muscular people have a higher proportion of body water because muscle contains almost three times as much water as adipose (fat) tissue.

a nourishing fluid. Even after you became a wonderfully created, beautifully organized, air-breathing body of approximately one hundred trillion cells, each individual cell had to remain next to water to remain alive. That water brings to each cell the exact ingredients it requires and carries away the end products of the life-sustaining reactions that take place within its boundaries. Water makes up about 60 percent of the body weight.

In the adult body, 6 percent of the water is replaced each day; in the infant's body 15 percent is replaced. Although up to four quarts of water may be taken into the body, another four quarts may be lost each day. Homeostatic mechanisms are so sensitive that the variation in body weight from change in the body fluids seldom exceeds one-third pound daily.

Water is a constituent of every cell of the body. It is present in varying amounts in different tissues. The total amount of body water is a function of age and body composition. In most adults, water makes up about 60 percent of total body weight and 70 percent of lean body mass (or fat-free tissue). Muscular people have a higher proportion of body water because muscle contains almost three times as much water as adipose (fat) tissue. Males have a higher amount of body water than females because they have proportionately more lean tissue and less fat. People lose water as they age, with a decline from 80 percent body weight at birth to 50 percent in old age, largely caused by a loss of extracellular water.

Water is present in two major compartments: the intracellular (within the cells) and the extracellular (outside the cells). These two compartments are separated by a semipermeable membrane that allows water to pass through readily. Some electrolytes or ions (particularly sodium, potassium, and chloride) can cross the membrane. The extracellular fluid can be further divided into the intravascular and intercellular compartments. The intravascular compartment includes the fluid in all parts of the vascular system (which are arteries, veins, and capillaries). It is separated from the intercellular (between cells) compartment (also called interstitial or extravascular) by the walls of these blood vessels. The intercellular fluid is responsible for carrying the nourishment to the individual cells and collecting any waste products to be taken back to the bloodstream.

The intercellular compartment acts as a buffer area. This occurs because its volume will adjust to prevent changes in the volume of either the intravascular or intracellular fluid. A third (transcellular) compartment includes the fluid that lubricates the joints and the fluid in the eyeball. The transcellular compartment represents a very small portion of total body water and is not usually involved in fluid shifts.

The movement of fluid from one compartment to another is controlled to a large extent by the concentration of minerals on either side of the membrane separating the compartments. Mineral elements in body fluids occur primarily as salts. These salts in solution separate into their component ions; one ion has a positive charge (cation) and the other a negative charge (anion). The charged ions are known as electrolytes. They account for the osmotic pressure that causes water to move from one compartment to another to establish a balance in the concentration of electrolytes on either side of the membrane. As the concentration of electrolytes increases, the osmotic pressure increases. When the osmotic pressure of fluid in one compartment becomes higher than that in the adjacent compartment, fluid is moved from the higher concentration until the pressure, or ion concentration, on each side of the membrane is equalized. When this occurs, the same number of molecules and ions per volume of fluid are present on either side of the membrane, the osmotic pressures are the same, the amount of fluid on either side remains relatively constant, and no fluid shifts back and forth.

Under most circumstances, the body is able to prevent an unfavorable shift in electrolyte concentrations so that there is no significant change in water balance among compartments. However, shifts do occasionally occur as the result of changes in electrolyte concentration in one of the fluid compartments. These shifts will be discussed further in the section on sodium.

Functions of Water

Water has seven main functions as it relates to vital body processes. The importance of a constant source of water is even more apparent when we consider the large amount of fluid that can be lost from the body in a short period of time.

Source of minerals.—Although water itself is made up of only two elements (hydrogen and oxygen), water may be a significant source of minerals such as fluorine, zinc, and copper. Up to 50 mg of calcium and 120 mg of magnesium per liter may be present in hard water but are removed in the ion exchange processes used to soften the water supply. Two quarts

Because of its ability to conduct heat, water plays an important role in the distribution of heat throughout the body and therefore in the regulation of body temperature.

of hard water may provide as much as 240 mg of magnesium, two thirds of the recommended intake. The use of hard water has been associated with decreased risk of cardiovascular disease. In contrast, soft water may contain up to 250 mg of sodium per quart, with high intakes a risk factor for hypertension. Because water is such a good solvent, it may also be the source of toxic elements such as lead or cadmium, pesticides, herbicides, and industrial wastes. Constant monitoring of the water supply is therefore essential to safeguard the health of the public.

Solvent.—The average male has approximately five quarts of blood. This intravascular water acts as a solvent for carbohydrates, proteins, fats, vitamins, and minerals. These nutrients as well as many hormones must be carried to all parts of the body for the individual cells to be adequately nourished and to function properly. Water is thus the transport vehicle for all the nutrients.

The spaces between cells (intercellular) have 12 quarts of fluid carrying nutrients that have left the blood vessels. This fluid also collects waste products and hormones or other substances that may be secreted by the cell. Within the cell, water serves as a solvent for nutrients that must be transported from one organelle to another and for waste products that must be eliminated.

Lubricant.—Another important characteristic of water is its incompressibility. Its molecules resist being crowded together. Thanks to this characteristic, water can act as a lubricant around joints. For the same reason, it can protect a sensitive tissue such as the spinal cord from shock. The fluid that fills the eye serves in a similar way to keep optimal pressure on the retina and lens. This is part of the transcellular compartment.

Temperature regulator.—Because of its ability to conduct heat, water plays an important role in the distribution of heat throughout the body and therefore in the regulation of body temperature. Some of the heat from the metabolism of carbohydrate, fat, and protein is required to maintain body temperature at 98.6° F. This is the temperature at which all enzymes operate most effectively. In fact, proteins in the brain will denature (break up) when body temperature reaches 105° F.

Subcutaneous fat acts as an insulating material, reducing the speed with which heat can be lost. This is an advantage in winter and a disadvantage in summer. Heat loss may also be affected by how close the blood comes to the surface of the skin. The blood vessels near the surface of the skin expand to promote heat loss in hot weather. In cold weather, they contract to minimize the possibility of heat loss. The distance between the blood vessels and the skin is the reason obese people suffer more in hot climates than nonobese people do.

Growth promoter.—For growth to occur, water must be present in all cells. Glycogen is about two-thirds water; fat tissue is one-fifth water; and muscle is close to three-fourths water. Growth would be impossible if water were not available.

Catalyst.—Water acts as a catalyst in many biological reactions within the cell. Water is also necessary for the reactions required to break apart, or hydrolyze, complex nutrients into their simpler component parts.

Acid-base balance.—The pH of the blood is kept between 7.35 and 7.45, just slightly on the alkaline (basic) side. To do this, the body uses the dilutional effects of total body water and the actions of lungs, kidneys, and blood proteins. Diet mildly affects the acid-base balance in the body. Foods high in protein also frequently contain much sulfur and phosphorus. These ions remain after the rest of the protein is metabolized and eventually form acids in the body, namely sulfuric acid and phosphoric acid. These acids can cause a slight decrease in the blood pH.

Most fruits and vegetables create a more alkaline effect. These foods contain sodium and potassium ions often attached to acids. When the food is metabolized, these ions remain and eventually form sodium hydroxide and potassium hydroxide, two bases. Although fruits contain acids, their metabolism results in the formation of bases. Small changes in blood pH (say to 6.9) will cause various health problems, even death. Water plays an integral part in maintaining the normal pH in the blood.

Water Needs

Water needs for adults are roughly estimated to be 1 milliliter per calorie in the diet. This works out to 10 cups for a 2,400-calorie diet. Water is lost in four ways in the body: (1) skin perspiration, (2) lung respiration, (3) urine, and (4) colon loss. The body normally acquires water in three ways: (1) Most people consume about 1 quart of water per day in various liquids. (2) Food supply (table 15.1) contributes another quart of fluid. (3) Water is a by-product of metabolism. For good health, water intake should equal water output.

Table 15.1
Percent Water in Foods (by Weight)

Category	Food	Percent Water
Meat	Eggs	74
	Beef	53
	Chicken	58
	Sardines	62
	Pork	42
Vegetables	Broccoli	91
	Carrots	88
	Corn	74
	Lettuce	95
	Peas	82
Dairy Products	Whole milk	87
	Cheese	40
	Cottage cheese	78
	Yogurt	89
Fruits	Tomato	94
	Apples	85
	Oranges	86
	Bananas	76
	Watermelon	93
Cereals	White bread	36
	Whole wheat	36
	Oats	3
	Rice	12
Beverages	Ice tea	99
	Coffee	99
	Cola (diet)	99
	Fruit drinks	99
	Milk (skim)	90.5
	Cola (regular)	90
	Milk (whole)	87
	Lemonade	87

Thirst.—Thirst is the first signal that the body registers when a person does not consume enough water. The brain (hypothalamus) signals the person that he needs to drink. The thirst mechanism is not always reliable, especially during illness or when participating in vigorous physical exercise. Athletes or vigorous exercisers weigh themselves before and after training sessions to determine their rate of water loss and thus their water needs. The weight loss should not exceed more than one pound from day to day. Children who are ill, especially those with fever, diarrhea, or increased perspiration, need to be reminded to drink plenty of fluids. Many physicians recommend drinking Gatorade™ or some similar drink that has potassium and sodium in its mixture when one has fever.

If the thirst message is ignored, the body registers a shortage of available water and begins fluid conservation. This defense mechanism occurs because the pituitary gland releases antidiuretic hormone (ADH) to force the kidneys to conserve water. As fluid volume drops in the bloodstream, blood pressure falls. The fall signals the kidneys to release an enzyme called rennin, which acts on a protein in the bloodstream to form the compound angiotensin I. Angiotensin I converts to angiotensin II if water is not consumed. That triggers the adrenal gland to release more of the hormone aldosterone, which signals the kidneys to retain more sodium and therefore more water. Remember that water always follows positive ions (especially Na). Thus low blood pressure, through this roundabout measure, causes increased water conservation in the body.

The effectiveness of ADH and aldosterone is limited. Fluid is constantly lost through the feces, skin, and lungs. Those losses must be replaced. Eventually, if fluid is not consumed, the body becomes dehydrated and suffers ill effects.

Dehydration.—If a person loses 2 percent of body weight in fluids, he or she will be thirsty. At a 4-percent loss of body weight, muscles undergo a significant drop in strength and endurance. By the time body weight is reduced by 10 to 12 percent, heat tolerance is decreased; and the person feels weak. At a 20-percent reduction, the person may lapse into a coma and soon die. Always allow many water breaks in your physical training. Don't try to see how long you can go without water.

On the other hand, excessive drinking of water can quickly overwhelm the kidney's capacity to excrete it. Water then accumulates in the body, causing headaches, blurred vision, cramps, and eventually convulsion. Try to find your happy medium.

The Major Minerals

The seven major minerals are minerals needed in amounts greater than 100 mg a day. They include calcium, phosphorus, magnesium, sodium, chloride, potassium, and sulfur. Three of these (sodium, chloride, and potassium) are known as the three body electrolytes. Now let us review the individual properties of the seven major minerals.

Calcium

Calcium holds the honor of being the most abundant mineral in the body. Its importance is gaining recognition, as evidenced by magazine articles on osteoporosis. Americans have been urged to consume calcium (offered now in everything from high-calcium bread to high-calcium soft drinks) to help prevent osteoporosis (weak bones), high blood pressure, and bowel cancer. In the clamor for more calcium, Americans have dramatically increased their consumption of calcium supplements. Should we increase our calcium intake? Let's review the facts.

Ninety-nine percent of the body's calcium is stored in the bones and teeth. The other one percent is in the blood and body fluids. Blood calcium is constantly changing and regulating itself metabolically. In fact, about a fourth of the calcium in the blood is exchanged with calcium every minute. Vitamin D and other hormones tightly control the blood's calcium concentration.

Ninety-nine percent of the body's calcium is stored in the bones and teeth. The other one percent is in the blood and body fluids.

Whenever the blood calcium concentration rises too high, these agents promote its deposit into bone. Whenever the blood concentration falls too low, the intestines will increase calcium absorption; or the bones will increase calcium release; or the kidneys will reduce calcium excretion to correct it. Thus the blood calcium concentration returns to normal.

Blood calcium is never affected by calcium found in food. This doesn't mean to say that blood calcium never changes. It does change; but it changes in response to changed regulatory control, not to diet. When blood calcium rises above normal, the result is known as *calcium rigor*. That is, the muscles contract and cannot relax. On the other hand, if blood calcium levels fall below normal, a condition called tetany results. This is characterized by uncontrolled contractions of muscle tissue due to a change in the stimulation of nerve cells. These conditions do not reflect a dietary lack or excess of calcium. These conditions are caused by a lack of vitamin D or by malfunctions in the endocrine glands (normally the parathyroid glands) that result in abnormal amounts of hormones that regulate blood calcium concentration.

On the other hand, a longtime dietary deficiency of calcium over the course of years can diminish the calcium reserves (normally 2.2 lbs. are stored in bones) found in the bones. The bones, not the blood, are depleted by calcium deficiency.

Calcium absorption.—Calcium absorption normally takes

place in the upper part of the small intestine (duodenum) because calcium requires a pH below 6 to stay in solution. Calcium absorption also depends on the vitamin D hormone *calcitriol.* Calcium absorption varies from about 25 to 40 percent of dietary intake but can increase to as high as 50 percent during pregnancy and at other times of high-calcium needs. Young people tend to absorb calcium better than older people. The lowest rates of absorption occur in post-menopausal women who do not receive supplements of the hormone *estrogen.* Estrogen therapy increases the synthesis of calcitriol, which increases calcium absorption.

Many factors increase calcium absorption, such as the acidic environment of the small intestine; the presence of calcitriol, parathyroid hormone, dietary glucose, and lactose. On the other hand, factors that limit calcium absorption include fiber, magnesium, or phosphorus in the diet and tannins in tea, also a vitamin D deficiency, menopause, diarrhea, and old age. Protein also affects calcium status but not by affecting absorption. Excess protein in the diet increases the amount of calcium excreted. This is why calcium recommendations in the U.S. and Canada (these countries consume more protein) are greater than for people in countries where protein intakes are lower. So try to maintain your protein intake at moderate levels (10–15%).

Most nutrient deficiencies make themselves known by way of symptoms that can be felt or seen, such as pain, skin lesions, tiredness, etc. But a developing calcium deficiency is utterly silent.

Calcium deficiency.—The average American diet does not contain an abundance of calcium, and low intakes are widespread in America. The urgency of obtaining enough calcium has to be learned through education because the body sends no signals saying it is deficient. Most nutrient deficiencies make themselves known by way of symptoms that can be felt or seen, such as pain, skin lesions, tiredness, and so forth. But a developing calcium deficiency is utterly silent. It becomes apparent only when a hip or pelvic bone suddenly breaks and will not heal. No evidence of a developing calcium deficiency can be found in a blood sample because blood calcium remains normal no matter what the bone content may be. Nor does depletion of bone calcium show up in an X-ray examination until it is so far advanced as to be virtually irreversible.

Calcium is essential for blood clotting.—It participates in a reaction whereby prothrombin (plasma protein) contributes to the synthesis of fibrin so that a blood clot can form. Without sufficient calcium in the bloodstream, blood will not clot.

Calcium is essential for muscle contraction.—It allows the proteins in muscles, actin and myosin, to interact properly during muscle contraction. If the blood calcium level falls below a certain level, muscles cannot relax after contraction. The body than stiffens and shows signs of tetany.

Calcium is essential for normal nerve transmission.—It permits the release of neurotransmitters as well as the flow of ions in and out of nerve cells. Tetany can also occur when nerve transmission fails because insufficient calcium is available.

Calcium is essential to prevent osteoporosis.—Osteoporosis is defined as an age-related disorder, characterized by decreased bone mineral content and increased risk of fractures. Women, and to a lesser extent men, have been urged to increase their consumption of calcium-rich foods to decrease their risk of osteoporosis. Osteoporosis can be further classified as Type I (post-menopausal), which appears in the years after menopause, and Type II (senile), which is found in people of advanced ages.

Some studies have shown that high calcium intake helps retard or prevent the progress of osteoporosis. Other studies have shown little benefit in calcium intakes above 500 mg/day. Other factors such as adequate estrogen, sunshine (vitamin D), and physical activity may be more important.

Besides contributing to bone strength, dietary calcium may reduce the risk of colon cancer. It appears that a high-calcium content in the stool can bind free fatty acids and bile acids found there. These compounds, when unbound, tend to irritate the colon. This irritation may increase cell turnover and, in turn, increase the risk of cancer. A daily dietary calcium supplement of 1,250 milligrams reduces the cell turnover in the colon. High calcium levels in the colon may also increase the tendency of cancer cells in the colon to clump together and decrease their tendency to metastasize (spread) to other areas.

Some studies indicate that taking supplemental calcium of 1 gram or more per day may also slightly decrease blood pressure. Careful studies show that about 50 percent of people register slightly lower blood pressure when they consume at least 1,000 milligrams of supplemental calcium per day. Systolic pressure is affected more than diastolic pressure. It is reasonable for a person with hypertension to experiment, in consultation with a physician, by increasing calcium intake to see if that produces a benefit worth the trouble and expense.

Because of the body's limited ability to absorb calcium, it cannot handle massive doses periodically but instead needs frequent opportunities to take in small amounts.

Recommended intakes of calcium.—The RDA for calcium is 800 milligrams per day for adults. The current RDA extends the 1,200-milligram level used in teenage years to age 25, in hopes that these higher calcium intakes will help women build and maintain a higher bone mass. Some authorities recommend that post-menopausal women who do not take estrogen replacements consume 1,500 milligrams of calcium daily.

The word *daily* should be stressed with respect to food sources of calcium. Because of the body's limited ability to absorb calcium, it cannot handle massive doses periodically but instead needs frequent opportunities to take in small amounts. The phrase *milk products* should also be stressed rather than *dairy products.* Butter and cream contain negligible calcium because calcium is not soluble in fat.

Good food sources of calcium.—The most abundant food sources of calcium in the U.S. diet are dairy products such as milk and cheese. One cup of low-fat milk has 300 mg of calcium. To obtain the RDA for calcium (800 mg/day), one must consume the equivalent of 2.7 cups of milk. By comparison, the RDA for calcium is also found in 1.9 cups of yogurt, 2.3 cups of almonds, 4.5 cups of broccoli, and 5.2 cups of cottage cheese.

People who do not like milk can use products made with milk, such as yogurt, cheese, and low-fat ice cream. All forms of milk, yogurt, and cheese allow about the same degree of calcium absorption. Bones in canned fish, such as salmon and sardines, also supply calcium. Actually, the most nutrient-dense calcium sources are green leafy vegetables. However, much calcium in these vegetables is not absorbed because of the presence of oxalic acid, which prevents calcium absorption. This makes nonfat milk the best overall source of calcium because of its high bioavailability.

Calcium supplements.—Most nutritionists recommend calcium supplements only as a last resort. There are three good reasons: (1) They are not foods. (2) They do not offer the variety of nutrients foods do. (3) Calcium is not absorbed as well from supplements as it is from milk. Most people take calcium supplements to prevent bone loss, but available evidence indicates that these supplements may not prevent bone loss. It may slow the rate of bone loss in post-menopausal women who do not receive an adequate calcium intake. But the final evidence from research on calcium supplements has not been reached. Until then, all we know with any certainty is that low calcium intakes from food, early in life, correlate with osteoporosis late in life. Calcium supplements are vastly inferior to milk for many reasons; but for the person who uses them, the following are some recommendations concerning them.

Calcium carbonate is the supplemental form usually recommended because it contains 40 percent calcium. Thus the dosage can be of smaller or fewer pills. For elderly people who have lost much of their stomach acidity, calcium citrate (which is acidic itself), might be a better choice. The lower percentage of calcium in that preparation, however, requires a greater number or size of pills. These supplements should be taken in divided doses with meals so that the acid produced by the stomach can aid digestion and absorption. In addition, calcium carbonate acts as an antacid and so interferes with the stomach's normally acidic environment.

Taking 1,000 milligrams of calcium in the form of calcium carbonate or calcium citrate is probably safe, but only long-term studies can confirm that. Consuming high dietary calcium foods does not present a risk, for these foods supply a natural balance of other minerals, in addition to calcium, decreasing the likelihood of mineral imbalance.

Toxicity of calcium.—The major risk from taking excess supplements is kidney stones. Research warns that calcium intake should not exceed 2,500 milligrams per day. Any more and extra calcium in the urine can increase the risk, especially in people who tend to form kidney stones. The body absorbs calcium less efficiently as calcium intake increases, but overzealous use of calcium supplements can overwhelm the control of absorption. Sticking to an intake of 1,500–2,500 milligrams poses no risk for developing this problem.

Phosphorus

Phosphorus represents 1 percent of the human body weight, and after calcium it is the most common mineral found in the body. About 85 percent of it is found combined with calcium in the crystals of the bones and teeth as calcium phosphate, the chief compound that gives them strength and rigidity. Phosphorus is also part of DNA and RNA, the genetic code material present in every cell. Phosphorus is necessary for all growth, because DNA and RNA provide instructions for new cells to be formed.

The body absorbs phosphorus efficiently and can increase

Magnesium helps relax muscles after contraction (especially the heart muscle). A magnesium deficiency causes an irregular heartbeat.

absorption from 60 to 90 percent as body needs vary. The high absorption rate plus its wide availability in foods makes phosphorus a lesser concern in diet planning than calcium. The active vitamin D hormone *calcitriol* enhances phosphorus absorption, as it does for calcium. Excretion by the kidneys is primarily responsible for maintaining body levels. This is unlike calcium, where changes in the rates of absorption are also important.

Functions of phosphorus.—Phosphorus plays many key roles in the cells' use of energy nutrients. Many enzymes and the B vitamins become active only when a phosphate group is attached. The B vitamins, you may recall, play major roles in energy metabolism. ATP itself, the energy carried by the cells, contains three phosphate groups and uses these groups to do its work. Phosphorus is critical in energy exchange. No deficiency disease is currently associated with a poor phosphorus intake, but a poor intake may contribute to bone loss in elderly women.

Food sources of phosphorus.—Phosphorus is one of the most difficult nutrients to limit in the diet because it is found in so many foods. Animal protein is the best source of phosphorus because phosphorus is so abundant in the energetic cells of animals. People who eat large quantities of animal protein, such as milk, cheese, and meat, have high phosphorus intakes. Cereals, bran, eggs, nuts, and fish are also good sources. About 20–30 percent of dietary phosphorus comes from food additives, especially those found in baked goods, cheeses, and processed meats, as well as in soft drinks (about 75 milligrams per 12-ounce serving).

RDA for phosphorus.—The average American takes in nearly twice as much phosphorus as calcium. Although the RDA for phosphorus is 800 mg/day, much more than this is consumed. The American diet provides 1,400–1,500 milligrams of phosphorus per day. Thus deficiencies of phosphorus are unlikely in adults, especially when considering its highly efficient absorption.

Toxicity of phosphorus.—An excess of serum phosphorus levels can cause the phosphate ions to bind calcium, which leads to tetany and convulsions. Inefficient kidney function can cause detrimentally high levels. However, there is no known toxicity in healthy adults associated with phosphorus consumption. Formerly, nutritionists believed that a high-phosphorus intake coupled with a low-calcium intake led to bone loss. Recent research casts doubt on the importance of the calcium to phosphorus ratio in the diet, as long as the RDA for calcium is met. If not met, then a high phosphorus intake may compound the bone loss from poor calcium intake.

Magnesium

The body of a 130-pound person has only about 1¾ ounces of magnesium. This barely qualifies it as a major mineral. Most of this is found in the bones (approximately 60%). Magnesium is best found in plant, rather than animal, products. This may explain why both U.S. males and females consume less magnesium than recommended. We absorb about 30–40 percent of the magnesium in our diets, but absorption efficiency can increase to 75 percent if intakes are low. As it does for calcium and phosphorus, the active vitamin D hormone calcitriol may enhance magnesium absorption.

Functions of magnesium.—Magnesium acts in all cells of the soft tissue, where it forms part of the protein-making machinery and where it is necessary for the release of energy. It releases energy by binding to ATP to form "active ATP." A magnesium ion bridges between the second and the last phosphate group on an ATP molecule.

More than three hundred enzymes use magnesium as a cofactor. Without magnesium, many enzymes would function less efficiently. Magnesium also helps relax muscles after contraction (especially the heart muscle). A magnesium deficiency causes an irregular heartbeat. In addition, it helps conduct nerve impulses and promotes resistance to tooth decay by helping to hold calcium in tooth enamel. However, a magnesium deficiency develops slowly because we have large tooth stores.

Good food sources of magnesium.—Whole grains, broccoli, squash, beans, nuts, and seeds are good food sources of magnesium. Dairy products, chocolate, and meat also contribute magnesium to the diet. "Hard" tap water often contains a high concentration of it. In fact, people whose drinking water has a high magnesium content experience a lower incidence of sudden death from heart failure.

RDA for magnesium.—The magnesium RDA is 350 milligrams a day for adult males and 280 milligrams for females. Adult men in America consume an average of 330 milligrams daily, while American women consume an average of 200

There is seldom a sodium shortage in the diet. Foods usually include more salt than is needed, and the body absorbs almost all that is eaten.

milligrams daily. Nutritionists are concerned with the low remaining intake for women, especially since many women have increased their calcium consumption in response to the fear of osteoporosis. Increasing calcium in the diet will cause a decrease in magnesium absorption. Women should choose some good sources of magnesium and eat them regularly.

Toxicity of magnesium.—There is no evidence that large amounts of magnesium have ill effects on healthy people, and large doses have been taken in the form of the laxative Epsom salts. Toxicity is associated with kidney failure because the kidneys regulate magnesium levels. A high magnesium level leads to weakness, nausea, and eventual malaise (bodily discomfort).

Sulfur

Sulfur is present in all proteins and plays its most important role in determining the contour of protein molecules. Sulfur helps the strands of protein to assume a particular shape and hold it. Some of the amino acids contain sulfur in their side chains. Sulfur helps link these amino acids together when two sulfur atoms bind to each other. This gives stability to many protein molecules. Skin, hair, and nails contain some of the body's more rigid proteins, and these have a high sulfur content.

There is no RDA for sulfur, and no deficiencies are known. We actually do not need to consume sulfur in our diets. Proteins supply the sulfur we need, so sulfur is naturally a part of a healthful diet. Only a person who lacks protein to the point of severe deficiency will lack the sulfur-containing amino acids.

The Electrolytes: Sodium, Potassium, and Chloride

Scientists call minerals like sodium, potassium, and chloride "electrolytes" because in water they can conduct electrical currents. Sodium and potassium ions carry positive charges, whereas chloride ions are negatively charged. Let's review each electrolyte and its role in nerve conduction.

Sodium

When most Americans think of sodium (Na), they also think of salt. This is understandable, for sodium combines with chloride (Cl) to form salt (NaCl). Sodium chloride, commonly called table salt, is 60 percent chloride and 40 percent sodium. One teaspoon of salt weighs 5 grams and contains 2,000 milligrams of sodium.

Much literature has been published concerning the intake of salt. Americans are at a dilemma concerning their sodium intake, for they both fear and crave salt. Americans love to splash it on their food for the taste but fear the consequences to their health. Some of this fear is warranted, and some is not. Let's examine sodium and see what role it plays in God's temple.

Functions of sodium.—There is seldom a sodium shortage in the diet. Foods usually include more salt than is needed, and the body absorbs almost all that is eaten. After absorption, it then becomes the major positive ion in the extracellular fluid and, therefore, a key electrolyte for retaining water in that compartment. In fact, sodium helps maintain fluid balance throughout the body's water compartments.

Nerve conduction would be impossible without sodium ions. Impulses are transmitted down the nerve membrane by sodium ions rushing into nerve cells. This reverses the positive charge of the cell membrane, which is called depolarization. During depolarization positive sodium ions rush in, generating an electrical current. The speed of depolarization of a nerve cell membrane is approximately the speed of a .38-caliber pistol shot. The electrical current travels from nerve cell to nerve cell. After the electrical wave passes through a nerve cell, sodium ions are pumped back out of the cell, and potassium ions are pumped back in. This process is called repolarization. When the ions regain their usual concentrations, the nerve cell is ready to "fire" again.

If the blood level of sodium drops, as it does during vomiting, diarrhea, or high perspiration, both water and sodium must be replenished to avert a medical emergency. This state can lead to muscle cramps, nausea, vomiting, and dizziness and later to shock and coma. The kidneys are the major organs to respond to this depletion. They release the hormone aldosterone which increases sodium retention.

Even in cases of severe rates of perspiration, sodium depletion in the body is unlikely because our diets contain ample sodium. One should become concerned when weight loss from perspiration exceeds six pounds. Even then, merely eating salting foods, not taking a salt tablet, is needed. Perspiration has two thirds the concentration of blood. For example, there are approximately two grams of sodium per liter of perspiration versus three grams of blood. If you lose more than six pounds of body weight through perspiration, you must regain this weight (within

1 to 2 lbs) before you exercise again. The danger of dehydration becomes prominent if sufficient fluid and sodium intake is not balanced.

Food sources of sodium.—Approximately one-half of all the sodium we consume is added during cooking or at the table. The other half is added during food manufacturing. Major contributors of sodium to the U.S. diet are white bread and rolls, hot dogs and lunch meats, cheese, soups, and spaghetti with tomato sauce, partly because these foods are eaten so often. Other foods especially high in sodium are tomato-based products in general; salted snack foods, french fries, potato chips; and sauces and gravies. Many condiments also contain large amounts of sodium, such as catsup, soy sauce, salad dressings, pickles, barbecue sauce, garlic salt, and relish.

Our sodium intake would be about 500 milligrams per day if we ate only unprocessed foods and added no salt. The typical American diet contains approximately 7,000 milligrams, which gives further evidence that cooking and food processing contribute most of our dietary sodium.

Approximately one-half of all the sodium we consume is added during cooking or at the table. The other half is added during food manufacturing.

An understanding of food labels should help one to control sodium intake. A number of descriptive terms are used on labels such as: "sodium free" (less than 5 milligrams), "very low sodium" (35 milligrams or less per serving), "low sodium" (145 milligrams or less per serving), and "reduced sodium" (a 75% reduction in sodium content). The terms *unsalted, no salt added,* or *without added salt* on labels describe food products processed without salt when it normally would be used. Sodium is also found in many medicines and tap water (especially softened water). These should be considered if sodium is to be restricted in the diet.

Recommended intakes of sodium.—No RDA for sodium has been established because of its widespread abundance in the American diet. The Food and Nutrition Board, however, has established safe and adequate dietary intakes. The minimum sodium requirement is 500 milligrams per day for adults, although we really only need about 100 milligrams. Americans consume much more than the minimum requirements of sodium in intakes of salt alone. For example, the average American intake of 7,000 milligrams of sodium per day translates to 18 grams of salt. A teaspoon of salt contains about 2,000 milligrams of sodium (a teaspoon of most dry food substances sold in markets equals approximately 500 milligrams). You may need to be more conservative when adding salt to your food.

Approximately 10–30 percent of Americans are sodium sensitive. For these people, high sodium intakes contribute to hypertension, and lower sodium diets (about 2,000 milligrams daily) often correct hypertension. Limiting daily sodium intake to 2,000 and no more than 3,000 milligrams would be wise. This may limit the risk of hypertension.

If you choose to lower your sodium intake, you can eventually adapt to a low-sodium diet. Your food, at first, will taste bland, but eventually (usually two weeks) you will perceive more flavor; and your tongue will have a lower salt threshold. The tongue's salt receptors will be triggered by less salt. By substituting garlic, lemon juice, and other herbs and spices, the adjustment to a lower salt intake will be made easier.

One more concern to prevent hypertension is the sodium to potassium ratio (Na/K). Estimates have shown that American males between 25 and 30 years of age consume 3,097 mg of sodium and 2,889 mg of potassium, or a ratio of 1.07. American women, on the other hand, consume 2,016 mg of sodium and 1,938 mg of potassium, or a ratio of 1.04. Most nutritional scientists recommend a ratio of 0.60. In other words, Americans should consume 40 percent more potassium than sodium to help keep blood pressure levels normal. At present, Americans are actually consuming more sodium than potassium, which may partially explain the fact that nearly one out of three Americans has high blood pressure.

Potassium

Potassium is the body's principal intracellular electrolyte. It performs many of the same functions as sodium, but it operates inside rather than outside cells. It is associated more with lowering blood pressure, not raising it as excessive sodium intake can. Cell membranes are relatively permeable to potassium (approximately 100 times more so than to sodium or chloride). If potassium were suddenly to leak out of the cells and not be pumped back in exchange for sodium, a medical emergency would occur. For example, if the cells were to give up to the blood only 6 percent of the potassium they contain, it would stop the heart.

During nerve transmission and muscle contraction, potassium and sodium briefly exchange places across the cell membrane. The cell then quickly pumps them back into place. This makes sodium and potassium critical in the transmission of messages along nerves and from nerves to muscles, as well as in the response of muscles, including the heart muscle, to those messages.

A potassium deficiency is more likely than a sodium deficiency because we generally do not add potassium to foods. Long bouts of vomiting and diarrhea deplete potassium stores. Also continually poor food intake, as may be the case in alcoholism or low carbohydrate diets, can result in potassium deficiency. When body potassium is depleted, its concentration in the blood and in the muscle cells falls; but its concentration in the central nervous system remains unchanged. The brain and nerves have a way of protecting themselves from changes they cannot tolerate. Apparently potassium is too crucial to their function to be allowed to vary. Blood and muscle potassium appear to be used as stores from which potassium can be released gradually to keep the nervous system's supply constant.

A low blood-potassium level is a life-threatening problem. Results often include a loss of appetite, muscle cramps, confusion, apathy, and constipation. Eventually, the heart will beat irregularly, decreasing its capacity to pump blood.

Food sources of potassium.—Good food sources of potassium are leafy green vegetables, milk, whole grains, dried beans, meat, and fruits (especially bananas). The major contributors of potassium to the U.S. diet include coffee, tea, milk, potatoes, and orange juice.

Recommended requirements and intakes.—The adult minimum potassium requirement is 2,000 milligrams per day. The American diet supplies approximately 2,000–4,000 milligrams daily. Persons with hypertension should adhere to the sodium-potassium ratio (0.60 Na/K). This means hypertensive individuals should include more potassium (40%) than sodium in their diets. Consumption of both minerals should not exceed 3,000 milligrams of each. The richest sources of potassium are fresh foods of all kinds (especially fruits, vegetables, and legumes). In contrast, most processed foods such as canned vegetables, ready-to-eat cereals, and luncheon meats contain more sodium and less potassium.

Toxicity of potassium.—When the kidneys function normally, excessive intakes of dietary potassium are not toxic. On the other hand, when kidneys function abnormally, potassium levels build up in the bloodstream and create a condition known as hyperkalemia. This condition can inhibit heart function by causing irregular heartbeats (arrhythmia). This eventually can cause the heart to stop beating.

Chloride

The chloride ion is the major anion (negative) of the extracellular fluids. Chloride can move freely across membranes and, therefore, can associate with potassium inside the cells.

In the stomach, the chloride ion is part of hydrochloric acid (HCl), which maintains the strong acidity of the stomach. The cells that line the stomach continuously expend energy to push chloride into the stomach fluid. One of the most serious consequences of vomiting is the loss of acid from the stomach, which upsets the acid-base balance.

A low blood-potassium level is a life-threatening problem. . . . Eventually, the heart will beat irregularly, decreasing its capacity to pump blood.

Chlorine is a poisonous gas. Public water utilities often rely on this gas to kill bacteria in water supplies. Consequently many water-borne diseases (typhus and typhoid fever) are rare in America. When chlorine reacts with sodium, hydrogen, or another metal in salt, it forms the negative chloride ion. Chloride is not poisonous and must be present in the diet.

A chloride deficiency is unlikely in the American diet because of the high consumption of salt (NaCl). The only way in which people can suffer a chloride deficiency is through frequent and lengthy bouts of vomiting, because stomach secretions contain chloride.

Good food sources of chloride.—Fruits and vegetables are naturally good sources of chloride. However, most chloride comes from the addition of salt to food. Recall that 40 percent of salt contains sodium, whereas 60 percent contains chloride.

Recommended chloride intakes.—For adults, the minimum chloride requirement is 700 milligrams per day. Assuming that the average American consumes at least 18 grams of salt daily, that yields 11,565 milligrams of chloride, an abundant intake of this ion.

Toxicity of chloride.—Recent research indicates that the chloride ion itself may cause the raising action of sodium, which can increase blood pressure. Together, then, the sodium and chloride components of salt are implicated in the high ratio of hypertension in America. One study suggests that chloride supplies a negative ion that allows the body to retain the positive sodium ion. Since chloride ions tend to remain in the body, they trap the positive sodium ions to balance the equation. One solution for hypertension is obvious; control your salt intake.

The Trace Minerals

A trace mineral is one for which our daily nutritional need is less than 100 milligrams. Trace minerals constitute less than 1 percent of all minerals in the body. If you could collect them all, you would have only a bit of dust, hardly enough to fill a teaspoon. Yet don't let the small amount fool you about their importance, for a deficiency of any of them may be fatal, and an excess of many is equally deadly.

> Today iron deficiency is one of the most common nutrient deficiencies worldwide. Iron is the only nutrient for which adult women have a greater RDA than men.

Information about trace minerals is perhaps the most rapidly expanding area of knowledge in nutrition. With the exception of iron and iodine, the importance of trace minerals to humans has been recognized only within the last 30 years. In fact, only four trace minerals (iron, zinc, iodine, and selenium) have recommended dietary allowances established for them. For five others, the Committee on Dietary Allowances published tentative ranges for safe and adequate daily intakes. Still others are recognized as essential nutrients for some animals but are not proven to be required for human beings. Many other trace elements are presently under study to determine whether they, too, perform indispensable roles in the body.

Iron (Fe)

Iron is probably the most widely known of all the essential minerals. Hardly a day goes by that a television ad doesn't depict our need for iron supplements. This public attention is understandable because iron is vital to cellular respiration. Every human cell—and, in fact, every living cell of every kind—contains iron. Iron is found in a variety of foods; but absorption is difficult, which causes it to become a problem nutrient for millions of Americans.

Iron was first recognized as a constituent of body tissue in 1713. Since that time, nutritionists have learned that the total amount of iron in the body measures 3–5 grams, varying slightly with age, sex, size, nutritional status, general health, and size of iron stores. Today iron deficiency is one of the most common nutrient deficiencies worldwide. Iron is the only nutrient for which adult women have a greater RDA than men. Virtually all iron exists in combination with protein and is responsible for the ability of every cell of the body to accept and release oxygen and carbon dioxide readily.

Iron can exist in two ionic states. Ferrous (reduced state) iron carries two positive charges (Fe++). Ferric iron (oxidized state) carries three positive charges (Fe+++). Due to its ability to switch back and forth between these two ionic states, iron is the ideal mineral to work with proteins involved in oxidation-reduction reactions. In every cell, iron is found in several of the proteins at the end of the energy metabolic pathways. These proteins donate the hydrogen from energy nutrients to oxygen, completing the extraction of energy for the cell's use.

Iron is concentrated in the blood, but some is present in every living cell. Over two thirds of the iron in the body is present in hemoglobin, the iron-containing protein molecule of the red blood cell. A small portion of iron exists as part of myoglobin, an iron-containing protein similar to hemoglobin but found in muscle. Iron is also present in the tissue enzymes, which are essential for cellular respiration, involving the exchange of oxygen and carbon dioxide.

The remaining one third of body iron is stored in the liver, spleen, and bone marrow. The amount of storage iron in the body varies (approximately 1,000 mg for men; 400 mg for women). Iron is stored as the soluble iron complex ferritin. Ferritin is present in the bloodstream in amounts paralleling storage iron.

Absorption of iron.—Several absorption mechanisms are used by the body to regulate iron absorption. This is important because the body cannot easily eliminate excess iron once it has been absorbed, and an overabundance of iron can be toxic. The body's iron absorption varies from 3 to 40 percent, depending on a variety of factors.

The form of iron in foods greatly influences its absorption. Iron that is still part of the hemoglobin (red blood cells) and myoglobin (muscles) in animal flesh is called heme iron. Heme iron is absorbed over twice as efficiently as the simple elemental iron, known as nonheme iron. Nonheme iron is also present in animal flesh, eggs, milk, vegetables, grains, and other plant foods.

The American diet is composed of about 10–15 percent heme iron, in which approximately 25–35 percent is absorbed. The rest of the diet is nonheme iron, of which about 2–20 percent is absorbed. This makes red meat (animal flesh) the best source of iron in the American diet, especially when you consider its iron content and the increased efficiency of absorption for the iron present in the heme form.

Reduce tea, especially at mealtimes, if your goal is to increase iron absorption.

To increase nonheme iron absorption, consume both heme iron and nonheme iron together. Eating meat with vegetables and grain products is the most efficient way to enhance the absorption of nonheme iron. Also, consuming organic acids, such as vitamin C, can increase nonheme iron absorption by changing the ferric form (Fe+++) to the ferrous form (Fe++). The ferrous form of iron is better absorbed. Consuming more foods rich in vitamin C will increase the serum iron levels in the body. If your iron levels are low, take an iron supplement with a glass of orange juice.

Several dietary factors interfere with the body's ability to absorb iron. In grain foods, phytic acid will bind iron and prevent its absorption in the G.I. tract. Also, oxalic acid (found in vegetables), can bind iron, reducing its absorption. Consuming more than 35 grams of fiber per day will cause the fiber components to bind iron, decreasing absorption. Tannins found in tea also reduce absorption. Reduce tea, especially at mealtimes, if your goal is to increase iron absorption. Finally, high-dose calcium supplements can also bind much iron.

Function of iron.—The major function of iron is to permit the transfer of oxygen and carbon dioxide from one tissue to another. Iron carries out this function primarily as a part of both hemoglobin in the blood and myoglobin in the muscles, but also as part of several tissue enzymes in cell respiration. The exchanges are involved primarily in the release of energy within the cell.

Iron plays a major role in the formation of blood. Hemoglobin is an essential component of the mature red blood cells, or erythrocytes, formed in the bone marrow. Erythrocytes begin in the bone marrow as immature cells known as erythroblasts. As these cells mature in bone marrow, they synthesize heme, an iron-containing protein, along with the help of vitamin B and the mineral copper. The heme unites with a protein called globin, and hemoglobin is formed.

The adult male has 15 grams of hemoglobin per 100 ml of blood, and the female has 13.6 grams per 100 ml. The total hemoglobin content of the 5 quarts of blood in the adult male is 750 grams. Because the average life span of erythrocytes is only 120 days, $\frac{1}{120}$ of the total amount of iron (20 mg) is released each day from old cells and is incorporated into the hemoglobin in the cells that replace them. Because it would be impossible to get this much iron a day from dietary sources, conserving iron is essential to survival.

Other functions of iron include:

1. Catalyzing the conversion of beta-carotene to vitamin A.
2. Producing iron-containing enzymes that fight infections.
3. Synthesizing carnitine, a vitamin-like substance needed to transport fatty acids.
4. Synthesizing collagen, the structural protein surrounding cells.
5. Producing antibodies.
6. Detoxifying drugs in the liver.

Recommended dietary allowances of iron.—The National Research Council recommends that adult allowances for iron be based on the assumption that an adult man must obtain approximately 0.9–1.2 mg of iron daily to replace body losses in urine, feces, and perspiration and that an adult woman needs from 1.4 to 2.2 mg/day to cover additional losses during menstruation. Because an average of 10 percent of ingested iron is absorbed, it has been recommended that men obtain 10 mg/day and women 18 mg/day from dietary sources. For women, this amount actually represents a narrow margin of safety and may fail to meet the needs of those with high menstrual losses of iron. The RDA could be as high as 32 mg/day.

During pregnancy, a total of 300 mg of iron is needed for the growth of the fetus. It is almost impossible for a pregnant woman to obtain the required amount of iron from food alone. As a result, it is recommended, in addition to obtaining 18 mg of iron per day from dietary sources, that a woman take a supplement that provides about 30 mg of elemental iron (which is equivalent to 150 mg of ferrous sulfate). Because of the constipating effect of iron supplements, however, physicians have found that women have difficulty complying with this recommendation. Larger supplements should not be used. Continued supplementation of a mother's diet for 2 to 3 months after delivery is encouraged to help ensure that iron reserves are replenished. Repeated pregnancies pose a special challenge to women to maintain adequate iron stores.

The American diet contains about 5–7 milligrams of iron per 1,000 calories. Thus men generally achieve a good iron status because a daily energy intake of 2,000–3,000 calories meets the RDA for iron. Most women, on the other hand, have difficulty eating 3,000 calories daily while maintaining desirable weight. They then have difficulty consuming 18 mg of iron daily unless they seek out nutrient-dense forms of iron for their diets, such as is found in fortified breakfast cereals. If that does not suffice, a

Some researchers postulate that poor iron stores may also decrease learning ability, work performance, and immune status even before a person becomes anemic.

supplement should be used to prevent iron-deficiency anemia.

Iron-deficiency anemia.—If body stores are used up or if the diet cannot compensate for losses, then iron deficiency sets in. Eventually, red-blood-cell and hemoglobin numbers fall so low that the amount of oxygen carried in the bloodstream is decreased. This condition is known as anemia. While there are many types of anemia, the major type found worldwide is iron-deficiency anemia. About 30 percent of the world's population is anemic, and about half of those cases are due to an iron deficiency.

To be classified as iron-deficiency anemia, the hematocrit (percentage of red and white blood cells and platelets to plasma), falls below 34–37 percent (normal is 40–52%). In addition, the hemoglobin concentration in the bloodstream falls below 10–11 grams per 100 milliliters of blood (normal is 13–15 grams). Probably about 8 percent of all Americans have iron-deficiency anemia. More Americans have an iron deficiency than have iron-deficiency anemia. About 30 percent of American women have scant or no iron stores. Their blood hemoglobin stores are still normal, but they have no stores to draw from in times of pregnancy or illness.

The clinical symptoms associated with iron-deficiency anemia include pale skin and brittle finger nails, which eventually turn up into a spoon shape. The person suffers fatigue, poor temperature regulation, loss of appetite, and apathy. Some researchers postulate that poor iron stores may also decrease learning ability, work performance, and immune status even before a person becomes anemic.

Iron-deficiency anemia has several causes. Poor dietary intake, chronic blood loss from heavy menses, ulcers, hemorrhoids, and colon cancer are the more common causes. The donation of one pint of blood represents a loss of 250 milligrams of iron. It generally takes several months to replace that iron, so limit blood donations to two or three times per year. Many people are iron deficient without showing symptoms of anemia. It takes a long time for iron-deficiency anemia to develop.

To treat iron-deficiency anemia, medicinal iron needs to be ingested. A good diet may prevent iron-deficiency anemia, but medicinal iron is a better cure. The iron treatment usually involves administration of 200 milligrams of iron as ferrous sulfate per day for 6–12 months. A vitamin C source should also be consumed with the supplement to enhance absorption.

Runner's anemia.—A special type of anemia that occurs in athletes is called runner's anemia. Three possible factors contribute to it: (1) Red blood cells are destroyed from foot strike as red blood cells pass through the foot during exercise (a condition called hemolysis). (2) Iron is being lost due to increased perspiration. (3) The increase in blood volume associated with athletic fitness may cause iron loss. Athletes with runner's anemia will experience poor sports performance because of early fatigue. Athletes should have their hemoglobin levels and other iron status indicators monitored, and they should attempt to meet their iron needs by either dietary means or iron supplementation.

Good food sources of iron.—The most nutrient-dense sources are spinach, oysters, liver, clams, peas, and legumes. Liver is the best source of iron but has recently fallen into disfavor because of its high cholesterol content.

Fruits and vegetables are fairly good sources of iron, but it is relatively poorly utilized. Vegetables provide three times as much iron in the American diet as fruits. Fruits and fruit juices are rated as poor iron sources, whereas potatoes and green stalks and leaves are good sources. Legumes are excellent sources. Fruit pulp contains twice as much iron as the juice. Canned fruits and vegetables cooked in iron containers will pick up additional iron, which is just as valuable as naturally occurring iron. Maybe it's time to return to iron pots and pans for cooking!

Although raisins are often recommended, they are not considered a good source of iron. In fact, raisins are high in calories. For example, one-fourth cup of raisins provides 109 calories and only 0.7 mg of iron.

Breads, either enriched or whole-grain, provide small amounts of iron per unit of weight. In fact, only about 5 percent of the iron in them is absorbed. The only good food group characterized as a poor source of iron is the milk and milk product group. The small amount of iron in milk is well absorbed but still makes an insignificant contribution to total intake.

Toxicity of iron.—Specialists once thought the body could not absorb too much iron. However, this theory was proven wrong when it was reported that the Bantu tribe in Africa suffered from siderosis, in which their iron reserves were found to be up to 30 times the normal 1,000 mg reserve. The absorbed iron, approximately 200 mg/day, came from kettles the tribe used to ferment beer.

Zinc is most critical in the healing process of wounds. Supplementary zinc is effective in promoting healing only when people have low intakes.

Siderosis is a condition in which iron accumulates in the normal storage sites of the liver, spleen, and even in the mitochondria of all cells. This causes a rise in the serum (blood) iron; and the bone marrow becomes hyperplastic, which means that it has too many cells. This excess of iron stimulates the growth of pathogenic organisms in the blood, resulting in an increased susceptibility to infection.

Another form of iron-storage disease that occurs in less than 0.1 percent of the population (about 22,000 Americans) is hemochromatosis. This disease is an inherited defect in which individuals absorb unusually high amounts of iron. This excess iron builds up to high levels especially in the bloodstream and liver. If not treated, excess iron is deposited in inappropriate tissues, contributing to severe liver and heart damage. A first sign of hemochromatosis is arthritis-like symptoms.

Zinc

Zinc has come to nutritional prominence as an essential trace element with wide clinical significance. Zinc is found in all parts of the body. In fact, zinc acts as the cofactor for more than 70 enzymes that perform specific tasks in the eyes, liver, kidneys, muscles, skin, bones, and male reproduction organs. A good rule to remember about zinc is "wherever protein is, there zinc is," for it helps with whatever jobs proteins do.

The human body contains 2–2.5 grams of zinc, with three fourths of this amount concentrated in the skeleton, from which it is removed slowly. High concentration of zinc is found in the skin, hair, testes, red blood cells, and proteins, all of which seem particularly affected by zinc.

Absorption of zinc.—Zinc is absorbed primarily in the upper part of the small intestine. Absorption appears to be regulated in the cells in the intestinal wall, which respond to zinc levels in the plasma. In the blood, zinc is bound to a protein and carried to the liver, where it is stored until needed. In the average adult, one-third to one-half of the 10–15 mg provided daily in the diet is absorbed. During pregnancy and lactation, absorption is increased twofold.

Absorption is decreased as the stores of zinc increase or when the diet contains large amounts of whole grains in which either phytic acid or fiber may bind zinc as an insoluble complex. Oxalic acid in some vegetables has a similar effect. Most American diets usually do not contain enough fiber to depress zinc absorption. High levels of calcium or copper also result in lowered absorption of zinc, so beware of consuming high levels of calcium supplements, for they could cause a problem with zinc absorption.

Functions of zinc.—Zinc has six major functions:

1. As part of enzymes, at least 120 of which have been identified.
2. Wound healing, growth, and protein metabolism.
3. Proper development of bone and sexual organs.
4. Proper immune function.
5. Insulin release and storage.
6. Prostaglandin synthesis.

As a result, zinc affects the following body functions:

Reproduction.—The mother has transferred about 150 mg of zinc to the fetus by the time of birth. Maternal zinc deficiency is clearly associated with low-birth-weight infants and is suggested as a cause of central nervous system problems. Zinc-deficient men have shown retarded gonadal development. Also, impaired sexual maturity in both sexes is another result of zinc deficiency.

Skin problems.—Zinc is most critical in the healing process of wounds. Supplementary zinc is effective in promoting healing only when people have low intakes. There is no added advantage from high levels of zinc. Zinc has been proven effective in reducing acne scars. Zinc is also successful in the treatment of an often fatal condition known as acrodermatitis. This condition usually appears within the first few months of life and is associated with the change in breast milk, which contains a zinc-binding protein that aids absorption. Skin rashes, diarrhea, and loss of hair are common symptoms in these infants.

Taste and smell defects.—Hypogeusia (diminished taste) and hyposmia (diminished smell) in a number of clinical situations are improved with zinc supplementation.

Growth.—Growth is severely stunted from zinc deficiency, reflecting its role in protein synthesis. A diet high in animal protein, supplemented by zinc, results in a rapid growth response.

Malabsorption disease.—Zinc deficiency can occur with malabsorption disease such as Crohn's disease.

Symptoms of zinc deficiency in adults include an acne-like rash, diarrhea, lack of appetite, reduced sense of taste and smell, hair loss, and poor growth and sexual development in children and adolescents. Poor learning ability may result. A persistent rash, especially in the presence of a poor diet, should alert a physician to evaluate zinc status in the person.

RDA for zinc.—Assuming a diet with 25 percent zinc absorption, the RDA is set for males at 15 mg of zinc per day and 12 mg per day for women. For women whose menstrual losses are negligible, 12 mg should be adequate unless the diet is devoid of animal food. During growth spurts, needs are slightly higher for both boys and girls (approximately 18 mg/day). For pregnant women, an additional 1 mg (first trimester), 2 mg (second trimester), and 5 mg (third trimester) of zinc is recommended to ensure the needs of the growing fetus and placenta. For lactation, an additional 10 mg is suggested to ensure that the mother can provide 1.6 mg of zinc, which is transferred in the milk each day. Formula-fed infants need 8 mg/day because zinc in cow's milk is less available.

Copper is needed in many of the reactions related to respiration and the release of energy. It is also important for proper immune system functions and blood clotting.

Good food sources of zinc.—Only recently has it been determined that the American diet may not provide enough zinc. The frequent incidence of hypogeusia, delayed wound healing, and growth failure, which are all signs of zinc deficiency, support the findings of low zinc intakes. The zinc content in the average American diet shows a mean content of 9 mg of zinc per day for women, and 14.3 mg for men. Zinc available in the food supply is estimated at 12.5 mg per person, suggesting that careful dietary planning is necessary if RDA is to be met.

The best sources of zinc are seafood and meat, which are expensive foods. Less expensive foods such as cereals and legumes contain significant amounts of zinc, but they also contain phytic acid that can interfere with intestinal absorption of zinc. In addition, up to 80 percent of the zinc in whole-grain cereals may be lost in milling. Absorption of zinc in leavened whole-wheat bread is enhanced 30–50 percent, compared with the availability.

Toxicity of zinc.—An excess of zinc through oversupplementation can cause a copper and iron deficiency. Research has shown that zinc supplements at approximately three to five times the RDA can reduce HDL cholesterol levels by about 15 percent. The reduction in HDL could cause atherosclerosis (hardening of the arteries) and heart disease. This shows why mineral supplements should not be consumed except under close scrutiny of a physician. Otherwise more harm than good may result. Zinc intakes over 2,000 mg daily also result in diarrhea, cramps, nausea, vomiting, and sometimes depress immune system function.

Copper

This trace element has frequently been called the "iron twin." The two minerals are metabolized in much the same way and share functions as cell enzyme components. Copper aids in iron absorption and metabolism.

Functions of copper.—The body contains about 75–100 milligrams of copper, which performs several vital roles. It helps manufacture hemoglobin and red blood cells. It is involved in the manufacture of collagen and the healing of wounds. It helps to maintain the sheath around nerve fibers. Copper's critical roles seem to have to do with helping iron shift back and forth between the ferrous and ferric states. This means that copper is needed in many of the reactions related to respiration and the release of energy. Finally, copper is important for proper immune system functions and blood clotting.

Copper deficiency is rare but not unknown. Symptoms of copper deficiency include anemia, low white-blood-cell count (specifically, the neutrophils), bone loss, increased serum cholesterol levels, poor growth, and heart disease. Excess zinc, as mentioned, interferes with copper absorption and can cause deficiency. Vitamin C supplements of 500 mg with each meal have been found to decrease copper status in young men. Whenever megadoses of vitamins or minerals are taken, interactions with other nutrients multiply.

Good food sources of copper.—Copper is primarily found in meats, liver, legumes, nuts, and whole-grain breads and cereals. Food tables can be misleading because soil conditions greatly affect the copper content of plant foods.

Recommended intake of copper.—Copper intake by Americans is low. U.S. males and females average 1.24 and 0.93 of copper per day, respectively, less than the estimated safe and adequate daily dietary intake of 2–3 mg. Several groups of people at the greatest risk for a copper deficiency include premature infants, people recovering from intestinal surgery, and absorption diseases. Also, using large doses of antacids may bind enough copper in the intestine to cause a deficiency.

Toxicity of copper.—The minimum toxic dose for copper is 100 mg. Copper can even cause vomiting at single doses greater than 10–15 milligrams. An inherited condition called Wilson's disease results in accumulation of copper in the liver, brain, kidneys, and cornea of the eyes. If not treated, mental degeneration is commonly seen in active cases.

Selenium

Selenium is a trace element that functions as part of an enzyme. The enzyme (glutathione peroxidase) acts as an antioxidant and, like vitamin E, can prevent oxidation of polyunsaturated fatty acids, providing an additional source of protection for them. Selenium's role as an antioxidant is complementary to that of vitamin E; neither can replace the other. Selenium's role in reducing free radical production gives it a potential for reducing cancer.

Some children living in a wide area across China developed a fatal disease of the heart muscle because they lacked selenium in their diet. This disease, coined Keshan disease, was reduced 80 percent by giving selenium to the children.

Kaschin-Beck disease is another disease occurring in eastern Asia that is related to selenium deficiency. Children develop joint stiffness at first, and then the disease progresses to growth retardation and severe joint problems.

The selenium content of plants such as grains is determined by the selenium content of the soil. In certain parts of the world, such as New Zealand, selenium intake is low because of the low amount of selenium in the soil. Regions in the U.S. also produce crops on selenium-poor soil, but Americans are protected from deficiency because of wide food distribution patterns and high meat intakes. Meats and other animal products are reliable sources of selenium because selenium is associated with the protein parts of foods.

Good food sources of selenium.—Good sources of selenium are found in fish, meat (especially organ meat), eggs, and shellfish. Grains and seeds grown in soils containing selenium are good plant sources. A recent survey found the major selenium contributors in the U.S. diet are tuna, beef, white bread, chicken, eggs, noodles, and milk.

RDA for selenium.—The RDA is 55–70 micrograms daily for adults. Probably 40 micrograms daily will satisfy our minimum needs. The American diet averages approximately 80–130 micrograms daily, which makes a selenium deficiency rare among Americans.

Toxicity of selenium.—Excess selenium intakes as low as 2–3 milligrams (35 times the RDA) can cause toxicity symptoms if taken for many months. Symptoms of toxicity include hair loss, nausea and vomiting, general weakness, and a garlicky odor of the breath. Also, cirrhosis of the liver can develop.

Some people feel that high intakes of selenium can prevent cancer. However, there is no evidence that intakes above recommended levels are beneficial.

Iodine

Dietary iodine is converted to iodide in the gastrointestinal tract. Iodide occurs in the body in an infinitesimally small quantity, but its principal role in human nutrition is well-known, and the amount needed is well established. Iodide is part of the thyroid hormone, which regulates body temperature, metabolic rate, reproduction, growth, the making of blood cells, nerve and muscle function, and more. This hormone enters every cell of the body to control the rate at which the cells use oxygen. This means that this thyroid hormone (thyroxin) controls the rate at which energy is released.

If dietary iodine intake is insufficient, the thyroid gland enlarges as it attempts to take up more iodide from the bloodstream, eventually producing a goiter. Goiters have occurred in people since 3,000 B.C., usually in women. Goiter affects about 200 million people the world over, many of them in Africa. In all but 4 percent of these cases, the cause is iodine deficiency. The remaining 4 percent (8 million) have goiter because they overconsume raw turnips, cabbage, and rutabagas. These vegetables contain compounds called goitrogens, which inhibit the function of the thyroid gland and, in turn, thyroid hormone synthesis. However, goitrogens are not an important cause of goiter, since they are destroyed by cooking.

An iodine deficiency during pregnancy may cause the infant to be born with growth failure and may develop mental retardation known as cretinism. An infant with cretinism has an IQ as low as 20 and a face and body with many abnormalities. Much of the mental retardation associated with cretinism in America has been averted because of the fortification of table salt with iodine.

Good sources of iodine.—Iodized salt, seafood, saltwater fish, and plants (especially plants grown near the sea) contain iodine. Sea salt in health food stores is not a good source since the iodine is lost during processing. A half teaspoon of iodine-fortified salt (about 2 grams) supplies the adult RDA for iodine. The ocean is the source of most iodine present in our diets. When seawater evaporates and rains on the nearby land, iodine becomes part of the soil. Plants that grow in that soil accumulate a higher percentage of iodine.

RDA for iodine.—The adult RDA for iodine is 150 micrograms daily. The minimum intake to prevent goiter is approximately 50 micrograms per day. Americans consume much more iodine (approximately 300 micrograms) than the RDA. There is no need for concern about insufficient iodine intake in America because of high sodium chloride intake with iodine.

Toxicity for iodine.—Excessive intakes of iodine can also cause an enlargement of the thyroid gland (toxic goiter), just as deficiency can. Levels up to 2–3 milligrams (13–20 times the RDA) per day appear to be safe. However, for people who eat a lot of seaweed (1% iodine by weight), the total intake can add up to 60–130 times the RDA. This goiter-like condition can be so severe as to block the airways in infants and cause suffocation.

Excessive intakes of iodine can also cause an enlargement of the thyroid gland . . . Much of the excess iodine comes from fast foods, in which iodized salt is liberally used.

Much of the excess iodine comes from fast foods, in which iodized salt is liberally used. Some excesses come from dough conditioners used in the baking industry. Also milk produced by cows exposed to iodine-containing medications and disinfectants is another source of iodine. Manufacturers are working to reduce unnecessary iodine use in dairies, restaurants, and bakeries.

Fluoride

In 1901, the beneficial effect of fluoride on the incidence of dental caries (tooth decay) was recognized. Researchers noted that dental caries in children with brown stains on their tooth enamels were relatively rare. Later the mineral fluoride was identified as the substance causing both the staining and the prevention of dental caries. Controlled fluoridation of water in parts of the U.S. began in 1945. Those who drink fluoridated water generally have 50–70 percent fewer dental caries than those who do not drink fluoridated water. The recommended amount of fluoride in the water is one part per million parts of water (ppm). If your water supply doesn't contain fluoride, talk to your dentist about the best means for children to obtain the needed fluoride.

Fluoride has its greatest effect on the body when bones and teeth are developing. Thus, consuming fluoride during childhood is important. Dietary fluoride during bone and teeth development aids in the synthesis of fluroapatite crystals, which make the teeth larger and more perfectly formed. Fluoride also inhibits the growth of bacteria that cause dental caries.

Good food sources of fluoride.—The best source of fluoride comes from drinking water that contains fluoride. Other good sources are found in seafoods, seaweed (kelp), tea, and fluoride toothpaste. No evidence shows that water fluoridation at present U.S. levels is harmful.

ESADDI for fluoride.—The estimated safe and adequate daily dietary intake (ESADDI) of fluoride for adults is 1.5–4 milligrams daily. This range is easily obtained in communities whose water supplies contain 1 mg per liter. This range of intake provides the benefits of resistance to dental caries without causing mottling (staining) of the teeth.

Fluoridation of water supply is a popular target among quacks and food faddists. Opponents claim that fluoridation increases the risk of cancer, heart disease, Down's syndrome, birth defects, allergic responses, kidney disease, and warts. Thousands of scientific studies have shown all of these claims to be fake. Fluoridation of the water supply has been found to be safe, effective, and beneficial.

Toxicity of fluoride.—In areas with highly fluoridated water (natural or added), severe mottling of the tooth enamel can appear. Mottled teeth are characterized by chalky white patches with yellow and brown staining. This enamel can become pitted. A fluoride intake greater than 6 milligrams daily can mottle teeth during the development stage in children. High-fluoride intakes in adults do not cause mottling. In addition, when fluoride intake reaches 20 milligrams daily during tooth development, the tooth structure is weakened and can crumble. This is called fluorosis.

Chromium

Chromium was first discovered in 1959 and was first associated with human dietary deficiency in 1966. It is now considered an essential element in human nutrition. There is much we do not understand about the mineral, but chromium deficiency may be related to both diabetes mellitus and coronary heart disease.

Chromium has been identified as part of the glucose-tolerance factor, which is required for optimal utilization of glucose. Chromium is believed to aid in binding insulin to the cell, which in turn allows glucose to be taken up by the cell.

Chromium deficiency is characterized by impaired glucose tolerance and elevated serum cholesterol and triglyceride levels. The mechanism by which chromium influences cholesterol metabolism is not known but may involve enzymes that control cholesterol synthesis.

Good food sources of chromium.—The best source of chromium is found in foods of plant origin, in which its level varies with plant species, soil, and season. Normally, vegetables provide from 30–55 ppm; whole grains and cereals, 30–79 ppm; and fruits, 20 ppm. The ultimate chromium level in foods is

Weakness and psychological and motor difficulties are manifestations of high tissue levels of manganese. Manganese toxicity occurs most often with iron deficiency.

closely tied to local soil content of chromium. To provide a good chromium intake, eat as many whole grains, rather than refined grains, as possible.

ESADDI of chromium.—The estimated safe and adequate daily dietary intake of chromium is 50 to 200 micrograms. Marginal to low chromium intakes in the elderly may contribute to their increased risk for developing diabetes mellitus. Some research shows that slightly higher intakes above the ESADDI may raise HDL cholesterol levels. More studies are needed to verify this effect.

Toxicity of chromium.—There is no evidence of toxicity from excessive dietary intakes of chromium. However, inhalation of chromium from industrial waste can be toxic, and the ingestion of excess chromium in drinking water has resulted in moderately acute toxicity. The effects of chromium are known to vary with the form available, and there are many uncertainties about the effects of excessive amounts and imbalances with other nutrients. Therefore, the use of chromium supplements should be discouraged.

Manganese

Be careful not to confuse the mineral manganese with magnesium. Manganese is considered an essential nutrient because of its many biochemical roles. Manganese is necessary for normal skeletal and connective tissue development. It acts as a catalyst in the synthesis of fatty acids and cholesterol. It is essential in the formation of urea, in which nitrogen is excreted. Finally, it plays a major role in the structure and function of the mitochondrion of the cell, which is essential for the release of energy.

No human deficiency symptoms are associated with a low manganese intake. Animals suffer alterations in brain function, bone formation, reproduction, and blood glucose regulation. If human diets were low in manganese, these symptoms would probably appear in humans.

Good food sources of manganese.—The best food sources of manganese are rice, oats, whole grains, beans, leafy vegetables, and nuts. The estimated safe and adequate daily dietary intake of manganese is 2–5 milligrams. Intakes of less than 0.7 mg are considered inadequate. The typical American diet contains approximately 3.6 mg of manganese per day, which is considered sufficient.

Toxicity of manganese.—Manganese is toxic at high levels, as evidenced by toxicity that appears in miners of manganese. Weakness and psychological and motor difficulties are manifestations of high tissue levels of manganese. Manganese toxicity occurs most often with iron deficiency.

Molybdenum

Molybdenum (mo-LIB-duh-num) is an essential element in human nutrition. The body contains approximately 9 mg of molybdenum which is concentrated in the liver, kidneys, adrenal glands, and blood cells. It is notable for its interaction with iron and copper, especially inhibition of copper absorption.

Molybdenum is an essential cofactor for several enzymes, including xanthine oxidase. This enzyme is involved in the formation of uric acid from purines and also aids in mobilizing iron from the liver reserves. Molybdenum may help in the prevention of tooth decay by promoting the retention of fluoride.

Although deficiency can be produced in animals, molybdenum deficiency in humans has not been observed.

Good food sources of molybdenum.—Molybdenum is readily absorbed (25% to 80%) and is excreted mainly in urine. Good food sources include beans, peas, meats, whole grains, and nuts. The estimated safe and adequate daily dietary intake is 0.15 to 0.50 mg for adults. The average American intake is approximately 0.2 mg, which makes deficiency unlikely.

Toxicity of molybdenum.—Toxicity is rare from an excess of molybdenum. Symptoms include weight loss, decreased growth, diarrhea, and anemia, which is associated with failure of the red blood cell to mature. High intakes of molybdenum may interfere with removal of copper from the blood or synthesis of the enzyme needed to transport copper.

[CHAPTER 16]

Understanding Weight Control

How do you feel today? Do you feel tired, listless, drowsy after a heavy meal, or sleepy in the afternoon? Do you lose your breath after climbing a flight of stairs? Do you collapse after mowing the lawn or playing 18 holes of golf? Do you get sick just looking at your bulging waistline in the mirror? Are you losing interest in your job, your schoolwork, your family, or your church activities? Are you as zealous in your worship of God as you used to be?

Many Americans can respond in the affirmative to the above symptoms. Many remark, "I just don't feel like I have any energy today!" Energy is a topic we talk about frequently, almost as if we could go out and buy it or get it from a pill. However, how we feel is not necessarily the best indicator of energy balance in our bodies. Energy balance is determined by two factors: calories that enter the body and energy that is used by the body. Overweight and underweight both result from unbalanced energy budgets. This chapter provides an overview of the energy equation and the factors that influence it, as well as methods to determine imbalance in the energy equation.

Energy In

Overweight people consume food energy in excess of expenditures and bank the surplus in body fat. Underweight people do not consume enough food energy and deplete body fat stores and possible lean tissue as well. The amount of body fat you might deposit in, or withdraw from, your "savings" on any given day depends on your energy balance for that day, or simply stated, the amount you consume (energy in) versus the amount you expend (energy out). You can reduce your fat deposits by withdrawing more energy from them than you put in.

Many factors influence our desire to eat. Hunger is a sign of the physiological drive to eat food. Appetite represents the psychological drive to find and eat food. Fulfilling both these drives should lead to a state of satiety, in which the desire to eat is extinguished for a short time. Together, these states of hunger, appetite, and satiety and the factors that regulate them greatly influence body weight. Let's examine some stimuli that influence our energy intake.

The Hypothalamus

The part of our brainstem which regulates hunger is called the hypothalamus. Our hunger increases or decreases depending on the stimulation (either chemical or electrical) of the nuclei cells in the hypothalamus. There are two major divisions of nuclei cells in the hypothalamus: the satiety division and the feeding division. When the satiety division is stimulated, we no longer feel hungry; and when the feeding center is stimulated, we become hungry. Most likely these divisions monitor the blood-glucose level for a signal. For example, a low blood-glucose level encourages feeding.

Research studies suggest that an underlying hunger for food is never totally absent. After a meal, glucose, fatty acids, amino acids, and other energy-yielding compounds increase in the bloodstream, which temporarily shuts off hunger. The satiety division in the brain registers that the satiation point is reached. Hours later, when the concentration of these compounds in the bloodstream begins to fall and liver metabolism slows, hunger returns because it is no longer inhibited by the metabolism of those energy-yielding compounds. Then the feeding divisions begin to dominate again.

Our appetite is regulated by such influences as the time of day, the availability of food, texture, taste, color, emotional state, and social custom.

Hormonal Regulation of Feeding

Our feeding behavior and satiety are controlled by hormones such as cholecystokinin (CCK), secretin, gastrin, and other hormone-like compounds. Cholecystokinin (CCK) appears to decrease hunger, while endorphin (the body's natural pain killers) and the hormones cortisol and insulin all lead to increased feeding. Actually, insulin probably affects both hunger and satiety. In summary, then, the body's hormonal balance influences the tendency to feel hungry or satiated.

Type of Meal Regulates Feeding

In animal studies, research has shown that a recent intake of carbohydrates greatly influences later food intake. When carbohydrate intake is reduced in animals for one day, they try to consume more carbohydrates the next day. On the other hand, if the animals consume a high-carbohydrate diet for one day, they tend to consume a diet higher in protein the next. Alterations in the protein or fat content of the diet have less effect. In humans, there is still debate about how powerful a high-carbohydrate meal really is in changing human feeding behavior. More research is needed before putting this information into practice.

The Set Point Theory

The set point theory maintains that each person has an ideal biological weight or set point. Once body weight reaches this point, a whole set of signals is produced that influences the person's food intake to maintain this weight. Some scientists suggest that the hypothalamus monitors the amount of body fat in humans and tries to keep that level constant over time. The protein, adipsin, produced by adipose cells may form the communication link between adipose cells and the brain that allows for this regulation.

Research has produced sound evidence that body weight tends to be regulated. For example, if one lowers his calorie intake, the blood level of a thyroid hormone (T3) falls, which causes the basal metabolic rate to fall. This causes the body to resist further weight loss as a protection against perceived starvation. The lower body weight decreases the energy cost of each future weight-bearing activity, and the total energy used by lean tissues falls because some of these tissues are also lost. Furthermore, the enzyme used by adipose cells and muscle cells to pull in fat from the bloodstream may increase its activity.

If a person consumes excessive calories, the metabolic rate tends to increase because the T3 hormone level increases. This causes resistance to further weight gain and, in theory, keeps body weight at a set point.

The set point concept is still controversial; even if it is valid, it is not yet possible to determine a person's set point independent of body weight. It can only be estimated from a person's weight over time. For example, a person who has weighed within a few pounds of 170 over the past several years is considered to have a set point of 170.

The set point theory may explain how the body might be able to choose whether to store or spend energy and may provide clues to the way the body maintains its weight. A person who overeats on a given day may metabolize the food less efficiently than usual and gain less weight. Whereas, a person who eats less than usual might conserve more that day and so lose less weight than expected. This might help to explain why gaining and losing weight are equally hard to do for a person at the set point weight and may also help to account for the mysterious plateaus at which both weight gainers and losers tend to get stuck. However, little evidence shows how set point operates. We must bear most of the responsibility for weight maintenance ourselves. The odds are against us, even though we may be helped by the set-point theory, of avoiding a weight gain in adulthood.

Regulation of Appetite

Our appetite is regulated by such influences as the time of day, the availability of food, texture, taste, color, emotional state, and social custom. After a meal, our appetite is satisfied and is reinforced by the pleasant feelings associated with satiety. Our food choice is usually determined by the taste of food and the physical feelings associated with a meal. Sometimes we find ourselves eating because of stress or depression. To help us overcome this depressed feeling, we eat because of the good feelings associated with eating.

Most of us eat primarily from appetite rather than from hunger. Most of us do not often experience real hunger, which will be experienced if you fast for a day. Chances are that you eat because of habit and custom, not from hunger. For example, many of us associate eating with watching television in our favorite easy chair.

Our appetite even changes while we eat. For example,

In summary, hunger is the physiological drive to find and eat food, whereas appetite is the psychological drive.

consider the last time you went through a cafeteria line. The first time you passed by the line you made mental choices of purchasing some meat, vegetables, salad, and a drink. When you went through the line, you probably changed your mind and added some chocolate pie, bananas and strawberries, or ice cream. Although this may be partly due to social custom, research with laboratory animals suggests that this action is also partly biological. As nutrients are absorbed or even mentally perceived, the liver and surrounding organs communicate with the brain and change subsequent food choices.

In summary, hunger is the physiological drive to find and eat food, whereas appetite is the psychological drive. Appeasing them both should leave you in a satiated state. Hunger is influenced by the brain, adipose tissue, liver, other organs, various hormones, and hormone-like compounds. Appetite is affected by social custom, time of day, food availability, taste, and other factors. Americans probably respond primarily to appetite cues, rather than hunger cues, in choosing what and when to eat. Keep track of what drives you to eat food during the next few days. Is it primarily hunger or appetite?

Energy Out

Now that we have learned some stimuli for consuming energy, let's look at how the body uses energy. The body uses energy for three basic purposes: basal metabolism, thermic effect of food, and physical activity. Let's examine each.

Basal Metabolism

The basal metabolic rate (BMR) refers to the rate at which the body uses energy to maintain itself during a state of complete rest. This includes maintaining a heartbeat, respiration, body temperature, and other metabolic functions. It does not include energy needs for activity or digesting food.

BMR can be measured by a technique called indirect calorimetry in which the amount of oxygen used by the body for 15 minutes is used. To determine a person's basal metabolic rate, he or she must lie awake in a warm room, as relaxed as possible, after fasting for 12 hours. Oxygen consumption is measured for approximately 15 minutes. From this, basal heat production is calculated on the basis of 4.82 calories of heat for every liter of oxygen used. Basal metabolism amounts to about 1 calorie per kilogram per hour in men, and 0.9 calorie per kilogram in women between 15 and 25 years of age. As we age, our BMR declines approximately 2 percent every 10 years after age 25.

BMR is influenced by a number of factors, one of which is body size and composition. A tall, thin person with a large body surface area will experience greater heat loss than short, muscular individuals. Thus the BMR of tall persons is greater. The BMR of muscular people is about 5 percent greater than for fat people because muscle tissues use more energy than fat tissue. Fat people have a lower BMR per weight than muscular persons of the same weight. The BMR of women is generally 5–10 percent lower than that of men, possibly owing to the greater accumulation of fat and lower lean body mass in women.

Other influencing factors on BMR include age, amount of sleep, function of the endocrine glands (especially the thyroid glands), state of nutrition, and fever. The highest BMR occurs in early childhood and at the growth spurt associated with puberty. The BMR declines with age at approximately 2 percent per decade. This means, if your diet remains constant, you will gain a considerable amount of weight as you grow older. For example, pretend you are 25 years old and in perfect caloric balance at 154 pounds eating 2,800 calories a day. If you continue to eat this same amount (2,800 calories a day) until you reached 75 years, you will gradually gain until at age 75 you would weigh 279 pounds. You must reduce your caloric intake as you get older. A good rule of thumb to follow is to reduce caloric consumption by 5 percent for each decade past 25 years of age. Thus, by age 35, you should be eating 95 percent of your caloric allotment at age 25; by 45 years of age, you would need to reduce to 90 percent; and so forth. However, people who remain active into their elderly years do not show such a great decline in basal metabolism because body mass is better maintained.

Various hormonal secretions from the endocrine glands regulate the BMR. The body's main regulator for the BMR is thyroxin, a hormone secreted by the thyroid gland. If there is a deficiency in the amount produced, a lower metabolic rate (30–50%) results, thus reducing the total caloric requirements. Conversely, overproduction of thyroxin increases metabolic activity and calorie expenditure. The male sex hormones (primarily testosterone) increase BMR by 15–20 percent, and the female hormones by slightly less. The growth hormone (somatotropin) may increase the BMR up to 20 percent. Epinephrine and norepinephrine (hormones secreted by adrenal glands) also influence the BMR, as do the hormones cortisol and insulin.

Energy cost for activity includes the amount of energy needed for all the muscles involved in the activity plus a small amount of energy to take care of the increase in heart rate and breathing that takes place during strenuous activity.

Sleep lowers the BMR by 10–15 percent; thus the amount of sleep is relevant. Sleeping more than 8 hours per day tends to lower the BMR. Climatic conditions also have an effect. The BMR can be lowered by as much as 10–20 percent in hot, humid, tropical areas. Infections and fever increase the BMR about 7 percent for each additional degree of increased body temperature.

With so many factors influencing the BMR, it is understandable why people vary in BMR and why some people can eat almost anything and never gain weight or vice versa.

Thermic Effect of Food

In addition to using energy for BMR, the body also uses energy for thermogenesis. Thermogenesis is the production of body heat in response to food intake and in the nonshivering response to cold.

Heat is produced when the food we eat is digested, absorbed, transported, metabolized, and stored. This is known as diet-induced thermogenesis or the thermic effect of food (TEF). The thermic effect of food refers to the stimulation in metabolism and therefore the production of heat that occurs 1–3 hours after a meal. Between 5 and 10 percent of the energy a person consumes will be used in this manner. To supply the body 100 calories, a person must eat 105–110 calories. The process of digestion, absorption, and metabolism uses the extra 5–10 calories to modify the nutrients so that they are more available for use. Thus, given a daily caloric intake of 3,000, the thermic effect of food would use 180–300 calories. The stimulation of heat production was greater when the diet had a high proportion of calories specifically from protein. Considerable evidence indicates that a diet high in protein does increase energy costs of maintaining the energy needs of the body.

The body also produces heat in response to cold. For example, hibernating animals maintain their body temperature despite the cold environment. Human infants are also able to do this, although to a much lesser extent. This ability may be due to the presence of brown fat. Brown fat differs from the usual yellow fat in that it contains more mitochondria, the energy producing bodies of the cell. These extra mitochondria generate more heat by burning more fuel, thus keeping the body warm. The extent to which adults have brown fat, if any, is still being studied. At this time the presence of brown adipose tissue in adults, and its links to the thermic effect of food, is open to question. Although it is unlikely that brown fat serves a pivotal role in weight regulation in adults, information is too sketchy to permit any definite conclusions.

Physical Activity

Energy cost for activity includes the amount of energy needed for all the muscles involved in the activity plus a small amount of energy to take care of the increase in heart rate and breathing that takes place during strenuous activity. Physical activity level is the biggest variable in energy use among people. Basal metabolism is roughly the same in most people (usually +25–30%, though greater differences occur), as are the energy expenditures for the thermic effect of food. Together, basal metabolism and the thermic effect of food represent about 60–75 percent of total energy use. The big difference in energy use among people is due to different activity levels. Some people are very active physically and others are very sedentary.

The actual cost of various activities has been determined by a series of tests that measure the amount of oxygen consumed and therefore the energy used in performing a specific activity (table 16.1). This table is fairly accurate for activities such as walking and running, in which moving the whole body accounts for 75 percent of energy costs. On the other hand, it probably overestimates energy costs for activities like sewing or piano playing. Before using the tables, recognize their limitations. Although the energy costs do represent the best average estimates available, they do not reflect the differences in efficiency when various people perform the same task. We also know that a 198-pound (90 kg) man requires more energy to walk a mile than a 132-pound (60 kg) man.

Many people are dismayed to learn how few calories are actually involved in some activities they consider relatively strenuous. For example, the energy cost of walking is only 4.0 cal/min for a 110-pound person or 60 calories burned while walking a 15-minute mile. Even more disturbing is the fact that intense mental work requires practically no more energy than daydreaming. Any extra energy costs could be attributed to tension in the muscles, associated with mental stress. However, the calories used in our daily physical activities can mount up. Using stairs rather than the elevator or parking in the outer area rather than close to the building can increase physical activity and hence energy use. Recent studies show that people who fidget and can't sit still use more energy (an extra 100 to 800 calories per day) than those who are generally relaxed.

Studies show that we do not eat so many more calories than people did at the turn of this century, but as a group we are considerably less active. This inactivity contributes to our increased rates of obesity over people of the early 1900s.

In summary, the body uses energy in three ways: the basal metabolism, the thermic effect of food, and physical activity. Normally, 60–75 percent of the energy used by the body comes from the BMR and thermic effect of food. The other 25–40 percent comes from physical activity, in which we have the greatest control over regulating our energy use. Obesity results when there is an energy imbalance between energy in and energy out.

The Balancing Act

In order to maintain proper weight, energy input must equal energy output. This sounds simple, but actually it is complex

Table 16.1
Energy Expenditure of Various Activities (cal/min/kg)

Activity	(kg) (lb)	50 110	60 132	70 154	80 176	90 198	100 220
Bicycling							
Leisure, 5.5 mph		3.2	3.8	4.5	5.1	5.7	6.4
Leisure, 9.4 mph		5.0	5.9	7.1	8.0	8.9	9.9
Racing		8.5	10.0	12.0	13.5	15.0	16.7
Basketball		6.9	8.1	9.8	11.0	12.3	13.6
Canoeing							
Leisure		2.2	2.6	3.1	3.5	3.9	4.4
Racing		5.2	6.1	7.3	8.2	9.2	10.2
Card Playing		1.3	1.5	1.8	2.0	2.2	2.6
Circuit-Training		9.3	10.9	13.1	14.8	16.5	18.2
Cleaning		3.1	3.7	4.4	5.0	5.5	6.2
Cooking		2.3	2.7	3.2	3.6	4.0	4.5
Dancing							
Ballroom		2.6	3.0	3.6	4.1	4.5	5.1
Choreographed		8.4	9.9	11.9	13.4	15.0	16.6
Twist		5.2	6.1	7.3	8.2	9.2	10.2
Digging Trenches		7.3	8.6	10.3	11.6	12.9	14.3
Eating		1.2	1.4	1.6	1.8	2.0	2.4
Food Shopping		3.1	3.7	4.4	5.0	5.5	6.2
Football		6.6	7.8	9.4	10.6	11.7	13.0

Activity	(kg) (lb)	50 110	60 132	70 154	80 176	90 198	100 220
Gardening							
Digging		6.3	7.4	8.9	10.1	11.2	12.4
Hedging		3.9	4.5	5.5	6.2	6.9	7.6
Mowing		5.6	6.6	8.0	9.0	10.0	11.1
Raking		2.7	3.2	3.8	4.3	4.8	5.4
Golf		4.3	5.0	6.0	6.8	7.6	8.4
Gymnastics		3.3	3.9	4.7	5.3	5.9	6.6
Ironing		1.7	1.9	2.3	2.6	2.9	3.3
Knitting, Sewing		1.1	1.3	1.6	1.8	2.0	2.2
Lying at Ease		1.1	1.3	1.5	1.8	2.0	2.2
Music Playing							
Conducting		2.0	2.3	2.8	3.1	3.5	3.9
Drums (sitting)		3.3	3.9	4.7	5.3	5.9	6.7
Horn (sitting)		1.5	1.7	2.1	2.3	2.6	2.9
Piano (sitting)		2.0	2.4	2.8	3.2	3.6	4.0
Violin (sitting)		2.3	2.7	3.2	3.6	4.0	4.5
Painting (inside)		1.7	2.0	2.4	2.7	3.0	3.4
Painting (outside)		3.9	4.5	5.5	6.2	6.9	7.6
Running, Cross Country		8.2	9.6	11.6	13.0	14.5	16.1
Running, Level Surface							
11 min. 30s per mile		6.8	8.0	9.6	10.9	12.1	13.4
9 min. per mile		9.7	11.4	13.7	15.4	17.2	18.9
7 min. per mile		12.2	13.9	16.2	17.9	19.7	21.5
6 min. per mile		13.9	15.6	17.9	19.6	21.4	23.2
5 min. 30s per mile		14.5	17.1	20.5	23.1	25.7	28.4
Skiing (Leisure)		4.9	5.8	7.0	7.8	8.7	9.7
Snowshoeing		8.3	9.8	11.8	13.3	14.8	16.4
Swimming							
Backstroke		8.5	10.0	12.0	13.5	15.0	16.7
Crawl, fast		7.8	9.2	11.1	12.5	13.9	15.4
Tennis		5.5	6.4	7.7	8.7	9.7	10.8
Typing		1.4	1.6	1.9	2.2	2.4	2.7
Volleyball		2.5	3.0	3.6	4.0	4.5	5.0
Walking							
Asphalt Road		4.0	4.7	5.7	6.4	7.1	7.9
Hillsides		4.1	4.8	5.8	6.6	7.3	8.1
Grass Track		4.1	4.8	5.8	6.5	7.2	8.0
Writing		1.5	1.7	2.1	2.3	2.6	2.9

because small imbalances can lead to large weight gains or losses over time. For example, suppose a person drinks one extra soft drink per day for a year. Assuming that energy expenditure stays constant and the soft drink contains 200 calories, the person will gain about 21 pounds in the course of the year.

200 calories
x 365 days per year
73,000 calories per year

3,500 calories= 1 lb of fat

73,000 calories per year
3,500 calories per pound
= 20.8 pounds gained in one year

Let's examine the energy balance formula in order to make some rational decisions about losing or gaining weight.

Energy Balance Formula

Caloric balance = calories from food – (calories from BMR
+ calories from physical activity
+ calories from thermic effect of food)

- Caloric balance occurs when the calories taken in equal those expended.
- Calories from food means the total number of calories taken into the body.
- Calories from BMR are those calories used while at complete rest.
- Calories from physical activity means the calories that are used during physical exertion.
- Calories from thermic effect of food means the calories used during digestion, absorption, and excretion.

If you are satisfied with your percentage of body fat and body weight, you should strive for caloric balance. This means your daily caloric input should equal your daily caloric output. Because the only way calories can enter the body is through the consumption of food, the type and quantity of food consumed determine the total number of calories that enter the body.

Calories leave the body in three ways. First, calories are burned up by our BMR. Second, calories are burned up by our daily physical exertion. Third, calories are used by the thermic effect of food. Let's analyze each part of the formula and determine how we can lose or gain weight.

Calories from food.—If you plan to lose weight, reduce the amount of calories consumed without sacrificing the basic nutritional needs such as vitamins, minerals, and proteins. Do not go on a crash diet, for a crash diet can harm your body's metabolism. Try to eat three small, well-balanced, low-caloric meals which contain the 45 known nutrients.

Calories from BMR.—As noted earlier, the BMR depends on several factors such as age, body size, gender, and function of the endocrine glands. Precise measurement of the BMR requires a trained specialist using special equipment. Exercise physiologists have developed a more simple, fairly accurate procedure for calculating the BMR, provided there are no endocrine or hormonal abnormalities.

One kilogram (2.2 pounds) of body weight burns approximately one calorie per hour in a male between 15 and 25 years of age. In women of the same age, one kilogram of body weight burns approximately 0.9 calories per hour. Age and body size also affect the BMR. As you get older, your BMR decreases in the number of calories used daily. BMR also decreases with a smaller body size. Women have approximately a 10-percent reduction in their BMR.

To determine your BMR, obtain from table 16.2 your calorie per kilogram of body weight at your particular age. Divide your body weight by 2.2 pounds to determine your weight in kilograms. Now multiply your body weight in kilograms by your age adjustment figure. The results show your BMR for one hour. To determine your BMR for 24 hours, multiply your one-hour BMR by 24. For example, compare the BMR for two men, ages 60 and 20, who both weigh 176 pounds:

As you can see, the 60-year-old man cannot eat as many calories as the 20-year-old man and expect to keep his weight constant. If the older man consumed a double meat hamburger, milk shake, and French fries, he would nearly equal his BMR

20-YEAR-OLD MAN	60-YEAR-OLD MAN
176 pounds/2.2 = 80 kilograms 80 kilograms x 1 age adjustment = 80 calories/hour 80 calories/hour x 24 hrs. = 1920 BMR/day	176 pounds/2.2 = 80 (kgs) 80 kilograms x 0.8 age adjustment = 64 calories/hour 64 calories/hour x 24 hrs. = 1536 BMR/day

for the day. As you can see, it is easy to gain weight as you get older, which makes it imperative to eat less or exercise more to burn up excess calories as you age.

Calories from physical activity.—Now that you have calculated your 24-hour BMR, add all calories in excess of the resting expenditure of energy for the various activities that make up your day. Daily calorie expenditures vary widely because of differences in job requirements and recreational endeavors.

Table 16.2
Determinants of Age Adjustment for Men and Women in BMR

Age	Men's Age Adjustment (calorie/kg body weight)	Women's Age Adjustment (calorie/kg body weight)
15–25	1.00	0.90
26–35	0.95	0.85
36–45	0.90	0.80
46–55	0.85	0.75
56–65	0.80	0.70
over 65	0.75	0.65

The harder the physical work, the more calories expended. It would be impractical to try to calculate your calorie expenditures exactly for the whole day, because you constantly change your activity level. Exercise physiologists have devised two methods to estimate calories expended during a 24-hour period. In the first method, determine the activity intensity level that best describes your daily activity from table 16.3.

After you have chosen your activity intensity level, multiply that percentage by your BMR for 24 hours, then add the result to your BMR. For example, to calculate the calories expended for the 60- and 20-year-old men described earlier, multiply each man's BMR by, say, 60 (daily intensity level) to determine the calories expended during physical activity. Then add the results to their BMR.

Table 16.3
Activity Intensity Levels for Men and Women

Intensity Level (%)	Classification
40	Sedentary—Very limited physical activity. Limited to walking and sitting (office workers, teachers, clergymen, etc.).
50	Semi-sedentary—Engaged in activities that involve standing and walking (policemen, housework, foreman, etc.).
60	Laborers—Manual physical work (lifting, pushing, etc.). Also include slight calisthenics, walking or jogging one or two miles, etc.
70	Heavy workers—Regular participation in vigorous physical activity (racquetball, tennis, swimming, running 3 miles or more, weightlifting, etc.).
80	Athletic training—Marathon running, swimming, cycling, intercollegiate sports. Very vigorous daily physical fitness program lasting more than 1 hour.

20-YEAR-OLD MAN	60-YEAR-OLD MAN
1,920 BMR x 0.60 activity intensity level 1,152 calories expended for physical activity 1,920 BMR + 1,152 calories needed for physical activity 3,072 calories expended for one day	1536 BMR x 0.60 activity intensity level 921.6 calories expended for physical activity 1,536 BMR + 922 calories needed for physical activity 2,458 calories expended for one day

The 60-year-old man needs to consume approximately 2,458 calories a day to maintain his body weight, whereas the 20-year-old man needs to consume nearly 3,072 calories a day. If they consume more calories than they expend, they will gain weight. If they consume fewer calories, they will lose weight.

Calories from thermic effect of food.—A certain number of calories is expended in the stimulation of metabolism and, therefore, the production of heat that occurs from one to three hours after a meal (thermogenesis). Each individual is different in the amount of calories expended through thermogenesis. Most nutritionists estimate that the average individual expends approximately 5 percent, some as high as 10 percent, of the calories consumed through the thermic effect of food. Therefore, if you consume 3,000 calories daily, you will expend 150–300 calories (5–10% of 3000).

Now that we have analyzed the formula, let us calculate our caloric consumption and balance our consumption and expenditure of energy. Use the example of the 60- and 20-year-old men who both weigh 176 pounds (80 kilograms) and eat approximately 2,800 calories daily. Substitute what we know about these men in the formula.

Caloric Balance = calories from food - (calories from BMR
+ calories from physical activity
+ calories from thermogenesis).

In order for us to lose one pound of adipose tissue (fat), we must create a deficit of 3,500 calories between calories consumed and expended. So if we divide each man's difference in calories consumed with calories expended, then we can see that the 60-year-old man will gain one pound of fat tissue (3,500/202) approximately every 17.5 days or about 21 pounds in a year. Whereas, the 20-year-old man will lose one pound of fat tissue (3,500/412) nearly every 9 days or about 42 pounds a year.

Let us calculate how much weight the 60-year-old man could lose if he went on a moderate calorie restriction diet of 2,000 calories daily and kept his physical activity the same.

20-YEAR-OLD MAN	60-YEAR-OLD MAN
2,800 (calories from food) –(1,920 (calories from BMR) + 1,152 (calories from activity) + 140)(calories at 5% thermogenesis) 2800 – (1920 + 1152 +140) 2800 – 3212 – 412 calories a day	2,800 (calories from food) – 1,536 (calories from BMR) + 922 (calories from activity + 140 (calories at 5% thermogenesis 2,800 – (1,536 + 922 + 140) 2,800 – 2,598 +202 calories per day

Caloric Balance = 2,000 calories
– (1,536 BMR
+ 922 activity level
+ 100 5% thermogenesis)
2,000 calories – 2,558
– 558 calories a day

If we divide 558 into 3,500 calories (needed to lose one pound), we see that this man will lose one pound of adipose tissue approximately every seven days or 52 pounds in a year. The best way to lose weight is to reduce your caloric intake moderately and increase your physical activity until you reach your desired weight. You should also note these precautions:

It's nearly impossible to obtain from your diet all the 45 known nutrients in their proper amount in fewer than 1,500 calories a day.

• Never try to lose more that 1 to 1½ pounds of adipose tissue a week, because severe caloric restrictions (crash dieting) could permanently lower your BMR. The body will perceive itself to be in a starvation state and lower its BMR in protection. Many Americans have lowered their BMR from crash dieting and wonder why they gain weight on 800 calories a day.

• Never consume fewer than 1,000 calories a day. The body needs at least this many calories to maintain proper glucose production from carbohydrate and fat. If these calories are not consumed, the body converts protein into glucose; and you begin losing lean body tissue.

• It's nearly impossible to obtain from your diet all the 45 known nutrients in their proper amount in fewer than 1,500 calories a day. In fact, most men and women need to consume 1,800 calories a day unless they are very small in stature. Choose your foods carefully if you lower your caloric intake below 1,800 calories. If you choose to consume fewer than 1,500 calories a day, do not stay on this diet more than 6 months, for your health could be affected.

Substitute your physical dimensions into the formula to determine whether you are maintaining or losing weight. If you expend more calories than you consume, you will tip the energy balance and will get rid of the excess fat in God's temple.

Determination of Body Composition: Are You Fat?

Many people are overweight and do not realize it because they base their judgment on the way they look in clothes. Some tall people look slim when they actually could be considered obese when measured by precise scientific instruments. The way you look in clothes does not determine your degree of fatness; rather it is total percentage of adipose tissue that you have on your body. For every pound of fat gained, nearly 200 miles of capillaries are needed to supply that one pound of adipose tissue. Hence, putting on 20 pounds of fat requires your body to produce enough capillaries to stretch across America. This excessive capillarization has a detrimental effect on the cardiovascular-respiratory system. Let's examine some ways in which we can determine our degree of fatness.

Height-Weight Tables

Possibly the simplest test for fatness is to stand naked in front of a mirror and closely examine your body. If you look fat, then you are fat. Another way is to compare your height to norms set up by insurance companies (see table 16.4). These charts are not always reliable, however, for insurance actuaries have devised desirable weights, not actual weights. These desirable weights are derived from people showing the average weight. In addition, the table's data are derived only from purchases of life insurance. This results in under-representation for poor people and many minorities. Another weakness in these charts can be shown by the example of the fat-determination studies done on the Dallas Cowboys football team. Running back Hershel Walker was determined to have 2 percent body fat, which is classified as excellent; yet the height-weight tables revealed that he was 30 pounds overweight. Strong individuals with much muscle development can appear fatter than they actually are. Also, overweight people will look at these charts and automatically determine that they have large frames, when many actually have small frames. Tables 16.4 and 16.5 can help you determine your frame size and true weight.

Skinfold Measurements

Another method of estimating fatness is by measuring the thickness of fatfold with a skinfold caliper. Because one half of the body fat is just under the skin and overlaying the muscles, the thickness of a pinch of skin and fat can be used as an indicator of total body fatness. This procedure is easily done by pinching the skin on the back of the upper arm (triceps area) and the top of the upper leg. The different thicknesses of these steps is due to the different amounts of underlying fat.

The fatfold should be firmly grasped between the thumb and forefinger. The depth of the fold is determined by the amount of fat present. The thickness of the fold is read in millimeters from the caliper dial and can be taken before and after an exercise program to assess fat loss.

The estimates of body fat percentages given in table 16.6 are fairly accurate. Readings taken properly should reveal a fat estimate within + 4 percent. The more obese an individual is, the less accurate the readings.

Underwater Weighing

The underwater weighing technique is usually more accurate than skinfold measurements but requires the use of expensive

Table 16.4
1983 Metropolitan Life Insurance Company Height and Weight Table

Men*				Women*			
Height	Small Frame	Medium Frame	Large Frame	Height	Small Frame	Medium Frame	Large Frame
5'2"	128–134	131–141	138–150	4'10"	102–111	109–121	118–131
5'3"	130–136	133–143	140–153	4'11"	103–113	111–123	120–134
5'4"	132–138	135–145	142–156	5'0"	104–115	113–126	122–137
5'5"	134–140	137–148	144–160	5'1"	106–118	115–129	125–140
5'6"	136–142	139–151	146–164	5'2"	108–121	118–132	128–143
5'7"	138–145	142–154	149–168	5'3"	111–124	121–135	131–147
5'8"	140–148	145–157	152–172	5'4"	114–127	124–138	134–151
5'9"	142–151	148–160	155–176	5'5"	117–130	127–141	137–155
5'10"	144–154	151–163	158–180	5'6"	120–133	130–144	140–159
5'11"	146–157	154–166	161–184	5'7"	123–136	133–147	143–163
6'0"	149–160	157–170	164–188	5'8"	126–139	136–150	146–167
6'1"	152–164	160–174	168–192	5'9"	129–142	139–153	149–170
6'2"	155–168	164–178	172–197	5'10"	132–145	142–156	152–173
6'3"	158–172	167–182	176–202	5'11"	135–148	145–159	155–176
6'4"	162–176	171–187	181–207	6'0"	138–151	148–162	158–179

*Weight in pounds (in indoor clothing weighing 5 lbs. with shoes with 1" heels).

Frame size is determined from ankle circumference, which should be measured with a tape measure at the smallest point above the two bones that protrude on each side (external and internal malleolus). Pull the tape measure as tight as possible.

Table 16.5
Determination of Relative Frame Size of the Human Body

Sex	Small Frame (inches)	Medium Frame (inches)	Large Frame (inches)
Male	< 8	8–9.25	> 9.25
Female	< 7.5	7.5–8.75	> 8.75

Table 16.6
Fatness Rating Scale

Classification	Men	Women
Very Lean	0–10	0–15
Lean	11–14	16–20
Marginal	15–17	21–24
Overfat	18–19	25–29
Obese	20 plus	30 plus

For men, a body fat less than 15 percent is considered healthy and above 20 percent is obese. For females, up to 24 percent body fat is considered healthy, and above 30 percent is obese.

laboratory equipment. This technique is based on the fact that muscles and bones are more dense than water, whereas fat is less dense. Therefore, the more a person weighs under water, the leaner he or she is. Weight under water reflects density, and this measurement is used in a mathematical equation to estimate body fat.

Bioelectrical Impedance

This technique uses a low-energy electrical current. Fat resists the flow of electricity. Thus the more fat storage a person has per inch of height, the more resistance. The subject lies on a table, with the limbs not touching the body. Current-injector electrodes are placed on the right hand and right foot. A harmless electrical current is generated and passed through the subject. Bioelectrical impedance analyzers convert body electrical resistance into an estimate of the percent of the body that is fat. The test takes only five minutes.

Precautions should be taken to ensure accuracy of measurement. Bioelectrical impedance valves are affected by recent food intake, recent exercise, recent alcohol intake, and the use of certain medications, such as diuretics. To get an accurate value, one must not have consumed alcohol within the last 24 hours, not have eaten within the last 4 hours, not have exercised hard within the last 12 hours, and not have recently taken medication that affects water balance in the body.

Android and Gynecoid Obesity

Another way to assess obesity is to calculate the distribution of fat stores in the body. Obesity can be categorized as android and gynecoid. Android obesity is usually found in males. The male appearance consists of a large abdomen (pot belly) and small buttocks and thighs (apple shape). High testosterone levels in men are thought to encourage upper body fat deposition. Fat storage in this area is easier to lose than in the thigh area.

Gynecoid obesity is the typical female obesity pattern which normally takes the appearance of a small abdomen and a much larger buttocks-and-thighs area (pear shape). The reason women tend to have this type of obesity is because the cells in this area contain more lipoprotein lipase, the enzyme that pushes fat from the bloodstream into fat cells. Also, the female hormone, progesterone, increases the action of lipoprotein lipase in the lower torso region. As you can see, there are biological reasons men tend to have android obesity and women tend to have gynecoid obesity.

Android obesity is associated with more heart disease, hypertension, and diabetes than is gynecoid obesity. The reason is that adipose tissue in the abdominal area tends to resist the action of insulin, which could increase the risk of developing diabetes mellitus. Developing diabetes mellitus then leads to an increased risk of developing heart disease and hypertension.

To determine whether you are becoming android obese, calculate your ratio of waist circumference (at the level of the umbilicus) with the circumference of your hips. A ratio greater than 0.9 in men and 0.8 in women indicates android obesity.

Classification

To answer the question, Am I fat? refer to table 16.6. Find your classification as indicated by your percentage of body fat tissue. The aim is for an optimal body fat, not just marginal. Table 16.6 classifies the percent body fat from lean to obese. For men, a body fat less than 15 percent is considered healthy and above 20 percent is obese. Women are allowed more fat because they carry more essential fat in breast tissue and other organs that have reproductive function. For females, up to 24 percent body fat is considered healthy, and above 30 percent is obese.

[CHAPTER 17]

Understanding Weight Management

Americans are literally digging their graves with their teeth; for every cell in our body is affected by what we eat or fail to eat. Many people deny their delicate, highly sophisticated cells the 45 known nutrients in their proper amounts. Consequently, many are obese and suffer from nutritional disorders that could be prevented by eating correctly. For example, the American Heart Association lists obesity as one of the major risk factors in heart disease and hypertension. The American Diabetes Society claims obesity is the leading cause of maturity-onset diabetes. The American Cancer Society estimates that 40 percent of all cancers may be due to nutritional abnormalities. Yet many Christians keep pouring abnormally high amounts of junk food, which has little nutritional value to the cell, into their mouths to be ground up by their teeth to be used by their bodies to operate their well-balanced, highly sophisticated, complex bodily functions.

When complications such as degenerative diseases occur, many Christians either blame God for their affliction, or they cannot believe God would let this happen to them. Do not blame God if you destroy His creation by overeating nonnutritional foods. Knowledge is the tool used to choose between right and wrong. The Bible tells us many times to become knowledgeable. In that light, let's examine what occurs to our bodies when we abuse food and treasure it above other priorities in our lives.

Obesity

Americans are overweight! More than 35 million Americans, representing 10–40 percent of the population in any age group, can attest to that statement. Weight control, although difficult, is important to many people for reasons of appearance as well as health. Many try dieting. In fact, at any given time 27 percent of men, 46 percent of women, and 75 percent of teenage girls are trying some type of weight-loss diet. Each new diet is promoted as the "ultimate diet" or the "diet to end all diets." Unfortunately, misinformation abounds; entrepreneurs everywhere are ready to capitalize on any approach that sounds plausible, regardless of whether there is any evidence of its effectiveness. Diets do not work 95 percent of the time.

This chapter will lead you through the issues of weight control. After reading it, you will be able to decide when diet books are telling the truth and when they are deceiving you.

Incidence of Obesity

National studies of Americans during the last 30 years show that many are overweight and obese. As you may recall in chapter 16, overweight is defined as 16–19 percent body fat for men and 25–30 percent for women. Obesity is defined as body fat greater than 20 percent for men and greater than 30 percent for women. These national studies revealed that 24 percent of adult men and 26.5 percent of adult women are considered

At least seven major health problems are associated with obesity. Some medical experts feel that obesity deserves to be termed our nation's number one health problem.

obese. Among the population of U.S. adults over 40 years of age, 80 percent of men and 70 percent of women are more than 10 percent overweight.

The U.S. Census Bureau has submitted figures showing that the average U.S. female is now 64 inches tall and weighs 142 pounds. This is 16 pounds above the recommended weight. The average U.S. male is 69.5 inches tall and weighs 173 pounds, 12 pounds above the recommended weight. As you can see, America is the land of the "fat cats."

Not only are American adults overweight, but national surveys also reveal that a large number of our children and teenagers are obese. Among American children and youth aged 6–17 years, 29 percent of the boys and 25.2 percent of the girls are considered obese. When comparing figures with those from 1963, the percentage of children 6–11 years old who are obese today is approximately 54 percent higher, and among youth 12–17 years of age it is 39 percent higher.

Health Hazards from Obesity

At least seven major health problems are associated with obesity. Some medical experts feel that obesity deserves to be termed our nation's number one health problem. Let's summarize each health problem.

Increased heart disease.—Approximately 80 percent of people suffering from heart disease are overweight. Not only do obese people have more of the typical risk factors for heart disease (high blood pressure and cholesterol), but they also experience more death from this cause.

Increased high blood pressure.—People who are obese are three times more likely to have high blood pressure than normal weight people. In fact, approximately 85 percent of people with high blood pressure are overweight or have been overweight. A BMI (body mass index, see chapter 6, page 34) of just 26 increases the risk of high blood pressure threefold for men and twofold for women.

Increased levels of cholesterol and triglycerides.—People who are obese have twice the risk of having high cholesterol and triglyceride levels than normal weight people.

Increased cancer.—The American Cancer Society has recently completed a study which involved more than one million men and women and found that obese males have a higher mortality rate from cancer of the colon, rectum, and prostate. Obese females were found to have a higher mortality rate from cancer of the gallbladder, bile ducts, breast, uterus, and ovaries.

Increased diabetes.—People who are obese have greater risk of acquiring diabetes than a nonobese person. A male with a BMI of 27 has four times the risk of diabetes, while a female has greater than six times the risk.

Increased arthritis.—People who are obese have double the risk of arthritis at a BMI 30 of a nonobese person.

Increased early death.—People who are obese are seven times more likely to die prematurely than nonobese people. Remember, "the longer the belt, the shorter the life."

Increased psychological hazards.—Most Americans adhere to the philosophy that "thin is in." Because of the strong pressures from society to be thin, obese people often suffer feelings of guilt, depression, anxiety, and low self-worth. Also, there is evidence of outright discrimination against the obese in college admission and in selection for many jobs. Whether or not the cause of obesity is psychological, the obesity itself has profound psychological implications. This burden may be the greatest negative effect of obesity.

As mentioned in chapter 16, the android form (body fat in stomach area) is associated with more heart disease, hypertension, and diabetes than is gynecoid obesity (body fat in hips and thighs). In other words, health risks are greater for those who have most of their body fat in the upper body. This body fat can be determined by looking at the ratio of waist-to-hip circumferences. A high ratio predicts elevated complications from obesity. In males, risk increases greatly when the waist/hip ratio rises above 1.0 and in females when it rises above 0.8. For example, if a male has a waist circumference of 42 inches and a hip circumference of 37 inches, the waist/hip ratio is 1.13 (42/37 = 1.13). This puts him at risk for the medical complications listed previously. If a female has a waist circumference of 35 inches and a hip circumference of 40, the waist/hip ratio is 0.88 (35/40 = 0.88), putting her at risk.

To determine your waist-to-hip ratio, do the following:

- Using a cloth tape measure, determine your waist circumference by measuring just above your umbilicus (naval). Pull the tape measure tight without causing an indentation in your body (i.e., don't cheat!).
- Measure your hip circumference at the largest point

The energy cost of many activities may seem small. However, walking one mile daily burns approximately 100 calories.

around your hips.

• Divide waist measurement by hip measurement.

Causes of Obesity

The three causes of obesity are increased calorie intake, decreased activity, and genetic predisposition. Let's quickly examine each.

Increased calorie intake.—The underlying cause of all obesity is the consumption of an excess of calories over a prolonged period of time. That is, an intake of calories in excess of calorie expenditure. However, this simple statement does little to explain why some people have so much more trouble maintaining a desirable body weight than others. Differences in genetics and activity levels are major explanations.

Decreased activity.—There is considerable evidence that the obese gain weight because their activity level is low rather than because their food intake is excessive. Studies done on obese children demonstrate that they consume approximately the same number of calories as nonobese children, but their caloric expenditure through activity is far inferior to the calorie expenditure of the nonobese children. The energy cost of many activities may seem small. However, walking one mile daily burns approximately 100 calories. For a 154-pound man, walking one mile daily for a year would account for nearly 10 pounds of body fat in a year. Almost all effective weight control programs involve exercise as well as diet.

Genetic predisposition.—Several studies have shown that hereditary factors are important in explaining why some people find it so hard to avoid obesity. Dr. Jean Mayer, a noted nutritionist, reported that 80 percent of the children with two obese parents became obese when reaching adulthood, compared with only 14 percent of the children with two nonobese parents. Another study comparing fraternal and identical twins found that, upon reaching adulthood, the body weights of identical twins were much more similar than the body weights of fraternal twins. Also, a study of adults who had been adopted before the age of one revealed that despite being raised by adoptive parents their body weights were still similar to that of their birth parents.

The reason appears to be that obese people use food more efficiently, have a tendency to store food quickly in the form of fat, and have much more difficulty mobilizing fat to meet energy needs. This does not mean that individuals who are unfortunate enough to inherit a tendency to obesity are doomed to be obese forever. It usually means, however, that they will be faced with a constant and often difficult struggle to overcome the strong tendency to accumulate fat. These people are more likely to produce more fat cells (hyperplasia) and to have larger fat cells (hypertrophy), or both. Many genetically obese people have an improper amount of an enzyme called lipoprotein lipase, which is the enzyme that permits their cells to pick up lipids carried in the blood. This may be one reason the person with a higher percentage of lean body, particularly muscle mass, can consume more calories than an overfat person. Muscles require much more calories than fat to be metabolized.

Studies done on infants as early as three months of age found that there is a lower energy expenditure in infants born to obese mothers compared to those born to lean mothers. Also, infants who become overweight by one year of age show lower energy expenditures compared to those who do not become overweight. Overweight adults also have a lower energy expenditure, both total and basal, than their nonobese counterparts. Since metabolic energy expenditure is controlled genetically, the trait is often inherited.

These studies demonstrate that some people are more prone than others to obesity due to genetic factors. Such people have to be unusually careful about their dietary and exercise habits to counteract these inherited tendencies.

Theories of Obesity

Several theories attempt to explain why people become obese. Let's examine some of the more popular ones.

Fat cell theory.—Small samples of fat can be safely and easily obtained for scientific study by slipping a small needle just beneath the skin and siphoning out some fat cells. When the fat is examined under the microscope, it's clear that there are numerous round fat cells. These small cells are practically invisible to the naked eye; it would take several hundred lined up in a row to make one inch.

By volume, roughly 90 percent of the cell is a single droplet of fat. The fatty acids that are present closely reflect fat that has been eaten over long periods. Thus people who tend to eat more vegetable oils than animal fat will have an oily adipose tissue containing fatty acids with many double bonds. Fat that is made by eating excess carbohydrate tends to be much more saturated, with fewer double bonds.

An average fat cell contains about a half microgram (one half-millionth of a gram) of triglyceride. To store the many pounds of fat present, it takes roughly 30 billion adipocytes (fat cells) in a normal, nonobese person. In all persons who become obese, these billions of cells tend to get larger. And the grossly obese are apt to have an even greater number of them. That is, morbidly obese people, who are more than double their desirable weight, are likely to have more and larger fat cells.

It is notable that with weight reduction the main change in adipocytes is a decrease in size. Fat cells, once filled with fat, do not disappear easily or at all in the adult state. Thus the formerly obese person persists in having a higher than normal cell number. Whether this increased number would ever disappear if the weight were kept down for many years remains arguable. Most evidence indicates that it would not.

We now know that the number of fat cells can increase in adult life with the likelihood varying from one part of the body to another. There is still evidence, however, that people with a large number of fat cells have more difficulty maintaining body weight than do those with fewer fat cells. These people seem to be able to lose weight up to the point where cell size reaches a normal level; but because of the larger number of cells, it is difficult to reduce beyond the point. For example, 95 percent of severely obese persons regain weight after weight loss compared to 66 percent of moderately obese persons. This is because reduced-obese persons have lower energy needs than a person of the same weight who was never obese.

In summary, the presence of extra fat cells has several important implications. Some obese people are likely to be heavy just because of the extra fat-cell mass, even when the fat cells contain only normal amounts of fat. Also, obese people with extra fat cells are going to find weight loss difficult because of biological pressures to keep the extra cells supplied with fat. In addition, obese people who have extra fat cells and have been obese since early in life may have to accept higher weight standards. Despite vigorous efforts to eat and exercise healthfully, body-fat levels in such people may still be higher than desirable.

Dietary theory.—This theory postulates that people overeat and therefore gain weight more readily when foods are available and when they are encouraged to eat them. Studies reveal that obese people tend to consume more calories than normal-weight individuals, while choosing larger portions of rich foods that are high in fats and sugars.

Most nutritionists believe that the abundance of tasty, calorie-rich foods, especially those high in fat, is the primary reason so many Americans are fat. The average American consumes approximately 40 percent of calories as fat, which is much higher than the 25–30 percent that is recommended. Animal studies have revealed that consuming 40 percent of calories as fat is too high if obesity is to be prevented. The most commonly used dietary means of inducing obesity in rats is to feed them a high-fat diet. When the fat content of the rat diet is increased to 40 percent, rats typically become obese. The rats appear to enjoy the extra dietary fat so much that they consume more calories than normal. Also, obesity can be produced in rats by feeding them supermarket foods such as chocolate chip cookies, salami, cheese, marshmallows, milk chocolate, peanut butter, and whole milk. These commonly eaten foods are favorites for late-night snackers. Rats become obese on such diets.

One reason dietary fat promotes obesity so easily in both rats and humans is that the body uses fewer calories to store dietary fat as body fat than it does for dietary carbohydrate. For example, if an individual consumes 100 extra calories from dietary fat, then only 3 calories are used by the body to transform the calories into body fat. However, 100 calories of extra carbohydrate requires 23 calories to make the transformation. To put it simply, excess dietary fat is more fattening than excess carbohydrate.

Another study substantiates this fact, for when obese women are given 2,000 calories of carbohydrate all at once (one huge meal), only 20 calories are actually stored as fat. The reason is that it is difficult for the body to turn the carbohydrate into fat; and when it does, the majority of the fat is used for metabolism. The message is plain: Pasta, potatoes, and bread do not make you fat nearly as much as the high-fat sauce, sour cream, and margarine used with them.

Another dietary explanation for obesity is found in a fairly common practice known as the "night-eating syndrome" in which a person eats relatively small amounts of food during the day but eats excessive amounts throughout the evening. This eating pattern stimulates the storage of fat for us during the period when intake is lower. Unfortunately, this fat is often resistant to being mobilized and contributes to the accumulation of more body fat.

Environmental theory.—Labor-saving devices have reduced the amount of physical activity that could help control obesity. Several studies have shown that obese people are much more successful than nonobese people in finding ways to reduce their energy expenditure. They tend to plan their time more efficiently to eliminate unnecessary activities and choose a lifestyle that is more sedentary than that of the nonobese.

Other studies have shown that many obese people are more likely to respond to external cues to eat rather than to internal hunger signals. They will eat food as long as it is in front of them but will not make an effort to get it. They will buy or consume food immediately after having eaten, in contrast to the nonobese, who are comparatively disinterested in food immediately after eating. According to these studies, obese people eat in response to the clock rather than to internal hunger sensations.

Treatment of Obesity

Americans spend more than 10 billion dollars every year for quick weight reduction treatments. These treatments and aids include special foods, exercise devices, appetite suppressants, formula diets, health clubs and spas, camps for children, behavior modification, individual counseling, and surgery. What they have in common is failure. For example, of those trying to lose weight, less than 5 percent maintain the weight loss for more than three years. Contrary to the claims in many ads, there have been no breakthroughs; and there are no easy solutions to weight control. The only realistic and sensible way for the obese person to achieve and maintain a healthy body weight is to cut calories, to increase activity, and to maintain this changed lifestyle for life. Let's focus on three important principles concerning weight loss for adults.

> A good weight-loss diet should include management of three types of activities: control of calorie intake, changing problem food choice habits, and increased physical activity.

Diet.—There is no diet that can be called a "magical diet" or the "ultimate diet," and there are no special chemical or magical constituents found in food that will cause or speed up weight loss. The truth is, no one needs to go on a diet; they need to *change* their diet. There are three important principles that must be understood before beginning a weight-loss program.

1. The body will resist weight loss. Thyroid hormone levels, and consequently basal metabolism, drop during weight loss. This drop makes it difficult to lose weight.

2. The goal of a weight-loss program should be to prevent obesity, since curing the disease is difficult. A weight-loss program should be considered successful only when its participants remain at their lower weight for three to five years. Dieting today often results in weight gain next month, which creates a yo-yo weight swing. We will discuss yo-yo dieting later in this chapter.

3. The weight loss should come from the fat stored in fat cells, not from muscle and other lean tissues. Rapid weight loss at the start of a diet program often represents fluid lost due to a decreased salt intake and loss of glycogen from the liver and muscles. Also muscle tissue may be lost as well. Most people are fooled when they weigh themselves after starting a fad diet. They have lost weight, but little of it represents fat loss. Diets that promise a loss of 10–15 pounds per week cannot ensure that the weight loss will be from fat storage alone. In fact, it is physiologically impossible to lose more than 2.5 pounds of fat from fat cells in a week.

Tips for selecting a weight-loss diet.—A good weight-loss diet should include management of three types of activities: control of calorie intake, changing problem food choice habits, and increased physical activity. Diets that focus on just eating fewer calories will not succeed. Specifically, look for the following characteristics:

1. The diet should include all the 45 known nutrients in their proper amounts. To do that, it should follow the emphases laid out in the food pyramid with a focus on lower-fat choices.

2. Rapid weight loss should be discouraged. A slow and steady weight loss should be stressed. A loss of 1 to 1.5 pounds per week of fat storage is ideal.

3. The diet should not have rigid rituals, such as only eating fruit in the morning or not eating meat after milk products.

4. The diet should contain at least 1,200 calories per day. Caloric consumption below 1,200 calories could possibly cause the body to lower its basal metabolism permanently. Also, because of insufficient carbohydrate in the diet, this low calorie consumption could cause the body to convert protein (lean body tissue) to glucose. Similar is the case in high protein-low carbohydrate diets. In addition, it is almost impossible to consume enough iron, especially for young women, if the diet calls for fewer calories than 1,500 per day. If the diet calls for fewer calories than this per day, it should recommend either fortified foods (for example, breakfast cereals) or a balanced vitamin and mineral supplement to supply iron.

5. No magical food can speed weight loss. If a diet suggests that there is (e.g., tofu, garlic, grapefruit), find another diet.

6. The diet should emphasize behavior modification to overcome problem eating habits. The diet should stress ways to make lifestyle changes that can reshape poor eating habits, along with ways to maintain weight maintenance to thwart further weight gain. This again is the "change your diet" idea.

7. The diet should not only stress good eating practices but also emphasize regular physical activity, stress reduction, and other healthy changes in lifestyle.

8. A sound weight-loss diet should allow you to participate

Regular exercise is an excellent way to lose weight. We use more calories in activity than at rest.

in social activities, such as eating at a restaurant or at a party. Teaching you to make wise choices in these situations will help ensure short-term and long-term success.

9. A diet should encourage the dieter to see a physician for a good physical checkup, especially if the dieter has previous health problems, such as heart disease or diabetes.

How to control calorie intake.—The best foods to eat when trying to lose weight are those high in carbohydrates. These should be predominately complex carbohydrates such as fruit, vegetables, grains, whole grains, whole-grain products, pastas, and so forth. Carbohydrates provide less than half as many calories as fat (1 gram of fat = 9 calories; 1 gram of carbohydrate = 4 calories). A weight-loss diet should include at least 150 grams of carbohydrate daily to prevent ketosis and reduce the risk of binging on large amounts of food, particularly sweets, because of intense hunger.

It is best not to reduce fat content of a diet below 20 percent of calorie intake. A diet too low in fat produces little satiety, so hunger returns quickly after eating. A diet that contains 30 percent calories as fat permits a person to incorporate most commonly eaten foods into the diet. Even subtle changes in food habits can produce desired weight loss. Changing habits appropriately is the key to both losing weight and maintaining a desirable weight.

Table 17.1 tries to answer the question, What foods should a good diet contain? It is probably best to eat during the hours of greatest physical activity, between 7 a.m. and 5 p.m. The absorbed fat heads right to the active muscles, bypassing the adipose cells. Conversely, a large dinner eaten after physical activity has ceased may leave excess fat in the bloodstream with no place to go but into fat storage. Watch out for those late-night snacks; exercise instead.

Consider these helpful hints for calorie distribution…

• While the adage, "Eat breakfast like a king, lunch like a queen, and supper like a pauper," is good, it may be impractical for most people. You can consume more of your calories earlier in the day. Eat breakfast that represents 30 percent of your daily corloic intake. Eat a large lunch that represents 40 percent of your calories. Then eat a smaller evening meal than usual that represents 30 percent of your caloric intake. Calories consumed earlier in the day tend less to become fat deposits.

• Don't eat within two hours of going to bed.

Normally, most people need to lose fewer than 50 pounds. By consuming a lower-calorie diet, these people should be able to achieve a desirable weight within one year. Remember, it took time to gain weight. It takes time to lose it.

Exercise.—Most people who want to lose weight hate the idea of exercise. But the lack of exercise is probably the major cause of their obesity. Obese people don't enjoy moving their bodies; for they feel heavy, clumsy, even ridiculous. Weight loss can occur without physical exercise; but when exercise is added to dieting, most of the weight loss will be from fat storage.

Regular exercise is an excellent way to lose weight. We use more calories in activity than at rest. Burning 200 extra calories per day can eliminate about 21 pounds of fat in a year.

Exercise makes several contributions to a weight-control program. Exercise alters body composition in a desirable direction, thereby altering metabolism and making daily energy expenditures slightly higher, even during rest. It also spends energy directly. Exercise also enhances the psychological benefits of looking and feeling healthy, and it reduces stress and stress-induced eating. Increased self-esteem accompanies these benefits, and this tends to support a person's resolve to persist in a weight-control effort.

Exercise has two other beneficial effects. First, the conditioned body is trained to use fatty acids rather than glucose as fuel. This means that after you have become conditioned, you will tend to burn more body fat during exercise than you did when you were out of condition. The best kind of exercise for burning fat is not severely strenuous but easy paced to moderate exercise of long duration (30 minutes or more). Second, regular, vigorous exercise will speed the metabolism slightly for a few hours up to a day. The basal metabolism is stimulated by about 5 percent for as long as a day.

Keep in mind that if exercise is to help with weight loss it must be active not passive exercise. Being moved passively, as by a machine at a health spa or by a massage, does not increase calorie expenditure. The more muscles you move, the more calories you spend.

Another thing to keep in mind is that the number of calories spent in an activity depends more on your weight than on how fast you do the exercise. For example, a person who weighs 125 pounds and runs a 6-minute mile burns 90 calories. That same person, walking a mile in 15 minutes, burns almost the same amount—83 calories. Similarly, a 200-pound person spends 140 calories on the 6-minute mile and only a little less,

Table 17.1 Foods That Are Appropriate for a Diet		
Minimum Servings	**Food Group**	**Some Suggestion**
4	Breads, cereals, and other grain products	Emphasize whole grain bread. Emphasize low-fat cereals. Emphasize rice and pasta. Be careful about sauces and gravy.
4	Fruits	Do not include avocados and olives. Don't add sugar or whipped cream. Eliminate fruit in syrups.
4	Vegetables	Include a wide variety; but avoid butter, margarine, and other sauces high in fat. Avoid fried vegetables.
2	Meat, poultry, and alternatives	Eat lean parts of meat, without skin; baked fish. Broil, roast, simmer; avoid foods that are breaded and fried. Eggs and legumes are good alternatives.
2	Milk, cheese, and yogurt	Skim or low-fat milk and cheese. Low-fat and nonfat plain yogurt.
Limit, but include at least one teaspoon of vegetable oil per day.	Fats, sweets	Avoid these. They provide calories and little else. Use spices and herbs instead of sauces, butter, and other fats. For dessert, try fresh fruit or choose baked products made with less fat and sugar. For example, angel food cake. Drink coffee or tea without cream or sugar.

132 calories, on the 15-minute mile. The rule seems to be that you don't have to work fast to use up energy effectively.

People sometimes ask about "spot reducing." That is, can you lose fat in particular locations on the body. Unfortunately, muscles don't own the fat that surrounds them. All body fat is shared by all the muscles and organs, so spot-reducing exercises that work only the flabby parts won't help reduce the fat located there. There is some good news though. Tightening muscles in trouble spots by way of a balanced exercise program will help the appearances of the fatty areas.

In summary, the benefits of exercise in controlling weight are:

- Appetite control.
- Stress reduction.
- Short-term increased energy output.
- Control of stress-induced eating.
- Increased self-esteem.
- Physical well-being.
- Burning of more fat during exercise by a conditioned body than by an unconditioned one.
- Long-term increase in BMR, with increased lean tissue.

Behavior Modification

In order for a weight-loss program to work, controlling energy intake is paramount. Another vital step is behavior modification. This means that each dieter must decide which behaviors contribute to obesity and find ways to modify those behaviors. To do this, a person should consider the events that cause him

Nutrition education involves understanding the principles of nutrition. Knowledge about problem foods in your diet can help you make appropriate substitutions.

to start eating, factors that influence food choices, and factors associated with the desire to stop eating. Psychologists often use terms like *stimulus control, cognitive restructuring,* and *self-monitoring.* This terminology helps place the problem in perspective and organize the intervention strategy into manageable steps. Let's examine some terminology.

Stimulus control involves controlling factors that encourage eating. To lose weight you must set about controlling stimuli that prompt you to eat inappropriately. This involves purchasing the appropriate foods, planning meals and exercise times, and altering food-related activities.

Eating behavior involves altering the way you consume food. For example, chew your food thoroughly, put your fork down between bites, and eat more slowly (overeaters eat faster than others).

Reward involves receiving praise along with positive reinforcement. Friends and family may provide praise and encouragement for you.

Self-monitoring is a key practice in behavior modification. Keep a record of your present eating and activity behaviors against which to measure future progress. Self-monitoring is an effective way to spot problems in eating habits, especially times of unconscious overeating.

Nutrition education involves understanding the principles of nutrition. Knowledge about problem foods in your diet can help you make appropriate substitutions.

Physical activity plays a vital role in behavior modification. Increase your physical activity. Park your car at the far end of the parking lot. Take short walks during the day. Take the stairs instead of the elevator, and always be alert to volunteer when given the opportunity to do extra physical activity. These strategies don't add up to many calories each, but over a year's time they become significant.

Cognitive restructuring involves changing one's frame of mind in regard to eating. For example, instead of using a difficult day as an excuse to overeat, substitute other pleasures for rewards, such as a relaxing walk with a friend. Set realistic goals, and think positively about your progress toward reaching them.

From all the behavior changes available, locate the ones that hinder you. Don't try to master them all at once. Set your own priorities. Pick one trouble area that hinders you most, start with it, and practice your strategy until it is habitual and automatic. Later you can select another trouble area and begin to work on it. Throughout the process, enjoy your new, emerging self.

Finally, maintaining weight loss may be more difficult than losing weight. A dieter can tolerate an occasional lapse. Planning a response to lapses should be part of the diet plan, including encouragement to stay calm when errors are made, to take charge immediately, and to ask for help. Without a strong behavior plan, a lapse frequently turns into a relapse. Once many poor food choices have been made, the dieter feels like a failure and tends to stray further and further from the plan. As the relapse lengthens, the diet plan eventually collapses; and the person returns to his original form. Dieting is difficult, and anyone who wishes to diet should be well aware of that. However, without a good behavioral plan, losing weight is even more difficult (see table 17.2).

Table 17.2
Behavioral Modification Principles of Weight Loss

- **I. Stimulus Control**
  - **A. Shopping**
    1. **Shop for food after eating.**
    2. **Shop from a list.**
    3. **Avoid ready-to-eat foods.**
    4. **Don't carry more cash than needed, and pay in cash not with credit or debit cards.**
  - **B. Plans**
    1. **Plan to limit food intake.**
    2. **Substitute exercise for snacking.**
    3. **Eat meals and snacks at scheduled times.**
    4. **Don't accept food offered by others.**
  - **C. Activities**
    1. **Store food out of sight.**
    2. **Eat all food in the same place.**
    3. **Remove food from inappropriate storage areas in the house.**
    4. **Keep serving dishes off the table.**
    5. **Use smaller dishes and utensils.**
    6. **Avoid being the food server.**
    7. **Leave the table immediately after eating.**

8. Brush your teeth immediately after eating.
9. Don't save leftovers.

D. Holidays and Parties
1. Plan eating habits before parties.
2. Eat a low-calorie snack before party.
3. Practice polite ways to decline food.
4. Don't get discouraged by an occasional snack.

II. Eating Behavior
A. Put the fork down between mouthfuls.
B. Chew thoroughly before swallowing.
C. Leave some food on the plate.
D. Do nothing while eating (e.g. read, watch television).
E. Take time for conversation while eating.

III. Reward
A. Solicit help from family and friends.
B. Help family and friends provide this help in the form of praise and material reward.
C. Plan specific rewards for special behaviors.
D. Use self-monitoring records as a basis for rewards.

IV. Self-Monitoring—Keep a Diary that Includes
A. Time and place of eating.
B. Type and amount of food.
C. Who is present.
D. How you feel.

V. Nutrition Education
A. Use a diet diary to identify problem areas.
B. Make small changes that you can continue.
C. Learn nutritional values of food.
D. Decrease fat intake; increase complex carbos.

VI. Physical activity
A. Routine Activity
1. Increase routine acts.
2. Increase use of stairs.
3. Keep a record of distance walked each day.

B. Exercise
1. Begin a very mild exercise program.
2. Keep a record of daily exercise.
3. Increase the exercise very gradually.

VII. Cognitive Restructuring
A. Avoid setting unreasonable goals.
B. Think about progress, not shortcomings.
C. Avoid imperatives like *always* and *never*.
D. Counter negative thought with rational statement.
E. Set weight goals.

Treating Morbid Obesity

Classification of morbid obesity refers to an individual who is at least 100 pounds over his desirable body weight. Estimates indicate that 5–10 percent of all Americans are classified as morbid obese. These obese Americans are seven times more likely to die from health problems associated with obesity than nonobese people. Many physicians recommend drastic measures to be taken in these cases if the more conservative approach (reducing calorie intake, increasing exercise, and modifying behavior) has failed. There are three main approaches to treat morbid obesity: surgical approach, dietary approach, and drug approach.

Surgical Approach to Treating Morbid Obesity

Intestinal bypass.—This type of surgery was once common in the 1970s. Since then, long-term health problems associated with the surgery have curtailed its popularity. This procedure connected the first foot of the jejunum to the last 4 inches of the ileum, bypassing approximately 12 feet of small intestine. This area contains most of the intestinal absorptive area, thereby profoundly reducing the body's capability to absorb nutrients and contributing to a rapid weight loss. However, severe physiological consequences from this surgery occur, such as electrolyte imbalances, gallstones, kidney stones, fat buildup in the liver, and anemia.

Stomach surgery.—This is the most common surgical procedure for treating morbid obesity. Commonly called "stomach stapling" (medical name: gastroplasty), the goal of this surgery is to reduce the size of the stomach to approximately 50 milliliters, capable of holding 3 ounces of stomach liquid. This prevents the dieter from overeating, for overeating solid foods would result in rapid vomiting. The success rate of losing weight with this procedure is encouraging. About 75 percent of patients eventually lose 50 percent of the body weight, and they can maintain much of that weight loss over time. This dramatic loss occurs because dieters are forced to do what was difficult to do before—eat less.

This type of surgery does have some negative effects. It's costly, it's normally not covered by medical insurance, and torturous months of discomfort must be endured while weight loss occurs. This procedure is analogous to jaw-wiring to prevent overeating, but it is considered more effective.

Gastric balloon.—This procedure calls for a balloon to be inserted into the upper portion of the stomach where it is supposed to stimulate satiety receptors, and thus reduce food intake. Because of the high cost of inserting the balloon and the danger of the balloon's deflating and passing painfully through the gastrointestinal tract, the medical community no longer recommends this procedure.

Dietary Approach to Treating Morbid Obesity

Extremely low-calorie diets.—If traditional dietary measures fail, treating morbid obesity with an extremely low-calorie diet is possible. This diet allows a dieter to eat 400–700 calories per day, often in liquid form. This will cause about a 3–5 pound weight loss per week, of which not all is fat loss but lean muscle tissue as well. Medical authorities recommend limiting this low-calorie diet to 12 weeks maximum. The dieter should then go off the diet for at least one month to minimize the loss of lean tissue. During the off period the dieter should eat a low-calorie but completely balanced diet. The dieter can then return for another 12 weeks of the extremely low-calorie diet.

Before going on this type of diet, these precautions should be heeded:

1. Never go on this diet without a doctor's care.
2. Use this diet only when more conservative approaches have failed.
3. The dieter needs to consume at least two grams of potassium per day because the heart tissue is destroyed and may eventually fail from an electrolyte imbalance of potassium and sodium.
4. Never stay on this diet for more than 3 months at a time for fear of sudden heart death. Nearly 60 Americans have died suddenly on this type of diet.
5. Participate in a behavior modification program designed to prevent weight regain once the diet is stopped.

Drug Approach to Treating Morbid Obesity

Treating morbid obesity has led to the use of a variety of drugs, usually with little or no success. Drugs include tranquilizers, which are supposed to reduce anxiety and therefore nibbling; phenylethylamines, which act by depressing the appetite but have serious side effects; bulking agents such as methylcellulose, used to give a feeling of fullness but which cause flatulence; and adrenaline and thyroxin, which increase metabolism but must be used only under medical supervision. Let's look at some of the more popular ones on the market.

Growth hormone releasers, largely proteins with high levels of arginine (an amino acid), are sold under a wide variety of names. They are to be taken at night when they will stimulate the secretion of growth hormone and increase metabolism and hence calorie use. These are of little to no value.

Amphetamines, which are available only by prescription (Dexedrine™), dull the appetite but are also addictive and have adverse effects on the heart and nervous system.

Treating morbid obesity has led to the use of a variety of drugs, usually with little or no success.

Phenylpropanolamine, the active ingredient in many cold remedies and over-the-counter products, is considered a safe and effective appetite suppressant by the FDA but should not be taken by people with high blood pressure, diabetes, or thyroid or kidney problems.

Starch blockers, now considered as illegal drugs, were formerly promoted to block the digestion of starch and thus reduce the calories available for absorption.

Arginine and ornithine, both amino acids, are promoted for their ability to stimulate the production of the growth hormone, which then causes the body to burn fat. They are of no proven benefit.

Spirulina, a protein powder produced from the growth of algae, is sold as an appetite suppressant based on its high content of the amino acid, phenylalanine. The FDA is not aware of any evidence that phenylalanine is safe and effective as an appetite suppressant.

Benzocaine, an active ingredient in dietetic candy, lozenges, and gum, is a topical anesthetic said to work by numbing the tongue, thus reducing the ability to taste foods.
No conclusive data support benzocaine's effectiveness as an anorexiant.

Cholecystokinin, a hormone involved in digestion in response to the presence of fat, has been claimed by producers of this drug to reduce hunger and cause sudden and dramatic weight loss. This drug has not been approved by the FDA for public sale for any purpose.

Grapefruit pills, with grapefruit extracts, diuretics, and bulk-forming agents, contain phenylpropanolamine, along with herbs or other ingredients. For years, grapefruit has been promoted by various people as having special fat-burning properties. Research has not been able to substantiate any of these claims. The FDA has not approved the sale of grapefruit pills and is unaware of any valid medical evidence that such products are safe or effective.

In spite of all the claims, no drug on the market is totally safe and effective in assisting in weight control for all people. The most feasible solution to the problem of obesity is prevention. The best programs for treating obesity include both exercise and dietary control, along with a good behavior-modification program.

Underweight

An underweight person is classified as someone who is more than 15 percent below the desirable weight for his height. Underweight individuals are confronted with health problems that may be just as severe as those which confront overweight individuals. Although they have a lower risk of hypertension, diabetes, and cardiovascular problems, they are much more susceptible to respiratory problems, ranging from the common cold to tuberculosis. In addition, they have difficulty conserving heat and maintaining a comfortable body temperature as environmental temperatures fluctuate. People who suffer from undernutrition tend to be a neglected segment of the population.

Treatment for Underweight Individuals

The treatment for underweight people involves creating a positive energy balance by increasing intake to exceed expenditure. The use of smaller, more frequent meals will in some cases help increase the total food intake, as will the addition of foods that provide as many calories in as small a volume as possible. It's hard to gain much weight eating raw carrots because they will fill one up before they offer enough energy. Calorie-dense foods hold the key to weight gain, the foods the successful weight-loss dieter avoids. Some high calorie-dense foods are butter, cheese, sugar, cream sauces, and gravies. These high-calorie foods are better used at the end of a meal because it is undesirable to create a feeling of satiety too early in the meal. Since many foods with high nutrient density are the same ones people should avoid to reduce the risk of cardiovascular disease, underweight individuals should heed the caution about the risks of long-term use of foods high in saturated fats and be encouraged to have periodic checks of their blood-cholesterol levels.

Exercise should also be included in the treatment of those underweight. Not only does moderate exercise stimulate the appetite (strenuous exercise depresses appetite), but it also fosters the development of muscle at the same time that extra energy is stored as fat. Participation in a good weight training program would develop muscle tissue and develop the desired type of weight gain.

In gaining weight, the weight gain should be made gradually, and the weight gain should be the result of a diet that is nutritionally balanced as well as calorie dense.

[CHAPTER 18]

DEVELOPING SELF-DISCIPLINE

The reason for long countdowns prior to spacecraft liftoffs is to get everything under control. The guidance system with all its scientific checks and counterbalances must be in order. If a spacecraft is to reach its destination, a great deal of care must be given to the guidance system. This is the case with humans, too; yet many Christians choose to live at full speed without any regard for traffic signals or road maps.

The writer of Proverbs issued a solemn warning on this point. "A man without self-control is like a city broken into and left without walls" (Prov. 25:28, RSV). In ancient times a city could not exist long without walls and fortifications. Such a city could be sacked and destroyed. Any person who is unable to control his own life is in the same precarious situation.

If you don't care what happens to yourself or what you become, who do you suppose will care? Who really should care, if you don't? If you don't care, what about the impact on your family and friends if you suffer a premature death or limiting illness/disease.

The Principle of Self-Control

"For God did not give us a spirit of timidity [weakness] but a spirit of power and love and self-control" (2 Tim. 1:7, RSV). The free-wheeling life sooner or later self-destructs. Disregard for the physical needs of the body soon brings despair. We are surrounded by the temptations of Satan and by our own inner weaknesses. Unless we determine to exercise self-control, we will find ourselves in the grip of the powers of darkness. The quality and future of our life is at stake. Self-control will determine whether we will look back on our life rejoicing or cursing the day of our birth.

The apostle Paul was the greatest missionary ever. On one occasion he shared his secret for being able to accomplish so much. "Well, I do not run aimlessly, I do not box as one beating the air; but I pommel my body and subdue it, lest after preaching to others I myself should be disqualified" (1 Cor. 9:26-27, RSV). He realized that he could ruin his future, his usefulness in the kingdom of God, if he failed to rule his own body and spirit well. If he wanted to do the best things in life, there were some lesser things he could not afford to do.

Paul used the world of athletics to speak of the necessary discipline needed for achieving his own personal goals. He noted that everyone in a race should run in an effort to win and that everyone who wants to master any sport must be serious about it, must pay the price of training.

Anyone who takes Christianity seriously, who tries to live the godly life, must recognize that such a task is not easy. The truth is, those who dare to follow Christ may find that many things do not always go better. To follow Christ is sometimes to travel upstream or to go against the tide. If life with Christ were the easy life, everyone would follow Him. However, the good life is a difficult yet rewarding life. Only those who are willing to rule their own body and spirit, to exercise self-control and discipline, can live it.

The person you become is directly related to whether you choose to exercise self-control over your life. Paul expressed his philosophy on this matter in 1 Corinthians when he wrote, "All things are lawful unto me, but all things are not expedient: all things are lawful for me, but I will not be brought under the power of any" (6:12, KJV). The apostle refused to become a slave to anything, including bad habits and evil temptations.

He refused to be a part of anything that was not expedient (did not make a contribution) or was enslaving.

Your personality develops only on the same ratio with which you grow in maturity. Maturity is a willingness to postpone fulfillment of present desires; and self-control governs the growth of maturity. People either learn to rule their own lives, to control themselves; or they take into their life everything that presents itself.

You will never discover the real you, never grow to be your unique self, until you are willing to exercise self-control. We can have more than human strength to rule our spirit, for our Heavenly Father will give us strength as we follow Him. The Christian life is the self-controlled life, guided and empowered by Christ. We can say with the apostle Paul, "I can do all things through Christ which strengtheneth me" (Phil. 4:13, KJV). The apostle also said in the same letter: "Being confident of this very thing, that he which hath begun a good work in you will perform it until the day of Jesus Christ" (Phil. 1:6, KJV).

> That is the bottom line of why we should exercise and take care of God's temple to the best of our ability—so we can serve Him longer and better.

For many of us to be happy, we may need to develop whole new lifestyles. We need to make a new commitment to God that we want to serve Him the best we can. This means we must "seek first his kingdom and his righteousness" in every facet of our lives (Matt. 6:33, RSV). We must also try to love our neighbor as ourselves (see Matt. 22:39). And finally, we must practice self-control over our lives by showing honor and glory to God with our bodies (see 1 Cor. 6:20). Only when we are in excellent physical condition can we serve Him longer and better.

You Can

I shared an office with a colleague and friend who had a sign displayed on our office wall which read in large letters "You can." I can't begin to tell you how that sign has changed many facets of my life. Every time I'm faced with a new challenge in my busy schedule, I immediately respond with excuses and rationalizations that I cannot possibly accept this new challenge. Then I look at that sign hanging on the wall, and confidence overshadows my laziness. The point is, "You can."

You can start an exercise program at any age. Thousands of senior adults can testify to that statement. Recently a senior-adult woman came up to me after a fitness seminar and remarked: "Look at me. I'm so old I can barely walk. How can I start exercising?"

My response to her question was, "Then start by barely walking."

Two years later I received a letter from her. She said: "I took your advice about walking. I'm now walking three miles a day. I feel better; my body is getting stronger; I can do more work for God. By the way, I won three people to Christ on my 88th birthday."

That is the bottom line of why we should exercise and take care of God's temple to the best of our ability—so we can serve Him longer and better. The Bible doesn't say that we are not to witness after we reach 65 years of age. We, as Christians, have the responsibility to serve God from our first breath to our last. May all of us strengthen our bodies through exercising so that we can become better servants for Him.

Many Christians use excuses such as "I'm too handicapped by some physical malady to begin an exercise program." Let me share an experience of the most courageous accomplishment I have ever witnessed in a sporting event. After completing a marathon run of 26 miles, 385 yards in my record time, I decided to watch other runners finish the marathon course. After watching for about five minutes, I saw the crowd giving a standing ovation to a pair of runners and sensed an emotion so strong that chill bumps covered my body and tears came to my eyes. These runners had run stride for stride for 26 miles, 385 yards together with unbelievable handicaps. The lead runner's feet were amputated at the ankle joint, and he had to run on a prosthesis. He held a rope in his hand and running behind him was the other runner holding the rope, who was completely blind. I looked at the pride of those runners crossing that finish line and again the words of that sign in my office entered my mind.

Christian, you can begin an exercise program even though you have a handicap. Your body may now be in poor physical condition; but through a slow, progressive exercise program, you can build it up and improve its efficiency. The only real excuse for not exercising is laziness. Many Christians don't want to put forth the effort it takes to strengthen the temple. Don't be lazy. Make a lifetime commitment to physical fitness, and enjoy some of life's happy fulfillments.

The Ideal Physical Fitness Program

The exercise program given in table 18.1 was developed from personal experience and is based on the latest research. To attain maximal benefits from exercise, plan a progressive program that meets your specific needs. The following suggestions can help form your exercise program.

Identify your own fitness needs.—The main health-related components of physical fitness are cardiovascular-respiratory (CVR) fitness, muscular strength and endurance fitness, flexibility fitness, and body composition fitness. You may have developed fitness in strength but may have neglected flexibility fitness. Check your fitness level in each of these four areas by reading the appropriate chapter and testing yourself. Now select a mode of training that can best improve your weakest areas.

Select a program that meets all of your fitness needs.—Marathon runners are not always physically fit because they may lack sufficient strength in their upper body which could lead to postural deviations. No single exercise can meet all of your needs. Select exercises in all aspects of physical fitness and especially make sure you have selected a program you enjoy. If you do not enjoy it, you may not carry it through to a meaningful result.

Select a regular time and place for your exercise.—Begin your workout at approximately the same time every day. Try not to allow any outside influence to interfere with this precious time. You may want to exercise at different places. Vary the route if you walk or jog. Set a goal for yourself. Great satisfaction comes from reaching that goal. Record your progress on a chart. Build your exercise program into your daily routine, and make it as much a habit as combing your hair or brushing your teeth.

Do not overexercise.—This can cause soreness or pain which will cause you to terminate your exercise program. Approach each exercise program with a positive attitude. Be thankful you are able to exercise.

Warm up and cool down before and after each exercise workout.—Approximately two minutes of easy jogging or three minutes of walking should precede an exercise bout to improve blood flow to the heart and muscles. Static stretching of the muscles prior to exercise can also reduce soreness and possible injury.

Cool down or slowly taper off after exercising.—Never stop exercising abruptly. After a jog or a bout of exercise, continue to walk and move around.

The ideal exercise program (table 18.1) develops all the health-related components of fitness. It strengthens the muscles

Table 18.1
An Ideal Exercise Program

Monday	**1. Do 5 minutes of flexibility exercises (described in chap. 8) before and after workout.** **2. Select your favorite mode of CVR exercise (walking, jogging, bicycling, swimming, aerobics, etc.) and perform for 30–40 minutes. Try to keep your working heart rate at the desired intensity level (60–70%) while exercising. (See chap. 5.)**
Tuesday	**1. Do 5 minutes of flexibility exercises before and after workout.** **2. Do 20–30 minutes of CVR training.** **3. Do strength training exercises for each body movement as described in chapter 7. Make sure you work each muscle at every major joint equally.**
Wednesday	**Repeat Monday's schedule.**
Thursday	**Repeat Tuesday's schedule.**
Friday	**Repeat Monday and Wednesday's schedule.**
Saturday	**Repeat Tuesday and Thursday's schedule.**
Sunday	**Day of rest. Go to church.**

We need to develop our lives as Jesus did. We need to develop our potential mentally, socially, spiritually, emotionally, vocationally, and physically.

and their various movements in a balanced manner. It also builds up flexibility in the joints and muscles; but, more importantly, it develops a sufficient amount of CVR fitness. This program also allows for the individual differences in fitness by permitting each person to develop at his own intensity, regardless of age or fitness level. For example, the highly fit person can train his CVR system (run, swim, bicycle, etc.) at an intensity level high enough to meet his needs. He may be able to run 7–8 miles in 40 minutes, whereas the unfit individual may be able to cover only 2–3 miles in 40 minutes. The key is to exercise at a pace that meets the requirements of the 60–70 percent intensity level for 30–40 minutes. Fitness in each of these physical fitness components will definitely improve God's temple, which will please you and show honor and glory to Him.

This exercise program usually takes 45–60 minutes to complete each day. By the end of 6 weeks you will definitely notice and feel a change in your body's physiology. Motivate yourself to stay with the program for at least 6 weeks, and by then you will definitely believe that exercise should be a part of your lifestyle.

We need to develop our lives as Jesus did. We need to develop our potential mentally, socially, spiritually, emotionally, vocationally, and physically. We should never neglect any one of these areas of potential growth, for complications will occur in other areas.

The Bible tells us that we are the body of Christ. We are what Jesus left on earth. He left us to represent Him to the world. His Spirit has come to dwell within us, and the world will know our God mainly by our representation of Him, which will be greatly enhanced if we develop fully this potential that He has created in us. Don't be lazy or use excuses like age or lack of time to fail to develop these six areas of growth. God wants you to be happy and have abundant life. He knows the only way for you to achieve this is for you to develop the unlimited potential that He has given you. Striving to achieve this potential will help you serve Him better and help you become a happy person.

My prayer for you is beautifully expressed by the apostle John. "I pray that in all respects you may prosper and be in good health, just as your soul prospers" (3 John 2).

Food Guide Pyramid

A Guide to Daily Food Choices

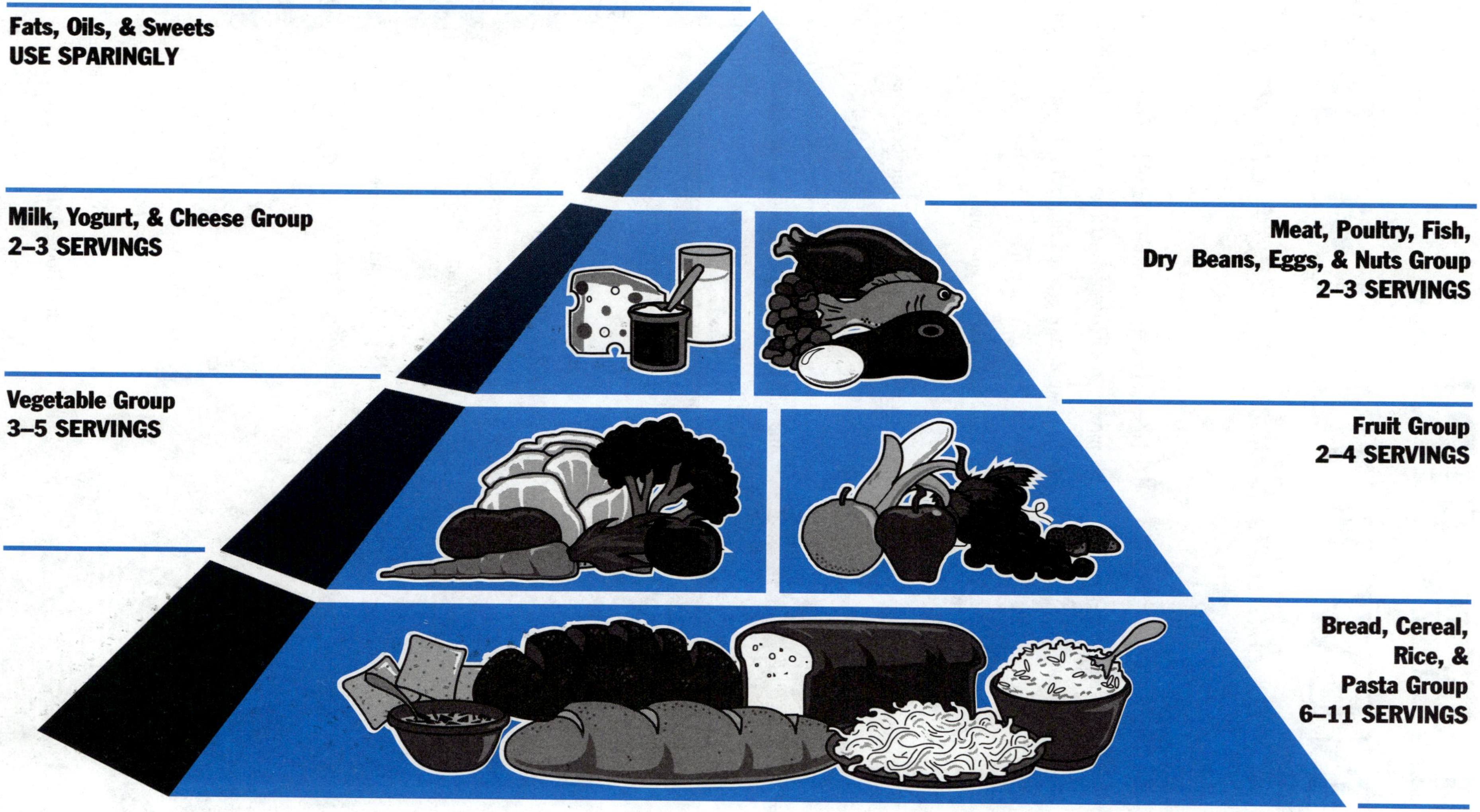